Contagion and Confinement

BARRON H. LERNER

Contagion and Confinement

Controlling Tuberculosis along the Skid Road

THE JOHNS HOPKINS UNIVERSITY PRESS
BALTIMORE AND LONDON

Printed in the United States of America on acid-free paper
9 8 7 6 5 4 3 2 1
The Johns Hopkins University Press
2715 North Charles Street
Baltimore, Maryland 21218-4363
The Johns Hopkins Press Ltd., London
www.press.jhu.edu
Library of Congress Cataloging-in-Publication Data will be found at the end of this book.
A catalog record for this book is available from the British Library.
ISBN 0-8018-5898-4

To my parents

None know—none can know, but they who have felt it—the burning, withering thirst for drink, which habit forms in the appetite of the wretched victim of intoxication.
—*Walt Whitman*

Disease is a speech of the psyche.
—*Saul Bellow*

Contents

Illustrations

Acknowledgments

Numerous people have assisted me at various stages of this book, and their help has been invaluable. To those not directly thanked below, your assistance is greatly appreciated.

First, I would like to thank the individuals who helped me obtain primary source materials. These include Karyl Winn and Gary Lundell at the University of Washington Archives, Pat Hopkins and David Hastings at the Washington State Archives, Frances Toone at the American Lung Association, Kathy Rexford at the American Lung Association of Washington, Stephen Blanket at the American Lung Association of New York, and Michael Garrick, Marlene Nottage, and Denise Anderson at the Washington State Department of Social and Health Services. Other archival collections that I used were those of the King County Medical Society and the Shoreline Historical Society. The late Wallace Lane and Joan K. Jackson were kind enough to share their personal papers. I would also like to thank the staffs of Fircrest and Kings' High School for enabling me to tour the old Firland Sanatorium facilities.

I interviewed numerous persons during this project, all of whom provided valuable information. They included Nick Hughes, Manny Wolinsky, Stewart Wolf, Kerr White, Arnold Linsky, Archibald Ruprecht, Jonathan Ostrow, Charles Lester, Sanford Lehman, Harold Laws, Waldo Mills, Helen Marshall, Richard Greenleaf, Marcelle Dunning, C. J. Martin, Donal Sparkman, Arthur Kobler, Kay Anderson, Charles Nolan, Wallace Lane, Otto Trott, Dorothy Northrop Hupp, Marion Amundson, June Elston, Edith Heinemann, Charlotte Rose, Burnice Calhoun, Polly Hertlein, Faye Cline, Marie Radoll, and George and Dorothy Gamble. Special thanks go to Walter Miller and Joan Jackson, who are certainly among the finest subjects a historian could ever want to interview. Both of them have helped to shape this book immeasurably. Joan and her husband, Stan Jackson, have lent both their moral support and their friendship.

Portions of the book appeared in two published articles: Barron H. Lerner, "Temporarily Detained: Tuberculous Alcoholics in Seattle, 1949 through

1960" (*American Journal of Public Health* 86 [Feb. 1996]: 758–66); and Barron H. Lerner, "Can Stress Cause Disease? Revisiting the Tuberculosis Research of Thomas Holmes, 1949–1961" (*Annals of Internal Medicine* 124 [Apr. 1, 1996]: 673–80). I wish to thank the American Public Health Association and the American College of Physicians for allowing me to use related material in this book.

Numerous individuals have contributed to this work, either after reading portions of the manuscript or having heard oral presentations, talks, or conferences. Special thanks goes to my dissertation committee, composed of James Whorton, Richard Kirkendall, Thomas Hankins, and Albert Jonsen. Colleagues first at the University of Washington's Clinical Scholars Program and later at Columbia University have offered trenchant criticism. In addition, my colleagues in Columbia's Division of General Medicine and Center for the Study of Society and Medicine have provided emotional support for this and other projects. Greatest thanks goes to David Rothman, who has read many versions of this book and provided countless helpful suggestions.

Others who have read all or portions of the manuscript are Judith Leavitt, Joel Howell, and Thomas Frieden. Helpful advice at various stages of the project came from Nancy Rockafellar, Nancy Tomes, Barbara Rosenkrantz, Martin Pernick, Chris Feudtner, Susan Lederer, Howard Markel, Nancy Dubler, Elizabeth Fee, Thomas Inui, and Sheila Rothman. I have greatly benefited from comments I received after presentations made at the American Association for the History of Medicine, the American Public Health Association, the University of Wisconsin-Madison, the College of Physicians in Philadelphia, the University of California at San Francisco, the State University of New York at Stony Brook, and several other venues.

Funding assistance for this project has primarily come from two sources: the Robert Wood Johnson Foundation and the Arnold P. Gold Foundation. The Johnson Foundation has been particularly generous, funding me both at the start of this book as a Clinical Scholar in Seattle and most recently as a Generalist Faculty Physician Scholar. Since my return to New York in 1993, the Gold Foundation has provided me with protected time to conduct research and to teach. I hope that the finished work contributes to the worthy mission of the Gold Foundation to foster the spread of humanism in medical education and practice.

Among those persons who have helped with the logistics of this project are Nancy Lundebjerg, Teri Copley, Victoria Donovan, and James Crowley. They all deserve special thanks. My wife, Cathy Seibel, helped to photocopy duplicate and triplicate copies of hundreds of note cards that I was certain would get lost during our move from Seattle to New York. My editor at the Johns Hopkins University Press, Jacqueline Wehmueller, has provided me with expert advice and enthusiasm.

It is to my family that I owe my greatest debt. My parents, Phillip and Ronnie Lerner, slogged through the manuscript, making helpful comments and finding typos. As always, they have given all of themselves to help me succeed. It is with great love that I dedicate this book to them. My children, Ben and Nina, provided much joy when I was not holed up in the basement working. My deepest thanks go to my wife, Cathy, who has provided expert editing and commentary and tolerated my near obsession with the historical figures and events depicted herein.

Contagion and Confinement

Introduction

[G.Z.] would rather go to jail than stay on [the locked ward]. Demanding a court hearing & to see Dr. ———. Using foul abusive—insulting language to doctor and to personnel about doctors. Was asked to be civil and patient. Will not attempt to understand why he is required to stay here over a year.
—*Nurses' notes, patient G.Z., 1968*

For the staff of Firland Sanatorium in Seattle, Washington, in 1968, the case of G.Z. was all too familiar.[1] G.Z. was a veteran diagnosed in the Midwest in 1956 with pulmonary (lung) tuberculosis. Over the next decade, he traveled around the country working as an unskilled laborer. Beginning in 1965, he was admitted to multiple hospitals on the West Coast, generally leaving against medical advice and then not taking his antibiotics after discharge. By his own account he was a heavy drinker, frequently going on sprees that lasted two or three days. During three admissions to Firland between 1967 and 1969, G.Z. went AWOL several times. He became drunk at the sanatorium on numerous occasions and spent much of his hospitalization on a locked ward. G.Z. was often uncooperative and belligerent. He also consistently resisted efforts by the staff to treat his tuberculosis.

Although most people with tuberculosis during the twentieth century did not present such a complex array of problems, patients like G.Z. were not uncommon. Pulmonary tuberculosis is at once an infectious and a chronic disease, a disease laden with medical, social, and public health repercussions. As such, it has presented unique challenges to those charged with control of the disease, forcing health officials, physicians, and nurses into such unfamiliar roles as counselor, confidante—and police officer.

This book is a social history of antituberculosis efforts in the United States after World War II, focusing on the efforts of Firland Sanatorium in Seattle, Washington. It begins with the premise that an understanding of tuberculosis requires more than simply knowledge of the tuberculosis bacterium and the pathology it causes. Rather, tuberculosis is, as the renowned microbiologist and philosopher René Dubos noted, a "social disease."[2] In attempting to define the meaning of the term *social disease* it is helpful to examine how physicians, other health personnel, and the lay public have historically understood both the cause of tuberculosis and strategies for its treatment.

The discovery of the etiology of tuberculosis is universally credited to the German scientist Robert Koch. Prior to the late nineteenth century, most observers believed that tuberculosis—or consumption, as it was often known—was a noninfectious disease acquired as a result of environmental conditions and hereditary predisposition. In a series of innovative experiments announced in 1882, however, Koch identified the tubercle bacillus (later named *Mycobacterium tuberculosis*) and demonstrated that its transmission from person to person was a prerequisite of the commonest form of the disease, pulmonary tuberculosis.[3] Yet Koch and other early commentators, such as William Osler, quickly stressed that an overemphasis on the causative role of the bacillus would be a mistake. Autopsy studies had revealed that nearly all members of certain urban areas were infected with the bacillus, but only some of them had developed the disease. Using what became a common metaphor, Osler argued that it was important to consider not only the seed (the bacillus) but also the soil (the patient) when analyzing why a given person had become tuberculous.[4]

By emphasizing the importance of the soil, commentators sought to reinforce a concept that had characterized medical thinking since the days of Hippocrates: the balance between health and disease was determined by an individual's general physical condition and his or her surrounding environment.[5] In the case of tuberculosis, therefore, any analysis of causation needed to take into account not only exposure to the bacillus but also an individual's nutritional status, living conditions, personal habits, and emotional state. Prevention of the disease warranted strict attention to these latter "social" concerns. "Let us not forget the importance to the possible host [of tuberculosis]," Osler noted in 1894, "of combating inherited weakness, of removing acquired debility, and of maintaining the nutrition at a standard of aggressive activity."[6]

If tuberculosis was thus caused by both medical and social factors, so, too, did treatment of the disease require attention to each of these elements. In the years prior to the development of antibiotics, popular therapies for tuberculosis routinely addressed both germ and patient. A primary goal of bed rest, for example, was to increase patients' overall strength, thus enabling their bodies to better fight the bacilli in their lungs. Physicians and sanatorium administrators gave close scrutiny to the living arrangements of discharged patients, at times entering patients into formal rehabilitation programs that provided jobs and housing. It is this concern with the social circumstances of patients—as opposed to merely the transmission and treatment of *Mycobacterium tuberculosis*—that this book equates with a social approach to the disease.

Having proposed to depict tuberculosis as both a medical and a social disease, a note of caution is necessary. Convincing recent scholarship in the history of medicine has employed the term *social* in a somewhat different manner. The scholars in question have argued that medical diseases should be considered not as objective scientific entities but rather as social constructs that reflect the social and cultural attitudes of those who employ disease terminology. In other words, it is incorrect to claim that the pathological findings that accompany a given disease exist independently of the social setting in which they are interpreted.[7] According to this theory of the social construction of disease, therefore, one should not—indeed, cannot—separate out the strictly medical aspects of tuberculosis.[8]

In a sense, this study corroborates the argument that all disease is socially constructed. At times, physicians in Seattle and elsewhere incorporated various social and cultural considerations into the very medical terminology they used to describe and understand tuberculosis. Yet, at the same time, this book's delineation of separate medical and social approaches to tuberculosis control can provide a valuable framework for examining how physicians, health officials, and society more broadly understood and conceptualized the disease. During the years 1945 to 1973, two distinctive strategies for controlling tuberculosis emerged. The first, while acknowledging the continued social problems of tuberculosis patients, stressed the causative role of the bacillus and the overriding importance of appropriate antibiotic therapy. The second viewpoint, embodied by Dubos and "social medicine" advocates such as Henry E. Sigerist, argued that purely medical interventions would ultimately be inadequate for the prevention and treatment of tuberculosis. Because "outside circumstances, such as poor living conditions, poor working conditions, [and] undernourishment" were the "chief cause" of diseases like tuberculosis, addressing these social problems was essential if the disease was to be controlled.[9] It is the interplay between these two visions of tuberculosis control that the following eight chapters explore.

This book is hardly the first history of tuberculosis to describe the disease as both medical and social. A number of American historians have studied the social aspects of tuberculosis, informing us about subjects as diverse as the cultural meanings of infection and contagion, the social experience of illness, and society's attitude toward the poor and the disadvantaged.[10] For example, in *The White Plague,* their 1952 history of tuberculosis, René and Jean Dubos cautioned against a reductionist view of the disease as a medical problem that science would ultimately solve. They argued that as a social disease, tuberculosis was in fact a marker of the persistence of societal problems such as poverty, poor housing, and malnutrition.[11]

Although historians generally have not disputed this assessment, they have disagreed about the extent to which control measures actually have tried to solve "the social problem of tuberculosis."[12] For instance, Barbara Rosenkrantz, Michael Teller, Barbara Bates, and others have argued that antituberculosis efforts have largely eschewed any type of social reform agenda.[13] Moreover, as medical science has grown in stature during the twentieth century, a narrow biological model of tuberculosis has increasingly taken hold.

In general, Rosenkrantz notes, "scientific diagnosis" has been favored over any "vague social theories" that have attempted to advance a broader etiology of the disease.[14]

One historian who has challenged this point is Georgina Feldberg. In her recent book, *Disease and Class*, Feldberg argues that physicians in the United States have consistently emphasized the relation of tuberculosis to patients' social circumstances. As a result, Feldberg concludes, preventive and therapeutic interventions have addressed not only the bacillus but the financial, nutritional, and employment status of patients. In this manner, physicians have attempted to ensure that patients had adequate bodily resistance to fight the disease.[15]

A major goal of this book is to reexamine this debate. Have efforts to prevent and treat tuberculosis truly taken seriously the notion that it is a social disease? Or has such a characterization of tuberculosis served as window dressing for strategies that have basically stressed control of the bacillus? The present volume revisits this historical debate from a perspective different from that of previous work. Specifically, it examines the medical and social aspects of tuberculosis control in the post–World War II "antibiotic era."

Most historians of tuberculosis in the United States and Great Britain have focused on the nineteenth and early twentieth centuries.[16] Because these years witnessed Koch's discovery, the inauguration of the public health campaign to control the disease, and the rise of the sanatorium movement, the emphasis on the turn of the century has enabled historians to develop convincing narratives about the origins of tuberculosis control efforts. At the same time, however, scholars have tended to treat the post–World War II era as a sort of denouement, in which the availability of antibiotics rendered moot the earlier provocative questions about the appropriate prevention and management of the disease. Curative medical therapy, according to these histories, enabled physicians and health officials to close sanatoriums and to achieve dramatic reductions in morbidity and mortality from the disease.[17] Yet such an account is misleading. Throughout the postwar era, tuberculosis remained a major health problem, particularly in poor urban communities. Thus even as the new drugs represented a major medical breakthrough, they simultaneously served to highlight the persistent social problems that prevented American health officials from achieving optimal control of tuberculosis.

The years 1945 to 1973, therefore, provide an especially promising opportunity to address the interface between the medical and social approaches to tuberculosis. In what ways did the sudden availability of antibiotics—the so-called magic bullets—initially promote visions of a medical "fix" to the complicated problem of tuberculosis? How did both health professionals and society at large respond when it became clear that the persistent social problems of patients would limit what the new medications could achieve? Finally, what did it mean, in the antibiotic era, to term tuberculosis a "social disease?"

In addition to its emphasis on the antibiotic era, this book supplements the existing historiography of tuberculosis in two other ways. First, it focuses on tuberculosis control measures in a West Coast city, Seattle, Washington.[18] Specifically, it describes how Seattle's antituberculosis efforts after 1945 both contributed to and benefited from the city's transformation from a western frontier outpost to a "network" city integrated with the rest of the country.[19] One particularly notable problem faced by health officials in West Coast cities like Seattle was the extensive population of male vagrants who lived on the region's "skid roads." Not only were these men prone to tuberculosis, but their heavy alcohol use and transient lifestyles often interfered with treatment efforts.[20] While other American cities had similar skid row populations, Seattle's Skid Road was distinctive, often representing the end of the line for migrants who had traveled west in search of work. To address the issues of alcoholism and noncompliance with antibiotic therapy, tuberculosis workers in Seattle after 1950 pioneered an elaborate program for Skid Road patients that combined rehabilitative services with the use of forcible detention. This program would continue until 1973, when Firland Sanatorium, long the centerpiece of Seattle's tuberculosis control efforts, finally closed its doors.

Although this book concentrates on tuberculosis control measures in Seattle and elsewhere on the West Coast, it also provides a perspective on similar efforts being undertaken across the United States. Postwar tuberculosis workers around the country quickly recognized that the mere availability of antibiotics would not solve the perennial problem of controlling tuberculosis among the poor. Many of the strategies they initiated to address these social problems, such as the provision of vocational training and psychiatric services, were also employed by sanatorium officials in Seattle. By using Seattle as a case study, this history aims to illuminate the broader issues that characterized tuberculosis control in America in the 1950s and 1960s.

The final novel theme of this study is its examination of how aggressive public health policies designed to protect the community from tuberculosis—specifically, forcible quarantine and detention—influenced both the medical and social strategies for combating the disease. Although other authors have discussed how health officials used the powers of public health to prevent persons infected with tuberculosis from spreading the disease, most of this work has focused on the early years of the twentieth century.[21] It was in the 1950s and 1960s, however, that involuntary isolation of tuberculosis patients reached its apogee. Seattle was particularly zealous in its use of quarantine and detention, establishing in 1949 a locked ward that ultimately became a model for others across the nation.

This book examines both the legal basis of Seattle's program of forcible isolation and its actual implementation. In doing so, it relies extensively on a review of the medical charts of patients hospitalized at Firland Sanatorium between 1949 and 1973. These records, which include medical progress notes, documents pertaining to quarantine and detention proceedings, and letters from patients and family members, shed light on the experiences of staff and patients involved in the process of forcible isolation.[22]

Through an examination of antituberculosis measures in Seattle prior to 1945, chapter 1 places post–World War II efforts in the city in historical perspective. The earliest strategies for controlling tuberculosis in Seattle, which began in 1909, typified Progressive reform both in the city and across the country. Those involved in antituberculosis work in Seattle sought to use scientific advances in the fields of medicine and public health to build a bureaucratic infrastructure capable of dealing with Seattle's leading cause of death. Tuberculosis control measures, such as the opening of Firland Sanatorium, simultaneously served medical, public health, and social functions: treating the disease, isolating the infectious, and providing the sick poor with shelter, food, and terminal care. Seattle officials paid particular attention to tuberculosis among Skid Road indigents and transients, whose rates of tuberculous infection were the highest in the city.

As financial conditions in Seattle worsened in the 1920s and 1930s, the once concordant medical, public health, and social goals of tuberculosis work came into conflict. Improvement and expansion of existing programs would not occur until the 1940s, when improved economic circumstances and the fortuitous acquisition of a 1,350-bed surplus naval hospital (known as the "new" Firland Sanatorium) greatly improved the ability of local health officials to find and treat cases of the disease. Yet, as chapter 2 describes, it was the discovery of potentially curative antibiotics that grabbed the attention and imagination of perennially frustrated clinicians, patients, and families. As at other sanatoriums across the United States, the 1946 introduction of curative drugs provided Firland physicians with a powerful medical therapy for tuberculosis that they had not previously possessed. The new chemotherapeutic agents were, as one Firland Sanatorium annual report noted, nothing short of "amazing."[23]

Yet, as chapter 3 demonstrates, the antibiotics—and the innovative resectional lung surgery that the new medications made possible—proved to be no panacea. Most importantly, however, physicians learned that patients did not necessarily comply with their prescribed therapy, frequently leaving the sanatorium against medical advice or not taking the medications after discharge. As had long been the case, this noncompliance with medical recommendations reflected the continued high rate of social problems—such as homelessness and unemployment—among patients with tuberculosis. In order to address these types of situations, tuberculosis workers at Firland and across the country undertook several innovations, such as hiring psychiatrists and psychologists to discuss patients' emotional problems during hospitalization and establishing extensive programs of social services.[24]

Such interventions support Georgina Feldberg's contention that American physicians have always conceptualized tuberculosis as a social disease—one that could not simply be approached as a medical problem that doctors could "fix." Yet at the same time, these measures highlighted an underlying tension in the treatment of tuberculosis. Some commentators at Firland and across the country sincerely believed that tuberculosis therapy should include social interventions designed to provide patients with a "proper way of life."[25] That is, they did not view their work as completed until the patient had the means to obtain a job, a home, and adequate nutrition. Others, however, paid attention to social circumstances only as a mechanism for getting patients to complete their course of antibiotic therapy. Throughout the 1950s and 1960s, physicians at Firland and other American sanatoriums struggled to reconcile these quite different visions of what it meant to prevent and treat tuberculosis.

One individual who conceptualized tuberculosis from an especially broad perspective was Thomas H. Holmes, whose career is detailed in chapter 4. Hired by Firland as a psychiatrist to help patients adjust to sanatorium life, Holmes embarked on an extensive research program designed to demonstrate that tuberculosis was both a social and a "psychosomatic" disease. Although he did not deny the role of the tubercle bacillus in causing tuberculosis, Holmes believed that poor social circumstances and emotional instability played an even more significant role in determining who developed the disease. By examining Holmes' radical epistemological philosophy, which played down the importance of bacterial infection in causing tuberculosis, chapter 4 highlights once again the complex ways in which tuberculosis has been understood during the twentieth century.

The need to understand tuberculosis as more than just a pathological infection of the lung was nowhere more apparent than in the case of Skid Road alcoholics. Long the bane of health officials in Seattle, the uncooperativeness of this largely white male vagrant population produced particular consternation once antibiotics had been introduced. Rather than getting cured, alcoholic patients who were noncompliant with outpatient drug therapy had high rates of relapse. As a result, health officials believed, they were likely to spread tuberculosis throughout the community.

As it did with tuberculosis, Firland approached the issue of excessive alcohol consumption from a broad perspective. During the 1950s, a group of physicians and laypersons from across the United States were attempting to transform the public's perception of alcoholism. Alcoholism, they argued, was not a moral transgression deserving of opprobrium but rather a medical disease requiring scientific treatment. Building on this notion, Firland Sanatorium developed a nationally renowned program of services to address the complex sociomedical problems of the tuberculous alcoholic. This program is analyzed in chapter 5. Inspired largely by Joan K. Jackson and Ronald Fagan, a research sociologist and a recovered Skid Road alcoholic, respectively, Firland staff attempted to frame tuberculosis and alcoholism as a single disease, "tuberculosis-alcoholism," that required a broad range of medical and social interventions.[26]

Yet, as chapter 6 demonstrates, health officials in Seattle did not anticipate that such a strategy would be sufficient to address the myriad social problems of the "recalcitrant" Skid Road alcoholic. In 1948, at the behest of tuberculosis control officer Cedric Northrop, the state of Washington had significantly strengthened the public health regulations that permitted Seattle health officers to forcibly isolate uncooperative patients who did not comply with antibiotic therapy. The central element of this program was the establishment of a locked ward at Firland in 1949. Although Ward Six was originally intended for the occasional "bad actor"[27] who threatened the public's health, Firland eventually detained nearly one-half of all hospitalized Skid Road alcoholics. This chapter examines the transformation of involuntary isolation from a strategy of last resort to a routine policy.

Retelling the story of detention at Firland and other sanatoriums after World War II provides the historian with a significant challenge. How are we to judge, from our present perspective, behavior that, in retrospect, appears excessive and inappropriate? At first glance, it might be tempting to characterize the events at Firland as another instance of the "social control" of a marginal, disadvantaged population of patients by an authoritarian medical profession. The historical literature is certainly full of examples of physicians overstepping their authority when attempting to protect the public health and to promote compliance with recommended therapies.[28]

Yet as chapter 7 reveals, the actual day-to-day implementation of coercive measures at Firland Sanatorium was considerably more complex. Forcible confinement—as well as Firland's intriguing use of prophylactic lung surgery as a type of social intervention—was one aspect of an intricate process of bargaining and negotiation among sanatorium staff, health officials, and a subset of extremely unreliable, uncooperative Skid Road patients. Quarantine and detention at Firland, moreover, were not static processes. Throughout the years of the locked ward's existence, patients and staff members raised objections to sanatorium policies. Eventually, in 1957, the Washington chapter of the American Civil Liberties Union investigated conditions at Firland. Although the ACLU's response was ambivalent, its efforts did eventually culminate in the establishment of a unique type of judicial hearing for patients detained on the locked ward. This book argues that, given the complex intertwining of issues of infectiousness, poverty, substance use, and stigmatization, a social control model is inadequate for assessing the quarantine and detention of tuberculosis patients in the 1950s and 1960s.

The main portion of the narrative ends with the closure of Firland Sanatorium in 1973. By the 1970s, rates of tuberculosis infection in Seattle and elsewhere had plummeted, and treatment took place almost entirely in the outpatient setting. Even if the incidence of tuberculosis in the United States had continued to decline throughout the 1980s and 1990s, the history of tuberculosis control in Seattle would have represented an important story. In addressing disease among the poor and underinsured, modern health professionals continually confront social problems when attempting to institute preventive or therapeutic measures. Moreover, as Allan Brandt has demonstrated in his history of venereal diseases, when the disease in question raises issues of morals and "proper" behavior, it is impossible to separate purely medical interventions from social judgments.[29]

Nevertheless, the resurgence of tuberculosis in the United States that began in the mid-1980s has explicitly returned to public consciousness the same issues that health officials in Seattle confronted between 1943 and 1973. Once again, tuberculosis preferentially affects the most disadvantaged members of society, such as injection drug users, the homeless, and recent immigrants.[30] In addition, as persons infected with the human immunodeficiency virus (HIV) are particularly susceptible to tuberculosis, the rise of tuberculosis has been intimately related to the appearance of the acquired immunodeficiency syndrome (AIDS). Like tuberculosis, AIDS has been conceptualized as a "social disease" that has both "innocent" and "deserving" victims.[31] Finally, as in the past, high rates of noncompliance with antibiotic therapies, which have facilitated the spread of drug-resistant strains of tuberculosis, have raised significant public health concerns.

As noted in the concluding chapter of the book, health professionals combating the return of tuberculosis in the 1990s have, in one sense, learned their history lessons well. Noting that tuberculosis remains a "visible symbol of contemporary social problems and inequities,"[32] they have again termed it a "social disease" that is caused in part by problems like poverty and homelessness. Recently initiated therapeutic strategies are not narrowly "medical" but seek to address issues of drug use, language barriers, and inadequate housing.[33] So, too, with respect to public health concerns, modern programs have designed policies with an eye to the lessons of the past. Many health departments, for example, have revised their quarantine statutes to permit the forcible isolation of noncompliant tuberculosis patients only when all "less restrictive alternatives" have been exhausted.[34]

Although such efforts are laudable, they may ultimately raise more questions than they answer. How should health departments balance attempts to ensure completion of antibiotic therapy with efforts to assist tuberculosis patients get housing, drug rehabilitation, or a job? Or should medical practitioners no longer feel obliged to address the complicated—and perhaps unresolvable—social problems of disadvantaged populations? Finally, if narrower programs that emphasize a medical solution to tuberculosis prove effective, of what value is the continued designation of tuberculosis as a social disease?

A series of related questions arise in the case of new public health initiatives designed to control the spread of tuberculosis. Is the coercion of tuberculosis patients invariably overused even when safeguards are established in advance? Does the use of coercive measures preclude concurrent efforts to rehabilitate patients who have numerous social problems? How should physicians and other health professionals treating noncompliant persons with tuberculosis balance their dual roles as caregivers and disciplinarians?

Indeed, such questions are hardly limited to tuberculosis or other public health problems. Modern clinicians are continually confronted with noncompliant patients who do not cooperate with prescribed therapies and who make excessive demands on the health care system.[35] Like their predecessors at Firland, practitioners today struggle to set appropriate limits for patients who are a danger not only to others but to themselves. How many heart-valve replacements should injection drug users receive if they continue to use illicit drugs? What should be done with a kidney failure patient who misses regular dialysis appointments and then demands emergency treatment? Are such noncompliant patients victims of a health care system that discriminates against the poor and disadvantaged, or do such persons ultimately bear some degree of responsibility for their uncooperative behavior?

This study of tuberculosis control in the United States from 1945 to 1973 does not definitively answer these questions. Nevertheless, by exploring the experiences of the staff and patients at Seattle's Firland Sanatorium, it does provide an important historical context for addressing the enduring nexus of disease, poverty, noncompliance, and the use of coercion.

ONE

Setting the Stage

The Origins of Tuberculosis Control in Seattle

Early municipal efforts to control tuberculosis in Seattle confronted three problems: the medical problem of treating the disease, the public health problem of preventing the spread of infection, and the social problem of addressing the suboptimal living conditions that predisposed poor and working-class persons to tuberculosis. Beginning in 1909, this ambitious strategy typified the city's Progressive reform movement, which combined the moral mission of cleaning up the Skid Road with the economic goal of building an efficient administrative framework for correcting urban problems.

The fact that tuberculosis simultaneously raised medical, public health, and social issues served to highlight its importance, but it also ensured that conflicts would arise over how best to implement these agendas. For example, should hospitals like Firland Sanatorium give priority to the treatment of persons likely to make a medical recovery from their disease or to the care of sicker patients who had nowhere else to spend the last months of their lives? To what extent should the King County Anti-Tuberculosis League and the Seattle Department of Health and Sanitation address the social problems that either predisposed persons to tuberculosis or interfered with their ability to take the "cure"? How aggressively were Seattle officials obliged to isolate uncooperative tuberculosis patients, particularly alcoholic vagrants from the Skid Road, whose behavior threatened the public's health?

These questions only became more difficult after 1920, when the end of Progressivism and then the Great Depression tempered enthusiasm for expensive reform measures like tuberculosis control. Nor would such conflicts disappear after World War II, when an infusion of money and the discovery of curative antibiotics led many commentators to predict that the complex problems raised by tuberculosis had finally been solved.

PUBLIC HEALTH AND REFORM IN EARLY SEATTLE

Founded in 1854 on the eastern border of the majestic Puget Sound, Seattle quickly became an important trading outpost. By 1880 the population of the city had reached 3,553 people. The largest industry in early Seattle was Henry Yesler's saw mill, built in 1853. Taking advantage of the city's waterfront location and the lush surrounding forestry, Yesler soon became a major exporter of lumber and timber.[1]

Major growth in Seattle did not occur until the 1890s. The city was rebuilt after a devastating fire in 1889, and the population surged when Seattle became linked to a transcontinental railroad, the Great Northern, in 1893. In 1897, as a result of the Klondike and Nome gold rushes, Seattle's port became the "gateway to gold" in Alaska.[2] By the first decade of the twentieth century, the city had a diverse manufacturing base, including twenty-seven lumber mills, numerous shipbuilding companies, printing and publishing concerns, foundries, and machine shops.[3]

By 1910, Seattle had become the "premier city of the northwest," having surpassed both nearby Tacoma, Washington, and Portland, Oregon, in population. The 1910 census listed Seattle's population as 237,194, making it the twentieth-largest city in the United States. As of 1916, Seattle was the leading port of the Pacific Coast, trading with the Orient to the west and to points east through the newly opened Panama Canal. In addition, four transcontinental railroads now had major routes coming to Seattle. As the city's population expanded, Seattle grew outward from its initial site at the inlet of Elliott Bay. By 1910, it had incorporated large areas of land, including Queen Anne Hill and Fremont, to the north, and West Seattle, to the south. The business district remained at the city's original center.[4]

The best-known section of Seattle, however, was the Skid Road. Unlike eastern cities such as New York, Seattle lacked the overcrowded, decaying slums and tenements that housed new European immigrants and promoted the spread of diseases like tuberculosis. Nevertheless, the arrival of thousands of single men, in search of Alaskan gold or seasonal jobs in the lumber industry or on the docks, ensured that a large transient population always resided in Seattle.[5] These men tended to congregate in an area abutting the waterfront just south of downtown, which came to be known as the "Skid Road." Originally, "Skid Road" had referred to the street on which loggers dragged their lumber on the way to Henry Yesler's waterfront sawmill. Applying grease to the road enabled the logs to skid, thereby easing the work of the oxen.[6] Although the road itself eventually took the name Yesler Way, the area directly to the south, which housed many of the loggers during the winter months, retained the original sobriquet. In subsequent years, a related term, "skid row," was used to describe similarly run-down portions of U.S.

cities, characterized by the presence of taverns, brothels, and flophouses. The classic skid row setting, however, remained western frontier towns that attracted large numbers of unattached vagrants.[7]

Life on the Skid Road has inspired many historical and fictional accounts. To understand Seattle, Murray Morgan wrote in his 1951 history of the city, it was necessary to understand the Skid Road: "While goldminers and gamblers, prostitutes and sports, softhanded cheechakos and horny-palmed river pilots from the Yukon roamed the newly cobbled streets, barkers shouted of the attractions to be seen in the basements. Every night at the corner of Second and Washington musicians from the People's Theater clashed in a resounding duel with a brass band from a rival establishment."[8] Screenwriters and novelists have also used the Skid Road as a backdrop. Numerous Hollywood films about the Alaskan gold rush contained scenes set in Seattle. In John Dos Passos's *The 42nd Parallel,* the Wobbly Mac and his friend Ike Hill come to Seattle in search of jobs, education, and women. Arriving on the Seattle waterfront, which "smelt of lumberyards [and] was noisy with rattle of carts and yells of drivers," they get drunk with two prostitutes, who promptly steal all their money.[9]

Everyday life on the Skid Road was considerably less romantic than in its fictional portrayals. Although work in the Seattle area grew plentiful as the city's economy expanded, many of the unskilled laborers could not find jobs in the winter. The work itself, moreover, was arduous, and the living conditions in logging camps or on farms in eastern Washington were squalid. Most importantly, wages paid to laborers during summer employment rarely provided for comfortable living during the off-season. As a result, a typical street on Skid Road revealed "men sitting on curbs and sleeping in doorways, condemned buildings, [and] signs that read: 'Beds, twenty cents.'"[10] Missions, run by the Salvation Army and other agencies, dotted the area, providing meals to the down-and-out and seeking to save their souls. The Skid Road consistently had Seattle's highest rates of infectious diseases like tuberculosis. As Morgan concluded in his history of Seattle, the Skid Road was the "place of dead dreams."[11]

The men who settled in the Skid Road area, like the rest of Seattle's residents, were largely native whites. Foreign-born men who lived on the Skid Road tended to be Norwegians and Swedes, many of whom had emigrated from midwestern states like Minnesota, Illinois, and Wisconsin. The Skid Road and its surrounding neighborhoods also became the haven for many of Seattle's nonwhites, who comprised only five percent of the city's population between 1900 and 1920. The largest minority, the Japanese, were often victims of racial discrimination, as were members of other nonwhite groups—including Chinese, African Americans, and Native Americans—who settled in Seattle.[12]

It is impossible to describe the Skid Road in Seattle without considering the importance of alcohol. Unemployment and idleness encouraged drinking, and entrepreneurs readily exploited the situation. The number of saloons in the area proliferated during the pre-Prohibition era. Most of Seattle's citizens had little good to say about saloons or their clientele. In 1915, Mayor Hiram Gill contrasted the good citizens of Seattle with "bums and hoboes dependent on alcohol."[13] What most bothered members of Washington state's active antisaloon movement, however, were the vice and degeneration that they believed accompanied the sale and ingestion of liquor. One of the leaders of Seattle's temperance movement was the fiery preacher Mark Matthews, whose Sunday sermons on "vice, sin, and the saloon" made clear the connections between liquor, gambling, prostitution, and the other transgressions that threatened the moral backbone of the city. Upon hearing the "full and steady roar" of the six-foot-five-inch Matthews, a writer for *Collier's* magazine commented: "Few men can paint black blacker than he."[14]

Naturally, much of the energies of the local chapters of the Anti-Saloon League and the Women's Christian Temperance Union focused on the Skid Road. In 1914 Washington voters passed Initiative 3, the state's first temperance law. The Women's Christian Temperance Union's successful battle for passage of the legislation had centered in Seattle and took its inspiration from the Skid Road. As a result of Initiative 3, the manufacture and sale of alcoholic beverages in the state of Washington was declared illegal. When the new law went into effect on January 1, 1916, Washington became one of twenty-three states to have passed prohibition legislation. Although voters across the state favored Initiative 3, 61 percent of Seattle's electorate voted in opposition.[15] This vote was one of several conflicting signals sent by Seattle voters regarding the issues of alcohol and the Skid Road.

Progressive reformers in Seattle did not focus solely on the problems of the Skid Road. For example, fifty local organizations joined together to form the Central Council of Social Agencies, which was dedicated to the elimination of problems like poverty and poor housing throughout the city. Meanwhile, Frank B. Cooper was molding a public school system that was "a superb example of progressive era urban schooling."[16]

The most elaborate reform movement in Seattle, however, centered on efforts to achieve municipal ownership of city utilities. A series of private companies were responsible for water supply, electric power, the street railways, and sewage and water disposal. This private ownership not only severely restricted city revenues but also promoted various types of corruption, such as bribery and graft. By eliminating both fraud and waste, reformers believed, municipal ownership would create a more efficient and economical Seattle. This effort to build a bureaucratic infrastructure within the city government exemplifies the type of Progressive reform described by historians of the "organizational synthesis" school.[17]

Thanks in large part to the efforts of the Municipal League, a coalition of reform-minded organizations, the municipal ownership campaign met with considerable success. By 1915 the city government had gained control of the so-called natural monopolies and had greatly improved services to the community. For example, the city constructed its first municipally owned street railway in 1914 and broke the monopoly of private businesses on the waterfront by opening the Port of Seattle.[18]

The municipal ownership campaign was intimately connected to issues of public health in Seattle. As the city's population rapidly expanded from thirty-four hundred in 1880 to twenty thousand by 1888, sanitary problems became more pronounced. Seattle's rudimentary sewer system, for example, was deemed worthless, as waste often flowed backward from Lake Washington into the city. Because services like trash removal remained in private hands, piles of garbage often lay rotting in many of Seattle's poorer areas.[19] By assuming control of the water supply, as well as the disposal of sewage and garbage, the city might not only produce more efficient and lucrative systems but might also ensure better health among its citizenry.

A series of initiatives by the city government addressed these sanitary problems. Seattle's sewage system underwent marked expansion between 1895 and 1908, enabling the city's refuse to be channeled into Puget Sound. Voters approved $1,250,000 worth of bonds in 1895, allowing Seattle to begin construction of a system that provided pure water for the city. Seven years later, voters financed the construction of a hydroelectric plant on the Cedar River and, thereby, the creation of Seattle City Light. Finally, in 1911, the Department of Health and Sanitation (formerly the Board of Health) assumed control of garbage collection in the city.[20]

While efforts to purify water and dispose of waste products had been part of public health efforts since the Great Sanitary Awakening of the mid-nineteenth century, new discoveries about the origin of disease were producing changes in public health practice. A group of European scientists, most notably Louis Pasteur in France and Robert Koch in Germany, had convincingly demonstrated by the 1880s that many common diseases were caused by microscopic particles known as germs or bacteria. Transmission of these bacteria to healthy persons, moreover, might cause the onset of disease. As elsewhere in the country, health officials in Seattle, such as Health Commissioner James Crichton, incorporated this new scientific knowledge into disease prevention strategies.

The discovery that microscopic organisms caused disease lent an important scientific imprimatur to public health work throughout Seattle. Crichton's frequent references to "scientific sanitation" typified the growing connection of science to municipal reform efforts across the country. As the Seattle public health historian Nancy Rockafellar has argued, the goal of creating a "healthful" Seattle was clearly at the core of Progressivism in the city.[21]

By 1910, public health efforts in the city appeared to be working. According to that year's census, Seattle's mortality rate—10.1 deaths per 100,000 population—was the lowest in the country. Crichton proudly publicized this figure in both the Health Department's *Annual Report* and its *Bulletin* issued for the general public. The low death rate, he wrote, was a triumph for the "great and progressive city of Seattle."[22] Indeed, the success of the Health Department was no accident. A 1913 survey revealed that Seattle spent more per capita on its health department than any other city in the country with a population greater than twenty-five thousand people. Once again, improved health in Seattle was tied to its overall development.[23]

FIGHTING THE WHITE PLAGUE

Despite these encouraging statistics, one major health problem remained. In 1911 tuberculosis was the leading cause of death in Seattle, responsible for over 13 percent of the deaths in the city. Moreover, the mortality rate from the disease had steadily risen over the previous four years. Despite its excellent public health record and low overall mortality, Seattle had done very little to address tuberculosis. Not until 1911, after a commission investigating the "proper control and final eradication" of tuberculosis in the city issued its report, did antituberculosis measures begin in earnest.[24] Like other Progressive Era reform efforts in Seattle, tuberculosis control was the result of a combination of economic and moral imperatives.

Although scientists discovered many new microorganisms during the 1880s, the most momentous finding was Robert Koch's 1882 identification of the bacterium that causes tuberculosis. By the late nineteenth century, tuberculosis, the "captain of all these men of death," was the leading cause of mortality in the Western hemisphere. Moreover, the disease often struck the relatively young: more than 50 percent of deaths from tuberculosis in the United States occurred in people between the ages of twenty and forty.[25] Not only did the disease cause prolonged illness and often death in this age group, but it also led to the splintering and impoverishment of entire families.

The term *tuberculosis* was derived from the discovery of small tumors, or "tubercles," in autopsy specimens of victims of the disease. The bacterium that caused tuberculosis, *Mycobacterium tuberculosis,* could infect almost every organ system in the body. For example, children were particularly susceptible to tuberculous meningitis, an invariably fatal infection of the tissues surrounding the spinal cord. As the disease progressed it led to paralysis of

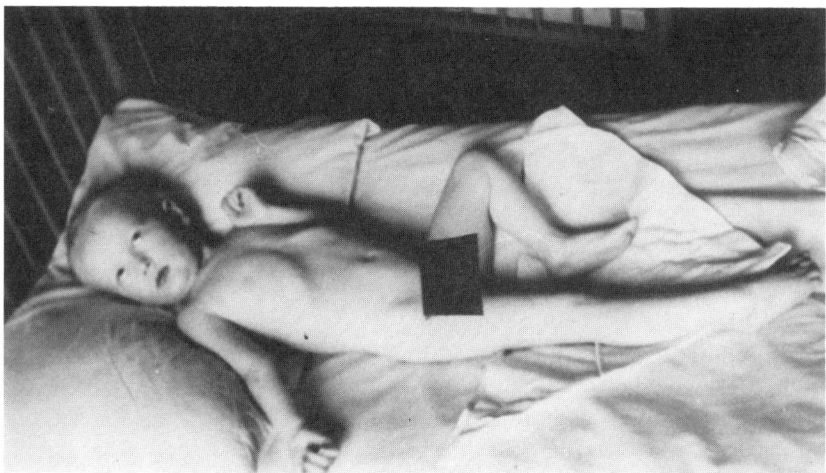

FIGURE 1.1 Child dying of tuberculous meningitis, described as "looking for the angels," 1938. Courtesy of Otto Trott, M.D.

the cranial nerves, causing the children's eyes to become fixed and dilated (figure 1.1). Helpless physicians could only tell distraught parents that their dying offspring were "looking for the angels."[26]

Other common forms of tuberculosis included infections of the kidneys and bones. Tuberculosis of the intestines, which was actually caused by a different bacterium, *Mycobacterium bovis*, generally spread through the ingestion of contaminated milk. Most commonly, however, tuberculosis attacked the lungs, where it caused the formation of cavities laden with tubercle bacilli. This form of the disease had been known as consumption in the nineteenth century: people were literally "consumed" by the disease, coughing blood and growing progressively wasted and short of breath.[27] Another common name for tuberculosis in the nineteenth century was phthisis, a Greek term for a wasting illness, and tuberculosis specialists well into the twentieth century continued to refer to themselves as phthisiologists.

While Koch's identification of the tubercle bacillus was of major importance, his work was seminal for another reason. His "thorough piece of medical investigation" demonstrated that tuberculosis was communicable, spread when uninfected individuals inhaled bacilli from an infected person's sputum. As with cholera and typhoid fever, physicians had long debated the contagiousness of consumption. Prior to Koch's experiments, most commentators believed that people contracted the disease as a result of hereditary and constitutional predisposition, as well as environmental factors such as miasmas.[28]

The knowledge that tuberculosis was communicable generated an emotional response among the lay public in Seattle. While it was commonly stated that "everyone at some time or another is just a little bit tuberculous,"[29] this belief did little to quell the terror instilled by a disease that was commonly equated with a death sentence. Recalling her service as a tuberculosis nurse in Seattle in 1913, Anna M. Moore wrote that "the public's attitude concerning tuberculosis in those days was one of great fear. . . . Sometimes it was difficult to get people to be examined when you were not supposed to mention the dread word, tuberculosis."[30] Fear of tuberculosis was so rampant that a term, *phthisiophobia,* was coined to describe it.

At times, fears were translated into action. In 1905, a Seattle man broke off his wedding plans after learning that his betrothed had a family history of tuberculosis.[31] Four years later, Washington became one of only two states to enact laws prohibiting marriage to people with tuberculosis. Indeed, the tuberculous were only one of several groups of persons forbidden to marry:

> No woman under the age of forty-five years, or man of any age, except he marry a woman over the age of forty-five years, either of whom is a common drunkard, habitual criminal, epileptic, imbecile, feeble-minded person, idiot or insane person, or person who has theretofore been afflicted with hereditary insanity, or is afflicted with pulmonary tuberculosis in its advanced stages, or any contagious venereal disease, shall hereafter intermarry or marry any other person within this state.[32]

This law revealed the explicit connection made between infectious diseases, such as tuberculosis and venereal disease, and a series of "inherited" conditions that were supposedly leading to the degeneration of the Anglo-Saxon race. Like other states across the country, Washington had an active eugenics movement that argued that individuals with mental illness, mental retardation, or criminal tendencies were "unfit" to marry and reproduce.[33]

Given the equation of tuberculosis with these other conditions, many Seattle residents had little compassion for the victims of consumption. The stigmatization of the tuberculous was exacerbated by the fact that the disease preferentially affected the poorer neighborhoods of the city. This is not to say that tuberculosis spared Seattle's wealthier citizens, who had begun to settle in First Hill and other prosperous sections of the city. Yet, as had been the case since the rapid advance of urbanization and industrialization in the nineteenth century, tuberculosis predominated among the poor, who were blamed for its spread. "Consumptives," according to the "Women's Round Table" section of the *Seattle Mail and Herald,* "seem to have an unconscious desire, which amounts to almost mania, to disseminate their terrible disease as far and widely as possible." Remarking on the "blood and sputum from their diseased lungs" found on the pavement, the author concluded that a healthy person "would a great deal rather see a ghost."[34]

Despite the fear that tuberculosis engendered, formal efforts to control the disease began more slowly in both Seattle and Washington than in the East and Midwest.[35] The earliest organization in the United States dedicated to the control of tuberculosis was the Pennsylvania Society for the Prevention of Tuberculosis. Founded in 1892 by a Philadelphia physician named Lawrence F. Flick, the volunteer group sought "to prevent tuberculosis by promoting the doctrine of contagiousness."[36] The society served a primarily educational role, instructing patients, families, and the general public on proper techniques to prevent the spread of the disease. In 1893, the Board of Health of New York City, at the behest of Hermann Biggs, established the country's first comprehensive program of tuberculosis control. Components of this campaign included making tuberculosis reportable, tracking down contacts of infected persons, and establishing dispensaries and sanatoriums to care for the sick. While tuberculosis affected all neighborhoods in New York, Biggs emphasized the need to control the disease where it was most prevalent: in the crowded tenement houses of the Lower East Side, which housed recently arrived Eastern European immigrants (figure 1.2).[37]

By 1898, Seattle had begun to adopt similar measures to control the spread of tuberculosis. The city passed an antispitting ordinance and added tuberculosis to the list of diseases that physicians were required to report to the Department of Health. Nevertheless, five years later, department officials admitted that compliance with mandatory regulation was minimal. In addition, well into the first decade of the twentieth century, Seattle had no facilities to house patients with infectious tuberculosis, aside from a few beds at the King County Poor Farm.[38] Consumptives remained at home, infecting their families and friends as they slowly died. It was the lack of a hospital that could provide care for the tuberculous that ultimately convinced a group of private citizens in Seattle to organize the Anti-Tuberculosis League of King County in 1909.

The role of a voluntary organization in initiating tuberculosis control measures in Seattle mirrored the pattern in Philadelphia and throughout most of the United States. The King County league quickly became affiliated with both a statewide organization, the Washington Association for the Prevention and Relief of Tuberculosis (later, the Washington Tuberculosis Association), and the National Association for the Study and Prevention of Tuberculosis (later, the National Tuberculosis Association).[39] League members were mostly Seattle businessmen, several of whom had a personal connection to tuberculosis. Typical was Horace C. Henry, a local railroad magnate who became the league's first president in 1910. Henry's son Walter had died of tuberculosis earlier that year.

The league was a direct descendant of nineteenth-century reform movements such as the Social Gospel and Charity Organization Societies (COS).

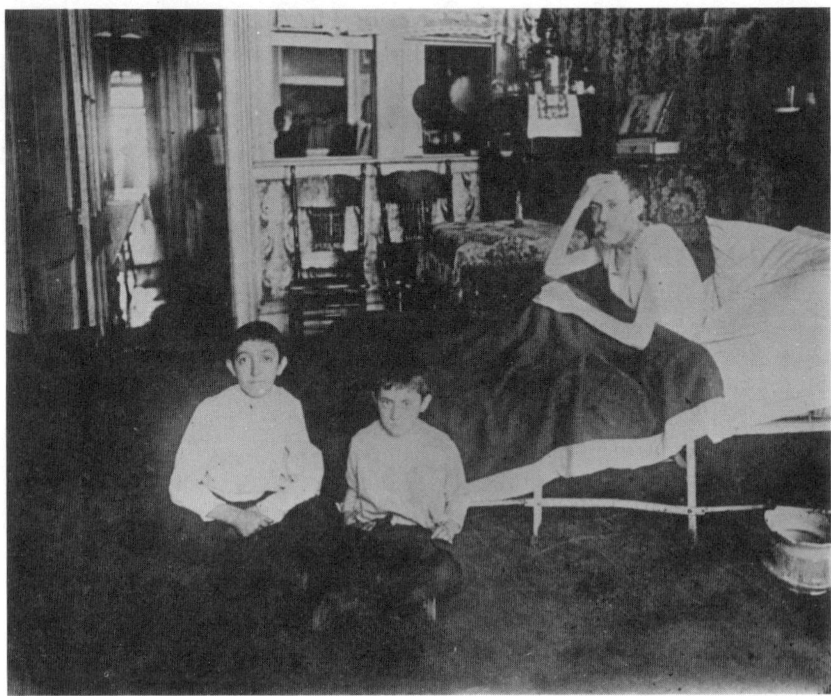

FIGURE 1.2 "TB in the tenements is a dangerous and communicable disease." Educational photograph, probably circulated by the Committee on the Prevention of Tuberculosis of the Charity Organization Society of New York, circa 1905. Courtesy of the American Lung Association of New York.

These groups had combined a strong emphasis on Christianity with the spirit of voluntarism, which encouraged economic self-sufficiency among the poor and explicitly discouraged relief measures.[40] Although tuberculosis work in Seattle, as elsewhere, was largely secular in nature, the league's motto, "God help us to help the helpless," bore more than a passing resemblance to the words of COS "guiding spirit" Josephine Shaw Lowell: "The best help of all is to help people to help themselves."[41]

As a result of the league's efforts, tuberculosis quickly became an important topic of discussion. Frequent articles appeared in Seattle newspapers in 1909 bearing such headlines as "What Is Seattle Going to Do for Her Consumptives?" and "City Must Take Care of the Sick." The league organized an annual observance of "Anti-Tuberculosis Sunday," held in churches each April.[42] Funding for league activities came through promotions such as "button days" and "tag sales" as well as a benefit carnival. In 1910 the league joined with the statewide organization to organize the first annual sale of Christmas Seals. In future years, Christmas Seals would become not only the league's chief source of fund-raising but also the characteristic symbol of the National Tuberculosis Association and its affiliates.

The league allocated its funding for several purposes. In addition to its publicity work, it began a formal program of visiting nurse services for tuberculosis patients in Seattle and King County. The league also helped to finance a free tuberculosis dispensary, which was in operation by 1911. As these activities were examples of the typical "demonstration projects" organized by voluntary agencies in the Progressive Era, the city Department of Health soon assumed the operation of nursing and clinic services in the city. The Anti-Tuberculosis League also earmarked a percentage of its funds for direct relief efforts, such as the provision of shelter and food to very ill tuberculosis patients and their families.[43]

Perhaps the most significant activity of the league in its early years was its role in the establishment of a public sanatorium in Seattle. Once again, the city had been slow to respond to a nationwide trend and was, according to one 1908 reference, the only city of its size without provision for the care of tuberculosis patients.[44] When the league finally broached the issue, the extent to which many Seattle citizens feared infection with tuberculosis became apparent. In the summer of 1909, thanks to a donation from the First Presbyterian Church, league members planned to erect a "tent colony" for the care of the tuberculous on Queen Anne Hill, overlooking Seattle. Upon arriving at the prospective site, however, the two wagons filled with tents, furniture, beds, cooking utensils, and food were met by a group of local women intent on preventing the establishment of the colony. In the words of William K. McKibben, the league's first executive secretary, each woman was "brandishing a broom stick, threatening death and damnation to horses and drivers and every terrible social worker in the wicked League."[45]

If the league's caravan had experienced an early example of "not in my backyard," it may have been a blessing in disguise. The local newspapers gave front-page coverage to the event, which elicited great sympathy for the work of the league as well as sixty offers of other potential sites to house the tent colony. Tents were ultimately erected at several of these locations.[46] League members knew, however, that tents were merely a temporary solution and that a permanent hospital was needed.

Planning for such a facility began in 1910, when league president Horace Henry donated $25,000 and a thirty-four-acre site twelve miles north of the city for the construction of a sanatorium. Henry dedicated his gift to the memory of his son. The location was particularly suitable, one commentator later noted, because of both its elevation and its "remoteness from the community's hysterical fear of the 'white plague.' "[47] In 1911 the Henry Sanatorium opened on the site, eventually housing thirty-five patients in a series of cottages.

Despite Henry's largesse, however, the operation of a city sanatorium was beyond the capacities of the league. Thus, in 1912, for a sum of one dollar, it deeded the land and cottages of the Henry Sanatorium to the city, with the stipulation that they be used in the fight against tuberculosis. The Health Department was grateful for the donation. A city commission charged with formulating plans to control and eradicate tuberculosis in Seattle had just issued a list of recommendations, which included the opening of sanatoriums and hospitals for the care of the tuberculous.[48]

Having received the league's gift, the city began to formulate plans to build and run a permanent sanatorium on the site. Given the rising death rate from tuberculosis that Seattle had experienced in 1911, Crichton believed it was an opportune time to place a bond issue on the ballot for this purpose. In March 1912, Seattle's taxpayers once again voted overwhelmingly to finance one of Crichton's public health projects, approving the $125,000 bond by a sixty-four-point margin (82 to 18 percent).[49] Completed in 1914, the new facility would be the centerpiece of tuberculosis work in the city for the next thirty-three years.

The tuberculosis control efforts detailed above typified Progressive reform in the city, inspired by a mixture of economic and humanitarian concerns. In the 1911 annual report of the Department of Health, Crichton emphasized that adoption of the tuberculosis commission's recommendations would ultimately save Seattle money:

> After having examined into the facts presented from different sources I am firmly of the opinion that, looking at the question simply as to dollars and cents, it can be readily proven that it is by far cheaper for a city or state to make ample appropriations to stamp out this disease quickly. . . . Looking at the question from the standpoint of the number of lives saved there is absolutely no doubt but that quick action and a well thought out plan of operation will save by far the greater number.[50]

Similar language characterized a 1909 State Board of Health report on tuberculosis control, which called for an "*efficient* system for the notification and registration of consumptives."[51] As the state went into the "tuberculosis business," the report continued, it was important to do so in an intelligent, economical, and comprehensive fashion.[52]

At the same time, it was clear that the plight of the tuberculous elicited great sympathy among Progressives in Seattle. This was not surprising, given the league's strong ties to nineteenth-century voluntarism. Although Seattle lacked the overcrowded tenements found in East Coast cities, there were still poor and homeless persons, particularly on the Skid Road. City health officials were most concerned with so-called terrace or block-front dwellings, which resembled the brownstones of eastern cities but had poor light and ventilation and contained little area for recreation. "From a housing and sanitary viewpoint," wrote one Seattle official in 1916, "I can hardly conceive of anything worse."[53]

King County Anti-Tuberculosis League members aroused public sympathy with their dramatic accounts of the lives of the indigent tuberculous who lived in such surroundings. "We had dug out poor wretches," wrote William McKibben, "coughing away their own lives and the lives of others in 5 cent flop houses under the downtown sidewalks."[54] League nurses, reported another writer, "discovered scores of sufferers hidden away in sardine lodging houses and other unsatisfactory shelters."[55] Use of this type of language was not limited to league members. Health Commissioner Crichton, while stressing the economic virtues of tuberculosis control, referred to its victims as "tubercular unfortunates" and described their affliction as the "Impoverishing Disease."[56]

The campaign to pass the $125,000 bond issue in 1912 had also demonstrated the public's concern for persons with tuberculosis. Newspapers and churches lent strong support, and Boy Scouts reportedly made "door knob calls" at every house in the city. Looking back at the 82 percent support given the measure, a 1928 Department of Health publication called the vote a "beautiful express[ion] by Seattle citizens . . . [of] philanthropic and humanitarian motives."[57] The stage was set for the opening of Firland Sanatorium.

EVOLVING GOALS AT FIRLAND SANATORIUM

The concept of the sanatorium dated back to 1854, when a physician, Hermann Brehmer, established the first such institution in the mountains of Germany. The first sanatorium in the United States, Edward Trudeau's Adirondack Cottage Sanatorium, opened in mountainous upstate New York in 1885. The primary goal of these early sanatoriums was curative. While there were differences in the "regimens" offered, treatment generally consisted of fresh air, good nutrition, and a carefully designed balance of bed rest and gradual exercise. By the first decade of the twentieth century, this prescription had been modified to some extent. The role of climate had become less important; sanatoriums and tuberculosis hospitals, particularly for the urban poor, were situated much closer to cities.[58]

Reflecting its location among a forest of fir trees, Seattle officials named the new sanatorium Firland. In 1914 James Crichton and his colleagues at the Seattle Department of Health named Robert M. Stith as Firland's first medical director. Stith, who had become the first physician-in-charge of the department's Division of Tuberculosis in 1912, was a midwesterner educated at the University of Pennsylvania School of Medicine. He arrived in Seattle in 1902 and quickly became involved with such public health issues as the purification of milk and water supplies. Stith's growing interest in tuberculosis control after 1910 stemmed in large part from memories of his mother's death from the disease.[59] Aside from a brief period of military service during World War I, Stith would remain as head of both Firland and the Division of Tuberculosis until his death in 1943.

The division coordinated a large number of community-based antituberculosis activities, including three clinics for diagnosing and monitoring patients, a visiting nurse service for care of patients in their homes, a screening program for food industry workers in the city, and a bacteriology laboratory for examining sputum samples of family contacts and persons with symptoms suggestive of the disease. (Sputum samples containing *Mycobacterium tuberculosis* confirmed the diagnosis of tuberculosis.) In diagnosing and following persons with tuberculosis, clinic staff relied not only on sputum examination but also on skin testing and, beginning in the 1920s, chest X-rays. Persons diagnosed with clinical disease by sputum or X-ray were either admitted to Firland or followed at home. Those with positive skin tests but no evidence of disease had most often been infected in childhood and had walled off the tubercle bacilli into dormant lesions. Such individuals required close observation but no active intervention.

When Firland first opened in 1914, it contained beds for 150 adults and 25 children. This total, however, was not nearly enough to hospitalize all of the 1,030 known persons in the city with tuberculosis, let alone another estimated three thousand persons with undetected or unreported disease. As a result, Firland always had a waiting list for admission.[60] Indeed, when the Tuberculosis Control Division of the King County Department of Health opened its own sanatorium, Morningside, for indigent patients who lived outside city limits, the new facility also generally had a waiting list. Patients who were able to pay for sanatorium care were hospitalized at two other facilities, the Pulmonary Hospital of the City of Seattle (later, the Riverton Sanatorium) and Laurel Beach Sanatorium.[61]

Firland had an impressive physical presence. Two of the buildings—the Administration Building and the Hospital for Adults (later known as Detweiler)—were particularly attractive, a combination of brick and English Tudor in an Elizabethan style (figure 1.3).[62] Although the Anti-Tuberculosis League no longer ran the institution, the stamp of the National Association for the Study and Prevention of Tuberculosis was everywhere: its characteristic red double-barred cross adorned the entire premises, from doorknobs to the sidewalk outside the Administration Building.

While relatively little is known about the composition of Firland's patient

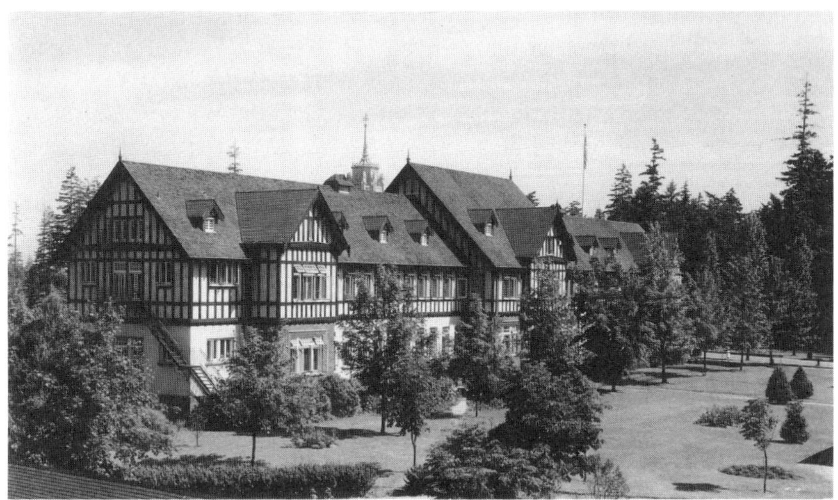

FIGURE 1.3 The Detweiler Building at Firland Sanatorium, circa 1930. This facility housed patients at bedrest. Author's personal collection.

population in this era, a list of professions contained in the Department of Health's annual reports reveals them to have been overwhelmingly working class. Roughly one-half of the patients were foreign born. In most years, an equal number of patients had "good housing," while the remainder were classified as living in "congested district[s] and poor housing." Among the latter group were the "wanderers," who constituted as much as 30 percent of patients in certain years.[63]

Hospitalization at Firland served two major purposes: it provided patients with medical treatment, and it isolated them from the community. Available medical therapy, however, was limited. In the case of tuberculosis, there was no "magic bullet" like Paul Ehrlich's recently discovered Salvarsan, an arsenical preparation that effectively treated certain cases of syphilis.[64] Nevertheless, physicians at Firland strongly advocated bed rest with gradual exercise, fresh air, and good nutrition. Bed rest, they believed, allowed for the rebuilding of muscle, the gaining of strength, and the healing of diseased lung tissue. Fresh air, particularly direct exposure to cold air in the winter, lowered the workload of the lungs and thus sped healing. A nutritious diet provided the body with strength to fight the tuberculosis germ.[65]

The second major value of sanatorium care was as a public health measure. The early sanatorium movement had largely stressed the curative nature of the institution. By the time of the Sixth International Congress on Tuberculosis in 1908, however, tuberculosis workers had begun to emphasize the value of preventive measures. The sanatorium contributed by removing infectious patients from the community. In addition, hospital staff used the inpatient setting to teach patients the proper techniques for preventing the spread of infection, both at Firland and following their discharge.[66]

While Stith most clearly delineated the medical and public health functions of the sanatorium, Firland also addressed the social problems of its poor and working-class patients. Persons unable to pay any portion of their hospital bill (generally more than 90 percent of those admitted) stayed at Firland for free. The cost of hospitalization was assumed by the city Department of Health; Washington State also contributed five dollars weekly for each indigent patient. Free admission of those with tuberculosis not only represented a service to poor or working-class households, but it also enabled other family members to return to work, thereby "remov[ing] considerable financial burden from the family."[67] Social agencies, such as the King County Welfare Department and the Community Chest Fund, also provided relief to many of these families. This service expanded when welfare allocations grew in the 1930s and 1940s.

Hospitalization itself also eased the burdens of patients and, indirectly, their families. Tuberculosis workers in Seattle and throughout the country refused to see their task as merely curing the patient of his or her medical disease. Rather, comprehensive therapy for tuberculosis included efforts to ensure that discharged patients remained both physically healthy and economically solvent. Among the mechanisms used to achieve these goals were sanatorium-based programs of vocational rehabilitation that sought to find less stressful jobs for patients who were sent home. In some parts of the country, officials established formal aftercare programs that provided supervised employment and intensive medical follow-up for recently discharged patients.[68]

Initially, the medical, public health, and social aims of Firland appeared to complement one another. In its early years, the sanatorium preferentially admitted severe cases of tuberculosis, many of whom had cavitary disease. In 1915, for example, 282 out of 289 admitted patients had either stage II (moderately advanced) or stage III (far-advanced) disease. Only seven had stage I (minimal) disease.[69] Not only were persons with advanced tuberculosis more in need of medical treatment, but physicians believed they constituted the greatest public health threat.[70] In addition, as Robert Stith noted, severely ill individuals generally had the most extensive financial and social problems: "The advanced case, the hopeless case, bedridden or nearly so, in poor surroundings, inadequate nursing or medical care, insufficient food, usually or often surrounded with a family of young children whose mother or older brothers or sisters must go out to work, is conceded to be the most prolific source of infection of tuberculosis."[71] Health officials continually stressed the humanitarian value of providing shelter and care to people gravely ill with tuberculosis, particularly those who were homeless or indigent: "The humanitarian appeal that such helpless, destitute, suffering creatures, as the majority of indigent advanced consumptives are, make upon the public, is and justly should be much more imperative than the demand of the comparatively self-supporting incipient."[72] Indeed, Stith noted that one of Firland's primary responsibilities was "to care for the advanced case until death."[73]

By the early 1920s, however, this apparent consensus regarding the sanatorium's medical, public health, and social functions had begun to break down. For example, in a reversal of traditional policy, Stith and his staff started to favor the admission of early—as opposed to far-advanced—cases of tuberculosis. This reassessment was driven by two major factors. First, physicians had increasingly come to believe that people with incipient tuberculosis actually represented a greater public health threat than those with advanced disease, who had presumably already infected their family members and friends.[74] Second, the waning of Progressivism and the resultant need to justify the efficiency of city expenditures had led Firland to emphasize its ability to cure tuberculosis.

By the end of the 1920s, the effects of this new policy were plainly visible. Whereas 60 percent of cases admitted in 1919 had been classified as far advanced, by 1929 this figure had decreased to 35 percent. In 1926, Health Commissioner E. T. Hanley went so far as to say that Firland should have "100 percent cures," adding that the admission of advanced cases "is exceedingly bad, psychologically, on the recovering individual."[75] Even Stith concurred, ruing the "very depressing effect" that extremely sick individuals had on "cases that have a chance for cure."[76] Given the limited number of beds at Firland, Stith added, patients with advanced disease "should not be in a sanatorium at all but in . . . the County Hospital."[77]

The growing push to admit more salvageable patients reflected not only evolving medical and public health concepts but also societal judgments about which persons were more deserving of expensive medical care. While some degree of financial assistance was provided to all patients and families that required it, Stith and his staff viewed patients who came from more-stable working-class families as better investments. Thus, mirroring the traditional welfare agency's distinction between "worthy" and "unworthy" poor, Firland showed preference to persons likely to experience both a medical and an economic recovery. This category included not only those workers with stable jobs but also mothers with small children. Admitting and curing working-class parents ensured that both they and their uninfected children would become "useful member[s] of society" who were a "benefit to their community."[78]

Such criteria of moral worth and citizenship implicitly excluded a population for whom tuberculosis was a particular problem: Seattle's extensive collection of Skid Road vagrants. While such persons were not systematically kept out of Firland, the growing emphasis on hospitalizing potentially curable patients who were "worth saving" served to discourage the admission of Skid Road denizens. In later years, Stith reiterated this philosophy in the form of two questions: "Should incurables and patients with a prospect of recovery be treated in close association? Should derelicts, bums, streetwalkers, and other objectionables be treated in close association with our respectable, useful citizens—bearing in mind that ambulatory patients must of necessity mix?"[79] As a result of Firland's changing admission policy, those considered incurable because of extensive medical or social problems increasingly spent their final days either at home or on the overcrowded wards of the city or county hospital.

Yet it was not only prohibitive admission standards that determined the composition of Firland's patient population but also the expected comportment of those hospitalized. As many historians have noted, tuberculosis sanatoriums of the early twentieth century were notoriously strict institutions, direct descendants of the paternalistic almshouses of the nineteenth century. Sanatoriums routinely generated extensive lists of rules and regulations that patients were expected to follow as they "chased the cure." Firland was no exception. Stith, who was known as "Pop," carefully regulated all aspects of patients' lives: how long they remained at bed rest, what they could read, and even to whom they could speak. Perhaps the best depiction of Firland was that of Betty MacDonald, whose thinly fictionalized account of her hospitalization at the sanatorium in the 1930s vividly captured the obsession with discipline. Typical was MacDonald's witty description of her futile effort to obtain a hot-water bottle from a nurse unaffectionately known as "Granite Eyes": "I said again, 'May I please have my hot-water bottle filled?' Granite Eyes said, 'It is a rule of the Sanatorium that hot-water bottles are never filled until October first.' I said, 'I'm cold. My teeth are chattering.' She said, 'October first,' and left. This was September twenty-eighth. Three days to go. Well, I could hold out if my teeth would."[80]

Although MacDonald reluctantly acceded to most of Firland's rules and regulations, a significant subset of patients regularly violated them. Such persons were subject to so-called disciplinary discharges. In 1916, for example, Stith sent home two patients because they continued to smoke in the hospital building "after repeated warnings."[81] Each year the Department of Health's annual report listed several persons who were asked to leave Firland prior to the completion of their therapy. Such individuals were termed "unsuited to sanatorium life."[82]

An even greater problem than disciplinary discharges, however, were discharges against medical advice. The percentage of patients who left Firland prior to an approved discharge was remarkably high. In one representative year, 1916, Stith approved of only twenty-seven of the ninety-six discharges. Part of the explanation for such high rates of early discharge was the patients' frustration with their medical therapy. Patients were hospitalized for months, often at strict bed rest, and at times showed no or only minimal improvement in their disease. For example, of the ninety-six patients discharged in 1916, only fourteen met National Association for the Study and Prevention of Tuberculosis standards for either "arrested" or "apparently arrested" disease.[83] None of the patients received the designation "apparently cured." Such statistics, combined with the dozens of deaths that occurred annually at the sanatorium, did not provide a strong argument for the efficacy of medical treatment. (Of course, physicians at Firland argued that premature discharges were a major reason why so few patients recovered.)

While Stith disapproved of all discharges against medical advice, he was particularly concerned with one group of individuals: those who steadfastly refused to follow necessary preventive measures and thus posed a threat to uninfected members of the community. Such persons routinely received the obloquy of health officials, such as Stith, who termed them "vicious and willful."[84] Stith had likely borrowed this terminology from his compatriots on the East Coast, who used similar language in a series of articles and speeches. In fact, in New York City, Hermann Biggs had opened Riverside Sanatorium in 1903 in order to detain "wilfully careless consumptives."[85]

Just who were these individuals who aroused so much ire among health officials? While uncooperative patients came from all walks of life, officials were most concerned with the so-called wanderers, who were also referred to as "tramps" or "rounders." The latter term referred specifically to persons who made the rounds of a particular community, living in lodging houses but frequently requiring admission to hospitals or jail. Although rounders might be tolerated in general, they caused considerable alarm when perceived as potential transmitters of tuberculosis. As Biggs wrote in 1904: "Homeless, friendless, dependent, dissipated, and vicious consumptives are those, which are likely to be most dangerous to the community. If not cared for in an institution, they are wandering from place to place, living in lodging houses or sleeping in hallways or wherever cover can be found; negligent as to the disposal of their expectoration, and disseminating infection in every place they visit."[86]

Given Seattle's extensive population of Skid Road transients, many of whom were alcoholics, health officials in the city focused considerable attention on consumptive rounders. In 1916, John Scott McBride, who served as Seattle health commissioner between Crichton and Hanley, identified two overlapping categories of individuals who raised particular concern. The first group, which he called the "wandering indigent," comprised poor tuberculous persons who traveled the country, in search of either a cure or work. The second group consisted of the "incorrigibles" who frequented the Skid Road. "What is the use of isolating 50 percent of our [tuberculosis] cases," McBride asked, "and leaving the other 50 percent to wander around lodging houses without any protection to those with whom they come in contact?"[87]

One potential solution to this problem, of course, was to institutionalize such individuals against their will, as Biggs had done in New York beginning in 1903. As in New York, Washington State law gave health officers "the power to remove to and restrain in a pesthouse or isolation hospital, or to quarantine or isolate, any person sick with any dangerous, contagious, or infectious disease until such sick person shall have thoroughly recovered."[88] Although Robert Stith called for the use of involuntary detention in his 1912–14 annual report, forcible isolation was not attempted in Seattle at this time. If the new emphasis on treating potentially curable persons from stable families served to exclude Skid Road patients from Firland, so, too, did the decision to limit the use of coercive public health powers. With chronic shortages of both funding and sanatorium beds, Seattle shifted the emphasis of its antituberculosis efforts away from the poorest of the poor. This situation would not change until after World War II.

WORLD WAR I AND BEYOND

Although they did not detain tuberculosis patients during the early years of the twentieth century, Seattle and Washington State officials were nevertheless establishing a precedent for the aggressive use of public health powers. In 1911, as part of their attempt to combat Seattle's well-deserved reputation as a wide-open frontier town, Health Commissioner McBride and Mayor Hiram Gill had instituted a quarantine policy for "persons afflicted with venereal diseases." Once war was declared in 1917 and the city filled with military personnel, venereal disease and its connotations of depravity became intertwined with issues of disloyalty to the war effort. There was an inability, Nancy Rockafellar has written, "to distinguish between sedition and vice—both activities came under the rubric of disloyalty."[89]

As a result, alongside Socialists and Wobblies arrested for spying and sedition, Seattle in 1917 and 1918 jailed more than five hundred "disorderly persons" suspected of having venereal disease. Health officials interned indefinitely those whose positive Wassermann tests indicated infection with syphilis. Those detained, particularly the men, were kept in overcrowded rooms with poor ventilation and minimal toilet facilities. Their food was contaminated by cockroaches, and they slept "with blankets that were dirty, bloody, and encrusted with the secretions of previous prisoners."[90] The policy was, as Rockafellar termed it, a "Quarantine Hell." Given the associations between liquor, vice, and transiency in Seattle, it should come as no surprise that many of those detained were either seasonal workers, pimps, or prostitutes who lived on or frequented the Skid Road.[91]

As both Rockafellar and Allan Brandt have detailed, the use of quarantine to control venereal disease during World War I occurred throughout the United States and particularly on the West Coast. Yet Seattle appears to have pursued this program especially aggressively. A 1918 bill introduced in the U.S. House of Representatives by Washington congressman John F. Miller used Seattle as a model for a proposed nationwide plan to "punish . . . immoral persons afflicted with venereal disease."[92] In the same year, the Washington state Supreme Court rejected a legal challenge to the quarantine policy, stating that in matters of public health, "all constitutionally guaranteed rights must give way."[93] Rockafellar has termed this decision the "high point of the authority of scientific public health in the twentieth century."[94] Nearly identical reasoning would be used in Seattle after 1949 to justify the detention of tuberculosis patients—even those who technically posed no public health threat.

Mobilization of troops for World War I had revealed the pervasiveness of tuberculosis among young American males. The armed services rejected roughly one hundred thousand men on the basis of active or inactive tuberculosis. Nevertheless, following the conclusion of World War I, tuberculosis control efforts across the country waned.[95] Seattle well exemplified this development. While funding for the Division of Tuberculosis Control remained roughly stable, even during the years of the Great Depression, much of the enthusiasm that had characterized earlier antituberculosis efforts had abated. A series of repeatedly proposed projects, such as the expansion and renovation of Firland and the tuberculosis clinic, were never carried out.

Several factors contributed to this stagnation of tuberculosis work. Although physicians had added a series of surgical procedures—such as artificial pneumothorax and thoracoplasty—designed to collapse lung cavities, the medical treatment of the disease in the 1920s and 1930s remained primarily supportive. Moreover, the value of public health measures remained far from clear. Even though the death rate from tuberculosis in Seattle had fallen from roughly 120 per 100,000 population in 1910 to only 60 per 100,000 in 1923,[96] it was difficult to prove that antituberculosis efforts were responsible for this decline. Indeed, a number of commentators, noting that mortality from the disease had begun to decline before the institution of tuberculosis control programs after 1900, argued that general improvements in living conditions best explained the falling death rate.[97] In addition, tuberculosis control was, to some degree, a victim of its own success. As tuberculosis had fallen from the first to the sixth leading cause of death in Seattle by 1924, health officials began to pay increasing attention to the prevention of more common, noninfectious conditions, such as heart disease and cancer.[98] Meanwhile, the King County Anti-Tuberculosis League, following the lead of the National Tuberculosis Association, turned its attention after 1920 to the prevention of malnutrition. While this strategy sought to prevent those exposed to tuberculosis from developing the disease, its primary aim was nevertheless the general promotion of good health and "fitness" among the children of Seattle.[99]

Yet it was the changing political climate in Seattle that most influenced developments in tuberculosis control in the 1920s and 1930s. The decline of Progressivism, coupled with economic depression (which, in Seattle, had begun well before the stock market crash of 1929) markedly tempered the earlier enthusiasm for expansive municipal planning ventures—particularly those of a strongly humanitarian bent. In such a frugal environment, descriptions of "wretches" and "sufferers" with tuberculosis, when used at all, no longer had the ability to rally taxpayers or to increase allocations from city coffers. Sensing this, health officials once again sought to portray antituberculosis efforts as an efficient use of tax dollars. For example, a pamphlet issued in 1934, "Mr. Seattle Taxpayer Goes Shopping," pointed out that city expenditures for public health, most notably tuberculosis, more than paid for themselves by saving lives.[100] Unfortunately for the Division of Tuberculosis Control, their own statistics—such as the high rates of both death and discharges against medical advice at Firland—called such claims into question.[101]

The attempt to portray the division as an efficient bureaucratic agency served to underscore how far tuberculosis work had moved from its origins as a social reform movement. Early antituberculosis efforts in Seattle, in the spirit of nineteenth-century public health work, had been an integral part of a vibrant reform movement that sought social change.[102] In other words, addressing the issue of tuberculosis had entailed consideration of the role that poverty played in predisposing the poor to the disease. Thus, the 1911 city tuberculosis commission had included the provision of housing and direct relief alongside its other recommendations for the eradication of tuberculosis in Seattle. Similarly, the King County Anti-Tuberculosis League's earliest efforts had involved the housing of indigent tuberculosis patients and the provision of money and food to victims of the disease.

By the 1920s and 1930s, however, this agenda had narrowed. The Division of Tuberculosis Control was a well-established city bureaucracy that sought to maintain the organizational framework that had been established to combat tuberculosis in Seattle.[103] Reflecting the policy of its national office, the Anti-Tuberculosis League shifted its emphasis away from the issue of poverty and increasingly emphasized educational programs and demonstration projects. It should come as no surprise, therefore, that tuberculosis control had no relation to the quite active political reform movement that blossomed in Seattle during the New Deal years. From 1931 to 1936, groups such as the Unemployed Citizens' League and the Washington Commonwealth Foundation promoted a progressive agenda, including the nationalization of banks and public ownership of utilities and natural resources.[104] Yet in contrast with the Progressive Era, the high prevalence of tuberculosis (and other diseases) among the poor remained separate from the reform agenda. Although certain commentators elsewhere in the country continued to urge that voluntary and governmental tuberculosis organizations advocate broader reform measures, the narrowing focus of Seattle officials typified tuberculosis control efforts in the United States after 1920.[105]

Given both the suffering and potential contagiousness of the tuberculous population in Seattle, organizing an elaborate campaign against the disease had made sense from the standpoints of medicine, public health, and social policy. But city officials quickly realized that limited resources would necessitate compromise. Thus, even as Robert Stith and his colleagues continued to depict tuberculosis as a social disease exacerbated by poverty, their decision to emphasize the care of medically and socially "viable" persons shifted attention away from the problem of tuberculosis in the poorest section of Seattle, the Skid Road. In the 1940s, economic recovery, the fortuitous acquisition of a larger sanatorium, and the discovery of antibiotics would revitalize tuberculosis control in Seattle. Yet the issues that arose in the interwar years—the extent to which tuberculosis control efforts should address patients' social problems and the proper use of coercive measures to ensure compliance with treatment—would persist.

TWO

The War Years

Dollars and Drugs Rejuvenate the Fight

Although the revival of tuberculosis control in the United States in the 1940s is typically associated with the discovery of antibiotic agents after World War II, acceleration of antituberculosis efforts in most areas of the country began with the economic recovery at the start of the decade. In Seattle, four major administrative improvements led to the rejuvenation of tuberculosis work in the early to middle 1940s: (1) the appointment of Cedric Northrop as Washington tuberculosis control officer; (2) the unification of tuberculosis control efforts in Seattle and King County; (3) the infusion of a large amount of state money earmarked for the hospitalization of the tuberculous; and (4) the acquisition of a 1,350-bed surplus naval hospital, which became the "new" Firland Sanatorium. With this new organizational framework in place, Seattle began an ambitious program to discover and hospitalize all previously undetected cases of tuberculosis in the city. Once again, officials emphasized that successful control of tuberculosis represented a solid economic investment for Seattle. In addition, antituberculosis efforts became an important source of civic pride for a city that was striving for a more prominent national reputation.

CEDRIC NORTHROP ARRIVES IN SEATTLE

"We have been congratulating ourselves," announced Surgeon General Thomas Parran in 1937, "because [tuberculosis] has been driven down six places among the causes of death." But, Parran cautioned, tuberculosis work needed to be reoriented. "We need new force—new driving power. We need to hitch up our 'galluses' for a last, long lift at the burden."[1] Only three years later National Tuberculosis Association (NTA) managing director Kendall Emerson reported that there had been a "renaissance" in tuberculosis work. Pointing to the fact that the *Journal of the American Medical Association* had published more than six times as many articles and abstracts regarding tuberculosis in 1939 as in 1933, Emerson concluded that "rebirth of interest in the control of tuberculosis has marked the fourth decade of the twentieth century."[2] By the end of the 1940s, most areas of the country had experienced a major resurgence of efforts to detect and treat cases of the disease.

While tuberculosis officials in Seattle agreed that control efforts needed to be accelerated, the city's slow economic recovery after the Great Depression meant that little funding was available. By 1938, Seattle's deficit, which had been growing throughout the 1930s, had reached $6 million, and the question was raised whether the city's annual allocation to Firland Sanatorium, some $225,000, might be revoked. In a suit challenging the legality of various city expenses, a judge had ruled that funding for Firland was "not among the mandatory duties of the city, or necessary to its corporate existence."[3] Although the Washington state Supreme Court eventually reversed this decision, the initial ruling had demonstrated that municipal support for tuberculosis control could not be taken for granted.

The actual success of antituberculosis efforts in Seattle during the first half of the twentieth century is difficult to gauge. After a steep drop in the death rate from tuberculosis between 1910 and 1923, mortality basically remained stable between 1923 and 1937, ranging from 55 to 60 per 100,000 population. After 1937, however, without any significant changes in Seattle's tuberculosis control program, mortality resumed its decline. In 1942 only 35.4 persons per 100,000 population died from tuberculosis, which represented a 35 percent decline from 1937.[4]

While the apparent dissociation of mortality and antituberculosis efforts potentially called into question the value of control measures, local officials used these heartening statistics to argue for more funding and expansion of the existing programs. As he had throughout his tenure as head of the Division of Tuberculosis Control, Robert Stith continued to point out deficiencies in the tuberculosis control program, particularly the shortage of sanatorium beds in the city. By now, however, Stith may not have been the best person to reinvigorate tuberculosis work. In 1940 he was sixty-six years old and had headed tuberculosis control efforts in Seattle for more than a quarter of a century. In addition, he remained as medical director of Firland, a responsibility that significantly limited the amount of time he could devote to public health issues. This type of dual arrangement was becoming increasingly uncommon in other large urban health departments, which generally hired full-time persons to direct divisions of tuberculosis control.

If tuberculosis control in Seattle needed new leadership, it was not long in coming. It came, however, at the state level, with the selection of Cedric Northrop as Washington tuberculosis control officer in 1941 (figure 2.1). Northrop had been offered the position at the suggestion of a former colleague, Kenneth Soderstrom, who had become the first head of tuberculosis control for the state in 1938. Washington had been particularly unaggressive in its attack on tuberculosis, being only one of eight states without a state

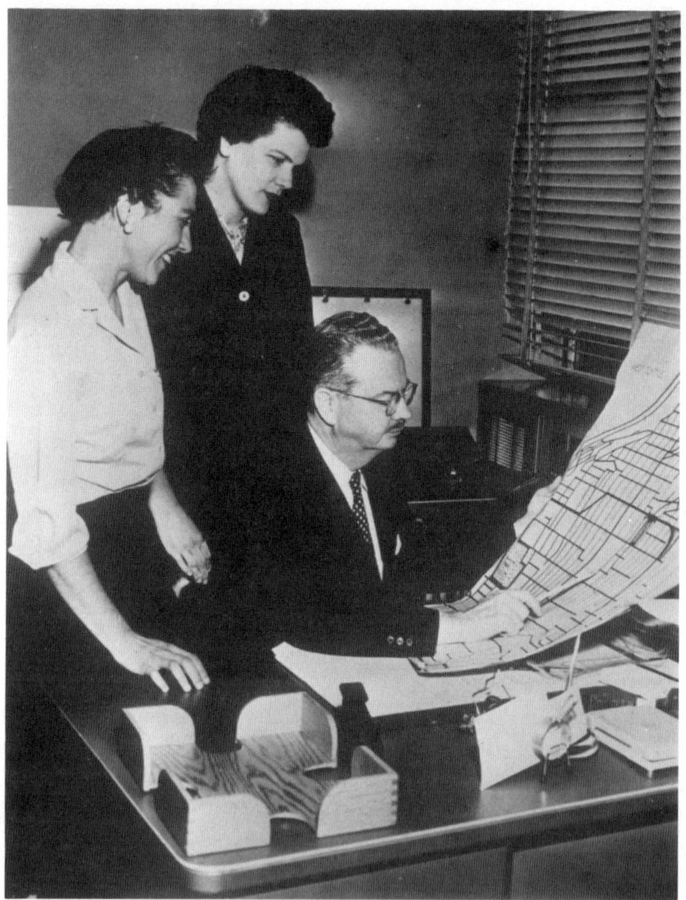

FIGURE 2.1 Washington State tuberculosis control officer Cedric Northrop consults with colleagues, 1960. Courtesy of the American Lung Association of Washington.

sanatorium and only having established a separate tuberculosis division in its Department of Health in 1938.[5] This attitude would change dramatically under Northrop.

Northrop's early career did not foreshadow the extreme dedication with which he would pursue tuberculosis control in Seattle and Washington. For one thing, he had received no formal training in public health. Northrop had grown up in Oregon and had attended medical school at the University of Oregon, graduating in 1936 at the age of thirty. After interning at Swedish Hospital in Seattle, he had completed his residency at Glen Lake Sanatorium in Minneapolis, Minnesota. Finally, in 1939, he had become superintendent of the North Dakota State Sanatorium in San Haven.

Perhaps the most important fact in Northrop's biography did not appear on his resume. While attending medical school in Oregon, he had contracted tuberculosis, spending nine months at the Portland Open Air Sanatorium. Like so many other physicians (and nurses) of his generation, Northrop had chosen to become a specialist in tuberculosis after having recovered from the disease. It was only during his years in North Dakota, however, that he decided to concentrate on public health work. As his widow, Dorothy Northrop Hupp, remembered, it was those "far advanced cases where you couldn't do a darn thing" that had spurred his interest in the prevention of disease.[6] Northrop had noted this factor himself when explaining why he left North Dakota for Washington. He had developed "a profound awareness that a physician who could prevent a case of TB was rendering more worthwhile service to the patient and his family and the community than the work of the greatest thoracic surgeon in America who operates on [the patient's] chest after [he] becomes ill."[7] Although prevention of tuberculosis and detection of early, asymptomatic cases by physical examination, skin testing, and chest X-rays had long been a focus of the antituberculosis campaign in the United States, these goals became increasingly prominent as overall rates of disease declined in the 1940s.[8]

Northrop's ultimate success in revitalizing tuberculosis control in Seattle and Washington stemmed largely from his utter devotion to his work. His former colleagues remember him as "extremely dedicated" and "tireless," repeatedly crisscrossing the state to lobby for more funding or to investigate the workings of city and county antituberculosis programs. Aside from indulging his one other passion—attending college basketball games—Northrop took little time away from his work. Indeed, he often remarked on returning home from an excursion to Spokane or Yakima that he needed to spend time "getting acquainted with the family." A tireless communicator, Northrop quickly became the major salesman for tuberculosis control in the region. He was also its scribe, preparing copious memorandums and reports as well as diaries detailing his activities. Northrop's style fit well with the longtime emphasis on promoting the efficiency of tuberculosis work in Seattle and strengthening its bureaucratic infrastructure.

Although Northrop had assumed a position in the state administration, he knew that much of the tuberculosis problem centered in Seattle. Moreover, with the coming of World War II, Seattle and King County were experiencing an influx of industrial workers as well as military personnel. After 1939, the awarding of defense contracts had led to a major expansion of the Boeing Airplane Company and shipbuilding industries in and around Seattle. Thanks in large part to the availability of jobs, the population of the city increased by 20 percent, to 480,000, between 1940 and 1943. This included a doubling of the African American population, most of whom had migrated from the South.[9] Northrop and his colleagues anticipated that the growing population of laborers in the city, who were likely to work excess hours and live in overcrowded dwellings, would contribute to an increased incidence of tuberculosis.[10]

The city's 1943 tuberculosis statistics confirmed these fears. The number of deaths, which had totaled 150 in 1942, had risen to 197. Of greater concern was that the death rate had jumped from 35.4 to 41.0 per 100,000 population. By contrast, most of the remainder of the United States experienced downward mortality during the war years.[11] Although city tuberculosis officials attributed this increase to the in-migration of persons who already had the disease, as opposed to greater transmission of tuberculosis in Seattle, they did acknowledge the seriousness of the situation. By this time, King County had opened a fifty-bed facility, named the Meadows, for custodial tuberculosis patients, but Firland and Morningside continued to have long waiting lists. Patients spilled over into public facilities such as the new county hospital, Harborview, which in 1943 was so overcrowded that it was forced to treat tuberculosis patients in its halls.[12]

It was at this time—June 1943—that Robert Stith died. City public health officials were daunted by the task of replacing such a legendary figure as Stith, but it was the patients and former patients of Firland who seemed the most devastated. An obituary in *Pep,* a magazine published by Firland patients, noted that "our doctor" had died. The obituary was simply entitled "Pop."[13] Stith's death signified the end of an era in Seattle. In his capacity as head of both the Division of Tuberculosis Control and Firland Sanatorium, Stith had examined almost every tuberculosis patient himself and had openly allocated local services based on concepts like "citizenship." Once separate persons assumed the two roles that Stith had held, such centralized, personalized assessments were replaced by a more fully bureaucratized system that devised more formal rules about hospitalization and public health concerns. Stith's individualized approach to patient care would not be entirely lost, however, particularly when Northrop and new city tuberculosis chief John Fountain began to confront the problem of recalcitrant tuberculosis patients after 1949.

Northrop had not waited for the news that tuberculosis was on the rise in Seattle and Washington to address what he perceived as major deficiencies. Building on the earlier efforts of his predecessor Kenneth Soderstrom and working with voluntary officials from the King County Anti-Tuberculosis League and the Washington Tuberculosis Association, Northrop helped to persuade the state legislature to pass a tuberculosis hospitalization law in 1943.

The law achieved three goals. First, it transferred the administration of funding for the seven county-run tuberculosis sanatoriums away from the state Department of Social Security and the county welfare departments and back to the Washington state Department of Health. This development did not directly affect Firland because the sanatorium was funded by the city. The law also established a mandatory 0.6 mill county property tax levy that was earmarked for hospitalization of the tuberculous. Finally, the law set up the State Tuberculosis Equalization Fund, through which the state was obliged to supplement funding for counties in which the 0.6 mill levy proved inadequate for the financing of tuberculosis hospitalization costs.[14]

The 1943 law had important ramifications for tuberculosis work in Seattle. The levy ensured that King County would, for the first time, contribute tax dollars to the care of Seattle citizens hospitalized at Firland. King County's unwillingness to finance care at Firland had long been a bone of contention between city and county officials.[15] Three years later, the county took a further step, assuming control of Firland. As a result, the city discontinued its annual allocation to the institution. Seattle and King County amalgamated their divisions of tuberculosis control in March 1947, and six months later they unified their health departments as the Seattle–King County Health Department, thereby completing the consolidation of antituberculosis efforts.[16] Also of great importance to Seattle officials was the fact that State Tuberculosis Equalization Fund money was likely to be heavily earmarked for Firland and Morningside Sanatoriums because these two institutions accounted for such a high percentage of tuberculosis hospitalization costs in the state.

Even with the passage of the new law, however, the major problem with tuberculosis control in Seattle persisted: the lack of adequate hospital beds. Even if money was now available to finance inpatient care, where were patients to be hospitalized? Northrop tackled this issue as well, suggesting a plan to enlarge Firland by enclosing the four large open porches, converting the old children's building, Josef House, into a facility for adult patients, and turning an old contagious diseases pavilion located on the grounds into a hospital for ambulant tuberculosis patients. A similar plan was eventually recommended by a 1943 joint city and county commission charged with studying the tuberculosis hospital situation. This arrangement would have increased the number of beds from roughly two hundred to at least three hundred.[17]

The notion that such improvements at Firland might be made during World War II was unrealistic. Funding was unavailable, and the wartime shortage of personnel—particularly nurses—made staffing an enlarged institution impossible.[18] By 1945, however, these problems appeared to be resolving. The war's end meant that military personnel trained as health care workers would be returning to the city. Moreover, that same year the state legislature allocated $3 million to serve as a nucleus for the postwar construction of tuberculosis hospitals throughout the state, including Seattle.

Northrop credited San Francisco tuberculosis specialist Henry Chadwick's critical 1944 report on tuberculosis control in Washington state as having persuaded the legislature to act.[19]

Chadwick had actually favored closing Morningside, markedly enlarging Firland, and converting it into a state sanatorium. While the idea of a state institution was again rejected, Chadwick's other plans began to appear realistic once Seattle and King County had merged their tuberculosis control divisions. Northrop, city and county officials, and the King County Anti-Tuberculosis League developed a plan in which Morningside would be closed and Firland expanded to roughly eight hundred or nine hundred beds.[20]

While World War II had interfered with certain aspects of tuberculosis control in Seattle, in other ways the war indirectly promoted antituberculosis efforts. During an era of active conflict, the familiar military metaphors that had long accompanied tuberculosis work in the twentieth century became even more popular. Just as the United States was waging war in Europe and Asia, so it was necessary, explained *Pep,* for patients at Firland to fight their tuberculosis: "Our immediate danger is the insidious forces in our bodies, the conquering of which, in the long run, leads to victory for the United States within the larger arena of war." [21]

On a more concrete level, screening of soldiers during World War II led, as it had in World War I, to a renewed appreciation for the degree of undetected tuberculosis in the general population. Approximately one hundred thousand (1 percent) of the roughly ten million military personnel who received X-rays were rejected because their films revealed cavities or other densities consistent with either active or inactive pulmonary tuberculosis. Chest X-ray screening, using a recently developed economical miniature film technique, was performed throughout Puget Sound at military installations, such as Fort Lewis and Fort Lawton. At the latter location, the army rented X-ray equipment that the University of Washington had been using to screen its incoming students for tuberculosis.[22]

Concern about the potential impact of tuberculosis on the war effort induced the U.S. Public Health Service to establish an Office of Tuberculosis Control in 1943. The new agency represented the first formal federal involvement in the control of the disease. Among the programs promoted by federal officials was the chest X-ray examination of workers in war industries. This program got under way in Washington in 1943 when the state Department of Health purchased a mobile X-ray unit, which Northrop believed was only the third or fourth such unit in operation in the country (figure 2.2). In one representative year, 1945, the department discovered 316 new cases of tuberculosis from roughly twenty-thousand miniature films taken.[23]

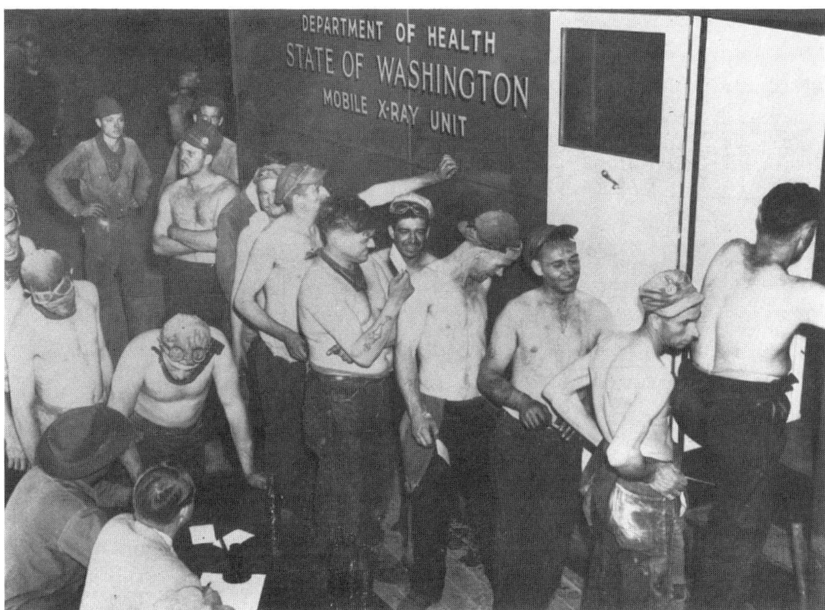

FIGURE 2.2 Employees of the Aluminum Company of America awaiting screening X-rays on mobile van, Vancouver, Washington, 1944. Courtesy of the American Lung Association of Washington.

POSTWAR MOBILIZATION

As the war drew to a close, tuberculosis control in Seattle remained in flux. Since Stith's death, several individuals had served as interim heads of Firland Sanatorium and the Division of Tuberculosis Control. With the unification of city and county tuberculosis services in 1947, a seven-member committee of city and county officials was appointed to find permanent replacements for the positions Stith had held. The committee ultimately chose John Fountain as the new director of tuberculosis control for the soon-to-be formed Seattle–King County Health Department. Fountain, a physician who also had obtained a master's degree in public health from Harvard University, had worked for the Washington state Department of Health and had served on the staff of Morningside Sanatorium.

Meanwhile, at Northrop's urging, the board looked to Minnesota to fill the new position of medical director of the King County Tuberculosis Hospitals (which included Firland, Morningside, and the Meadows). During his residency in Minnesota, Northrop had become familiar with the state's successful tuberculosis control program as well as one of its major leaders,

Roberts Davies. Davies' biography was similar to that of many of his peers. As a medical student at the University of Minnesota, he had developed bilateral pulmonary tuberculosis and had remained at bed rest for over eighteen months. After he recovered, Davies completed his training and in 1937 took a position on the staff of Nopeming Sanatorium, located in St. Louis County, Minnesota (which included Duluth).[24]

During a ten-year stay at Nopeming, Davies helped to organize a highly successful countywide tuberculosis control program that emphasized the provision of an adequate number of sanatorium beds and the mass X-ray surveying of the entire population. By identifying and hospitalizing all active cases of tuberculosis, the program produced a 90 percent decrease (that is, a "virtually complete disappearance") in the number of new cases.[25] Northrop agreed with this strategy and cited it in his efforts to convince tuberculosis officials in Seattle to offer the position to Davies in 1947.[26]

Merely hiring Davies brought Seattle no closer to attaining what Davies termed "the prerequisites for a successful campaign of tuberculosis eradication."[27] The projected expansion of Firland carried a $6 million price tag, a cost the state was not willing to finance. Although the King County Anti-Tuberculosis League had purchased a mobile X-ray van in 1944 and had begun screening certain segments of the population with miniature films, a comprehensive community-wide X-ray survey made little sense if no beds were available to hospitalize those diagnosed with tuberculosis.[28]

Shortly after Davies' arrival, however, tuberculosis workers in Seattle learned that the federal War Assets Administration had declared a local 1,350-bed naval hospital as surplus property. Northrop and Davies quickly realized that the facility, located seven miles north of the city, was a near panacea. With the provision of more than a thousand beds to hospitalize the tuberculous of Seattle and King County, the first step in Davies' plan of eradication could be achieved immediately.

To facilitate the acquisition of the naval hospital by King County, Northrop and Davies contacted one of Washington state's U.S. senators, Warren Magnuson. Magnuson, who was serving the first of his six terms, was sympathetic to the transfer but was caught in a difficult bind. The Veterans' Administration, which technically had first rights, had expressed interest in the facility for the hospitalization of ill and disabled veterans. Members of the American Legion in Seattle ardently petitioned Magnuson to throw his support behind this plan.

Although Magnuson received a great deal of pressure from veterans' groups, the argument from those advocating conversion of the hospital into a tuberculosis sanatorium was even more compelling. Mortality from tuberculosis had continued to increase in Seattle during World War II, reaching a peak of 44.8 per 100,000 population in 1945. The rate of new cases annually was also on the rise. By May 1947, more than 135 persons with active disease were waiting for sanatorium admission; many had been listed for six months or more. An estimated eight hundred to a thousand additional cases remained undiagnosed. Public officials, including Washington governor Monrad Wallgren and Seattle mayor William Devin, stressed to Magnuson the severity of the tuberculosis problem.[29] But the concern was not limited to elected officials and health agencies. As demonstrated in a collection of letters sent to Magnuson, the tuberculosis situation in the late 1940s was generating the greatest "public resentment"[30] in Seattle since the start of antituberculosis efforts in 1909.

The letters recalled the humanitarian motivations that had led to the initiation of tuberculosis work in the community in 1909. A representative letter was written by members of a local union of plumbers and pipe fitters: "[Tuberculosis] is something that strikes every group in society, rich or poor. . . . We, as your constituents, representing over 2,000 families, very earnestly urge you to exert all your influences with the Navy Department so that these facilities become available immediately because while this delay is going on, people are dying."[31] A manager of a local realty company concurred. "You could do no greater humanitarian service," he wrote, "than to lend your efforts to making available this idle hospital to the City of Seattle."[32] Another letter writer stated that he sympathized with those receiving suboptimal care because he was a former "lunger."[33] At times writers used specific cases to bolster their arguments. The secretary of the Central Labor Council informed Magnuson that a "little girl" in one of his apartments had been on the waiting list for a hospital bed for more than three months.[34]

What does not come through in these letters is a concern over the potential infectiousness of persons on the waiting list, although this issue remained of great importance. A 1943 study of a hundred tuberculosis deaths in Seattle by a University of Washington nursing graduate student, Thorbjorg Arnason, described the "dismal picture of the home conditions" among those on the waiting list, many of whom lived with large families in "crowded quarters." Moreover, Arnason found, only thirteen of the hundred deaths had occurred in a sanatorium. This statistic indicated that the majority of persons in her study "presented a danger as a source of infection for tuberculosis in the community: first, in the home, to family and associates; second, in hotels and rooming houses, to other lodgers and associates; third, in lunch rooms and restaurants, to other customers; fourth, at places of work, such as the grocery and the shoemaker's shop."[35]

Caught between the competing needs of the tuberculous and the veterans, Magnuson helped to broker a compromise in which the large naval facility was to serve as both a veterans' hospital and a sanatorium. Ultimately, however, the Veterans' Administration backed out of the arrangement because

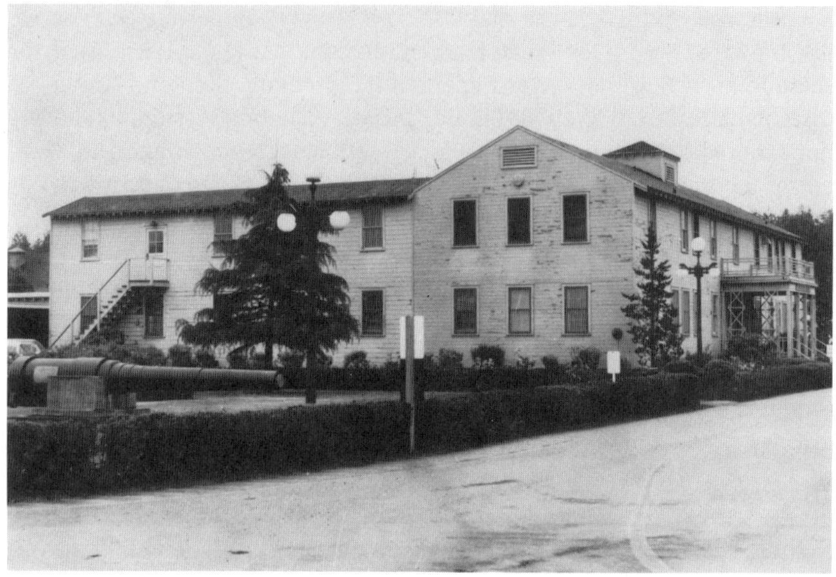

FIGURE 2.3 The Administration Building of the new Firland Sanatorium. This picture dates from the late 1950s. Courtesy of the American Lung Association of Washington.

its appropriation for fiscal year 1948 did not appear adequate to operate the proposed institution.[36] As a result, the naval hospital became Seattle's new tuberculosis sanatorium (figure 2.3). When health officials finally obtained the lease to the facility in November 1947, many observers believed that Seattle was "sounding the death knell for tuberculosis."[37]

Although he anticipated shortages of staff, Davies was eager to open the new hospital. By October 1947, the waiting list for a sanatorium bed in Seattle had reached 207 persons, the largest number in the city's history. The transfer of approximately 450 patients from Firland, Morningside, and the Meadows, which occurred on November 25, 1947, was described as "the greatest mass movement of patients from one tuberculosis sanatorium to another in the history of any United States civilian hospital."[38] Over the next several weeks, patients on the waiting list and those hospitalized at Harborview Hospital were admitted to the new sanatorium, which assumed the familiar name of Firland. Meanwhile, the three old sanatoriums were closed.

Not everyone in Seattle approved of the new developments. In a letter to the *Seattle Times*, one woman decried the "abandonment" of the original Firland for the new facility, whose run-down barracks were admittedly no match for the magnificent architecture and bucolic surroundings of its predecessor: "The county has moved the patients to the shed-like structures of the naval hospital. This place is surrounded by a high barbed wire fence instead of the beautiful parklike grounds of [the original] Firland."[39]

For city health officials, however, the number of sanatorium beds was considerably more important than where they were located. The acquisition of the naval hospital meant that Seattle and King County had seven beds per annual tuberculosis death, well over the National Tuberculosis Association's recommended ratio of three beds per annual death. By 1950, with the construction of a new sanatorium in Selah and an addition to Edgecliff Sanatorium in Spokane, Washington had twenty-three hundred sanatorium beds and had become only the fourth state in the country to abolish waiting lists for the tuberculous.[40] Well into the 1950s, even after the introduction of antibiotics, persistent waiting lists in cities like Detroit, Cleveland, Chicago, New York, Oakland, and Boston and in states like Tennessee and Florida continued to cause, in Cedric Northrop's words, "much heartache."[41]

SEATTLE AREA CHEST X-RAY SURVEY

Possessing an adequate number of beds for its tuberculosis patients, Seattle could now embark on the second arm of the strategy that Davies had used so effectively in Minnesota: X-ray screening of the entire population for undetected cases of the disease. Building on its successful wartime experience with X-ray screening, the King County Anti-Tuberculosis League had continued to operate its mobile unit after the war; between June 1944 and July 1948, it took a total of 103,810 miniature films in neighborhoods, industries, and schools.[42]

What particularly interested tuberculosis officials in Seattle was the possibility of conducting a community-wide survey of the type Davies had engineered in Minnesota. Emil Palmquist, who had become the director of public health for the joint city-county health department, eagerly solicited the assistance of the U.S. Public Health Service (PHS) for this task. With the conclusion of the war, one of the major responsibilities of the PHS's newly formed Division of Tuberculosis Control was to coordinate mass X-ray surveys of selected cities across the country. The role of the PHS was to donate a large number of mobile X-ray machines to these cities and to supply advisory personnel. Additional funding came from local sources. By 1948, the PHS had taken close to one million X-rays in three cities: Minneapolis-St. Paul, Milwaukee, and Washington, D.C.[43]

Although the PHS expressed interest in coming to Seattle at the end of 1948, one major problem remained: financing the survey. Representatives of the PHS estimated that $80,000 to $100,000 of local support would be needed to X-ray four hundred thousand of the city's roughly half million residents over the age of fifteen.[44] The logical source of this money, according to Palmquist, was the King County Anti-Tuberculosis League. The league's counterpart, the Hennepin County Tuberculosis Association, had supplied $62,000 of the $77,600 needed to help conduct the survey in Minneapolis-St. Paul in 1947.[45] Yet when Palmquist, John Fountain, Cedric Northrop, and representatives from the King County Medical Society, the PHS, and the National Tuberculosis Association proposed this arrangement to league representatives in early 1948, the league demurred. Not only was it not inclined to finance the survey, but some of its members also questioned the value of the survey in the first place.[46]

In listing her reservations regarding the X-ray survey, league executive secretary Honoria Hughes cited problems encountered in Minneapolis, such as the poor follow-up of patients with abnormal films. Yet the league's reluctance to participate in what appeared to be a crucial step toward the control of tuberculosis in Seattle really spoke to two other issues: the long history of distrust between the King County league and governmental officials and the increasingly ambiguous role of the voluntary association in public health work.

Aside from Robert Stith, the two figures who had dominated early tuberculosis work in Seattle and Washington were both women: Hughes and Bethesda Beals Buchanan, the longtime executive secretary of the Washington Tuberculosis Association. Hughes, born into an Irish working-class family in Montana, became executive secretary of the King County league in 1933; Buchanan, a University of Washington graduate originally from Iowa, was the driving force behind the establishment of the state association.[47] Dynamic and somewhat headstrong, Hughes and Buchanan got along neither with each other nor with city and state tuberculosis officials. Yet both women had proved to be indefatigable advocates for tuberculosis control, pioneering educational programs, running the annual Christmas Seal drive, and lobbying the government for increased funding.

Hughes and Buchanan saw their roles in a traditional voluntaristic light. Their agencies were supposed to develop a series of demonstration projects, which, if ultimately successful, would be turned over to governmental agencies. Examples of projects begun by the King County league included the original city tuberculosis dispensary, Firland Sanatorium, and a program of social and vocational services. Despite these seemingly successful partnerships, however, major tensions existed between the largely female volunteers and the male physicians who staffed governmental agencies. Because control of the work shifted from voluntary to government agency and from female to male, successful projects became associated with both government and with men. Although many of these efforts had originated in the voluntary sector, demonstration projects, to some degree, always remained "women's work."[48]

Buchanan and Hughes also resented what they saw as attempts by governmental tuberculosis officials to use Christmas Seals money to finance their own projects. Thus, the request that the King County Anti-Tuberculosis League finance the bulk of the Public Health Service's proposed X-ray survey in Seattle reopened an old wound. Hughes and her colleagues basically argued that because the PHS survey was a governmental project, it should not primarily be financed by Christmas Seals. Voluntary associations, noted league member Frederick Exner, must not "support financially the work of the Health Department or otherwise subsidize the City Government with funds raised by private subscription, since the Government is not a suitable object for charity."[49] Hughes also feared that a large outlay of league money to the survey would result in the curtailing of traditional league programs, such as its health education work.

In the end, the NTA prevailed upon Hughes and the King County league to change its mind about financing the survey. By April 1948, the league had begrudgingly agreed to donate $61,000 toward the effort. The remainder of the funds—approximately $40,000—came from the Seattle City Council, the King County Commissioners, and the Washington Tuberculosis Association.[50] Once the Anti-Tuberculosis League was on board, the city addressed the issue of how best to organize the survey, scheduled to begin in September 1948. Mayor William Devin named an executive committee, which included Emil Palmquist and Anti-Tuberculosis League president Wayne Dick. Lawrence Bates, an insurance salesman and former president of the Municipal League, served as executive chairman. Bates quickly began to mobilize what Devin would later term "probably the most successful community venture in our history."[51]

Ultimately, 398,309 individuals received seventy-millimeter miniature X-rays between September 9 and December 18, 1948, a total that represented almost 80 percent of persons above the age of fifteen in Seattle. As a result, 402 persons with active tuberculosis were admitted to Firland Sanatorium over the next two years. Nearly 150 persons were employed on the project, and more than three hundred community agencies participated. More than twelve thousand Seattle residents volunteered as X-ray hostesses, statisticians, and health educators, who provided information about the survey. Individual physicians gave their time to read rolls of miniature X-rays using machines called "illuminators."[52]

Over the fifteen-week period, seventeen mobile X-ray machines were positioned throughout Seattle, at department stores such as the Bon Marché and Frederick and Nelson, at the University of Washington, and at the Pike Place Public Market. At the behest of the survey's Public Information Division, the city's newspapers provided extensive publicity on the daily schedule of X-ray units. Radio stations featured spots with Betty MacDonald that promoted the endeavor. In addition, volunteers distributed posters, pamphlets, and buttons bearing slogans such as "O.K.—Let's X-Ray" and "I've Had My Chest X-Ray." At a planning meeting in August, one volunteer mentioned her intention to get the crooner Bing Crosby to perform a special program in honor of the survey. There were some things, however, that the survey advisory committee could not achieve. "Bing Crosby, incidentally," read the minutes of the next meeting, "will not be available as was hoped."[53]

An important factor propelling the survey was the memory of the recent World War II victory. The executive committee selected a military facility, the New Field Artillery Armory, as its operations headquarters. Mayor Devin suggested that the official slogan of the survey should be "Join the Battle—X-Ray Seattle."[54] The executive committee organized the survey with what can only be termed "military" efficiency, producing hundreds of charts and documents and sending out thank-you notes to each of the more than twelve thousand persons who participated in the survey. X-ray hostesses were instructed to "pin the 'I've had my chest X-ray' button to the clothing of the person who has just been X-rayed. DO NOT HAND IT TO HIM."[55]

The X-ray survey also became an important symbol of Seattle's civic pride and community spirit. During World War II, largely due to the role of the Boeing Airplane Company in supplying planes to the Allied cause, Seattle had finally emerged as a national city. In the eyes of both the media and city officials, completion of a successful X-ray survey was a means to gain further recognition. A parade including palomino horses, the naval station band, and four of the mobile X-ray machines kicked off the survey on September 8. Mayor Devin received a well-publicized chest X-ray early in the survey.[56]

When the success of the survey became apparent, Seattle trumpeted its efforts. "8,309 X-Rays Set Day Record Here," read one September *Seattle Times* headline. In a November article entitled "X-Ray Campaign in Seattle Is Near Record," the *Times* noted that the city had taken more films than Minneapolis. By the conclusion of the survey, Seattle had X-rayed a higher percentage of persons aged fifteen and over than had Minneapolis, Milwaukee, or Washington, D.C.[57] Devin and other city officials continually reiterated the importance of the community effort that had made the survey "the greatest single public health activity ever undertaken on the Pacific Coast."[58] "I know of no previous undertaking in which so many thousands of our citizens joined forces toward a single objective," Devin remarked. "Many of those volunteers learned, perhaps for the first time, the satisfaction which comes from helping to build a finer community."[59] The mayor established a trophy, an Alaskan totem pole, which he promised to award to any city that surpassed Seattle's percentage of citizens X-rayed. Numerous cities took up the challenge. Between 1944 and 1952, the Public Health Service obtained screening chest X-rays on 5.8 million persons in seventeen U.S. cities.[60]

Even as Seattle's concern with its national image generated enthusiasm for the survey, a persistent small-town atmosphere also contributed to its success. Seattle in 1948 closely resembled the typical post–World War II American city described by William O'Neill in *American High.* The city's residents still largely worked and shopped downtown, not yet having begun the pilgrimage to the suburban areas that would soon expand to the north of the city and across Lake Washington to the east.[61] As a result, the survey's X-ray machines, strategically situated in downtown department stores and other businesses, reached a large percentage of the population. The X-ray hostess manning the machine at Bartell's Drugs, moreover, might have been the daughter of a neighbor in Capitol Hill or a former classmate from Lincoln or Garfield High School. Seattle officials would try to recapture this small-town milieu in the 1950s and 1960s by attracting residents downtown to "civic-minded ventures" such as the annual Seafair festival and the 1962 World's Fair.

The character of the survey also reflected the changing political climate of the city. By 1949, Murray Morgan states in *Skid Road,* the long history of social reform that had begun in Populist and Progressive Seattle was just a memory. Politics in the city at this time was best exemplified by the rise of the conservative Teamsters' union, under the control of Dave Beck. As Morgan mournfully notes, Seattle had become a middle-class town, "a town of high wages and white collars, a prosperous town dominated by a fat, bland, tough labor leader named Dave Beck."[62] The notion that tuberculosis was associated with poverty, or that the survey represented an effort to improve the lives of the tuberculous poor, appeared nowhere in discussions of the campaign. The crucial importance of surveying the tuberculosis-prone Skid Road population was duly noted, but mostly in the context of devising strategies to reach persons who were generally "not subject to participation in affairs outside their own section." When the X-ray machines arrived on the Skid Road in November, a headline in the *Seattle Post-Intelligencer* read, " 'Skid' Civic Pride Reaches Heights for X-Rays."[63]

Despite its best efforts, the staff of the X-ray survey was unable to reach 20 percent of the targeted population. A certain percentage of these individuals included Seattle's extensive population of Christian Scientists, who generally were unwilling to participate.[64] Moreover, for those whose screening X-rays were abnormal, the evaluation process had just begun. The roughly fourteen thousand persons who had abnormal miniature films received a letter in the mail instructing them to return to the "Retake Clinic" in the Armory for a fourteen- by seventeen-inch X-ray study. Such individuals were often difficult to track down, particularly if they lived a transient existence on the Skid Road. If the repeat X-ray indicated either active or inactive tuberculosis, the survey staff sent a letter to the patient's private practitioner or, if the patient lacked a physician, to the city tuberculosis clinic. Follow-up then became the responsibility of the physician or clinic.

The results of the survey—7,166 cases of "suspected" tuberculosis, 1,206 actual cases, and 402 hospitalizations at Firland—appeared to please everyone in Seattle except one person. Frederick Exner was a radiologist who had grown up in Iowa and, like Roberts Davies and Cedric Northrop, trained at the University of Minnesota. Exner became active in public health work after arriving in Seattle in 1935 and served as the president of the Anti-Tuberculosis League in 1949 and 1950. Despite his public health activities, Exner embodied the conservative politics of the American Medical Association at this time, remaining a staunch foe of "bureaucratic" and "socialized" medicine. He is perhaps best remembered for his fight against the 1950s plan to fluoridate Seattle's drinking water, a plan he termed a "hoax" that encouraged public health "dictatorship."[65]

Exner was a "skilled parliamentarian" who knew how to acquire power. He became president of the King County Medical Society in 1956 by stacking the organization with his supporters. As president of the Anti-Tuberculosis League, he was a constant thorn in the side of the Seattle–King County Department of Health, stressing the importance of voluntarism and the need to "prevent abuse and overexpansion of governmental function."[66] "If you mentioned the word 'Exner' to [Cedric Northrop]," recalled Seattle phthisiologist Walter Miller, "he would turn purple [and] his blood pressure would double."[67]

In the case of the X-ray survey, Exner charged that the U.S. Public Health Service, both in Seattle and elsewhere, was propagating "man-killing lies." According to Exner, promotional campaigns associated with the surveys incorrectly implied that a negative screening film indicated that a person had no chest disease whatsoever—neither tuberculosis, nor cancer, nor heart problems. As a result, Exner claimed, at least one woman in Seattle was dying of cancer.[68]

Although Exner's invective was excessive, his claims had some validity. In Minneapolis, at least, publicity had suggested that screening X-rays could demonstrate that an individual had "no tuberculosis, no cancer, no enlarged heart."[69] Yet in Seattle there had been sensitivity to this issue. Promotional campaigns did not mention diseases other than tuberculosis, and X-ray findings suggestive of other diseases were handled like those indicating tuberculosis: private physicians or the Health Department were notified of possible pathology and encouraged to pursue an additional workup.

Exner's criticisms were very much in the spirit of other commentators of this era, such as Henry Garland, whose writings described the limitations of the X-ray technique for making clinical diagnoses. Exner continually stressed that while radiographs could suggest pathological conditions, actual diagnosis and treatment remained the role of the "licensed doctor."[70] At the same time, however, he emphasized the role of the experienced radiologist (preferably) or phthisiologist in reading both the miniature and regular-sized films.[71] Because of his "tumultuous, vigorous, unhappy" personality,[72] even valid claims raised by Exner ultimately received little attention. For both public health workers and the citizens of Seattle, the 1948 X-ray survey represented a crucial step in the ongoing effort to control tuberculosis in the city.

THE FUNDING PUSH

Frederick Exner's attempts to point out exactly what the X-ray survey could and could not accomplish served to highlight a fundamental issue about the changing prevalence of disease in Seattle and the country as a whole. Although the survey unearthed a large number of persons with active tuberculosis (and many more with evidence of old tuberculosis), the disease was clearly on the decline in Seattle, representing only the seventh leading cause of mortality in 1948. Meanwhile, even taking into account Exner's reservations about X-ray technique and the need to confirm diagnoses suggested by X-ray, thousands of survey films did reveal evidence that was suggestive of heart disease or cancer—the two most common causes of death in Seattle. In total, survey films identified 2,464 persons with suspected heart disease and 3,495 persons with possible cancer or other diseases.[73]

The information generated by the X-ray survey about nontuberculous disease attracted a great deal of interest from public health officials.[74] Efforts to prevent chronic diseases, which had begun in the 1920s, were accelerating markedly. In the voluntary sphere, existing organizations, such as the American Cancer Society and the American Heart Association, expanded, each raising several million dollars annually by the late 1940s. Meanwhile, dozens of other agencies formed to raise funds to fight medical conditions such as diabetes, multiple sclerosis, Parkinson disease, and kidney disease.[75] Locally, articles appeared in Seattle newspapers, publicizing fund-raising and promotional efforts to "conquer" and "battle" heart disease, cancer, and other conditions. On the governmental level, there was also growing concern about chronic diseases. The Washington state Department of Health organized a Chronic Disease Control Section in 1949. The section's programs, which initially emphasized the prevention of rheumatic (heart) disease and the early detection of cancer, were aided by federal grants from the newly established National Cancer Institute and Heart Institute.[76]

Yet despite the fact that chronic diseases had become the "great killers," financial support for tuberculosis work in Seattle from the late 1940s until the

1960s continued to dwarf funds allocated to other public health programs. Throughout the 1950s, the King County Anti-Tuberculosis League raised growing amounts of money for tuberculosis work. The Seattle–King County Health Department, although evincing concern about diseases of aging, devoted a much higher proportion of its efforts to tuberculosis control.

It was at the state level that tuberculosis control received its most overwhelming support during this era. If tuberculosis work in Seattle in the 1920s and 1930s had been characterized by chronic funding shortages, the years after 1945 were notable for a massive infusion of support from a state government that had been notoriously penurious in its support of both tuberculosis control and public health work in general. From 1949 to 1955, between 60 and 70 percent of all state public health money was spent on tuberculosis hospitalization.[77] If the money obtained from the mandatory county millage and other tax revenues was included in the reckoning, roughly 85 percent of all public health funding in the state actually went to tuberculosis control.[78] Although the need for prolonged hospitalization made tuberculosis more expensive to control than other diseases, 85 percent is still a remarkable figure given the relatively low mortality from tuberculosis in Washington state at this time.

How did such a successful fund-raising campaign become established? As noted above, increased state involvement in the funding of tuberculosis hospitalization had begun when the state legislature allocated $284,339.41 for the 1943–45 biennium as its first Tuberculosis Equalization Fund payment. Although each county raised money for tuberculosis control from its mandatory 0.6 mill levy, it became clear that this income would be inadequate to cover hospital costs in counties, such as King, with a high number of tuberculosis patients. Moreover, with the acquisition of the naval hospital, and an anticipated occupancy rate of more than one thousand patients, the amount of Equalization Fund money allocated to King County would require additional augmentation.

It was initially unclear whether the state legislature would be willing to fund such increases. Fortunately for the tuberculosis control program and its major advocate, Cedric Northrop, there was a sympathetic ear in the office of the governor, Arthur B. Langlie. Born in Minnesota in 1900 to parents of Norwegian descent, Langlie had spent most of his childhood in Bremerton, just west of Seattle. After earning a law degree from the University of Washington and working at a local law firm, he became affiliated with a new political movement in Seattle known as the New Order of Cincinnatus. Named for a Roman statesman who had emphasized public service, the "conservative, reformist, and moralistic attitudes"[79] of the New Order were attractive to Langlie. Langlie, in turn, was attractive to the Cincinnatans, who chose him to run for mayor of Seattle in 1938. Running as an independent candidate promising to fight labor corruption and to cut taxes and government expenses, Langlie was easily elected.

Langlie had little impact on tuberculosis control during his two-year tenure as mayor, but this changed when he was elected governor in 1940. "Startled and convinced"[80] by statistics revealing the inadequate number of tuberculosis beds in the state, Langlie had strongly supported the 1943 legislation establishing the mandatory mill tax and the Equalization Fund. Although Langlie was defeated in his bid for reelection in 1944, his successor, Monrad Wallgren, presided over rapidly accelerating allocations to the Equalization Fund, which totaled $4,299,828 for the 1947–49 biennium.[81]

The true test of state funding for tuberculosis control came after Langlie was reelected governor in 1948, at a time when "heavy financial demands [were] being made upon the state treasury."[82] In a special message to the legislature in February 1949, Langlie warned that the inflationary "easy credit, easy spending days" of the Wallgren era were over. Langlie was particularly concerned that voters in 1948 had passed the Citizens' Security Act (Initiative 172), an ambitious piece of legislation that mandated the state to provide medical benefits to all residents on relief. This program provided one of the country's most comprehensive health support systems. Even though spending on the poor was cut in 1949 with the passage of Initiative 178, the large expenditures generated by the Citizens' Security Act forced the state to go on deficit spending for the final year of the 1949–51 biennium.[83]

When Initiative 172 first passed, the state legislature made several attempts to control costs. For example, the biennial allocations to both the state public school system and the University of Washington were cut back substantially. In an effort to generate income, Langlie had even come out in favor of a flat 2 percent state income tax, an idea he had long opposed. (The legislation did not pass.)[84]

Despite these widespread cutbacks, the state Department of Health, in preparing its budget for the 1949–51 biennium, had requested $7.9 million for the Tuberculosis Equalization Fund. This figure represented an increase of almost 85 percent from the $4.3 million received during the previous biennium. In March 1949, the legislature announced that its allocation to the Equalization Fund would total only $6.5 million. Despite the fact that the fund had received a substantially larger outlay in an era of cost containment and cutbacks, tuberculosis workers in the state reacted with alarm. Concern was particularly great in Seattle and King County, which was slated to receive at least half ($4 million) of the requested allotment of funds.[85] The $1.4 million deficiency threatened plans to fill the new 1,350-bed Firland Sanatorium with cases detected by the 1948 mass survey and future screening programs.

Reluctantly, Roberts Davies and his Firland colleagues devised several contingency plans, in which they debated which services would be cut back and how to decide which two hundred to four hundred patients were to be denied hospitalization.[86] Meanwhile, tuberculosis workers throughout Seattle and the state began an ardent campaign to get the $1.4 million restored. (A similar effort two years previously had succeeded in attaining additional Tuberculosis Equalization Fund allocations.) The King County Anti-Tuberculosis League, for example, alerted thousands of its supporters to the funding deficit and encouraged them to contact their legislators.[87]

When such efforts proved unsuccessful, Cedric Northrop organized a campaign to obtain money from Governor Langlie's emergency fund. Although money from this fund had previously gone only to emergencies within actual state departments, offices, and institutions, Northrop organized governmental and voluntary tuberculosis workers, the county commissioners, and other groups to urge Langlie to allocate $750,000 of the available $2 million for the hospitalization of tuberculosis patients, primarily at Firland. Given the well-developed organizational infrastructure of the tuberculosis control program, Northrop was able to coordinate an extremely effective appeal; meetings were held with Langlie and his associates to arrange the transaction.[88] In pursuit of the funding, as throughout his tenure as state tuberculosis control officer, Northrop was like a "terrier." As Northrop's longtime colleague Walter Miller recalled, politicians would say, "Give Cedric what he wants; just get him off my back."[89]

With the state's (and Seattle's) tuberculosis control program at the "crossroads,"[90] Langlie gave his blessing: in February 1950, he agreed to allot the $750,000. Although this amount did not restore the entire $1.4 million operating deficit, it proved enough to keep Firland running at full capacity through 1951. Langlie's decision also had important symbolic value. At a time of severe financial constraints, he gave tuberculosis hospitalization a special status. Over the next decade, during which time the state's economic situation remained tenuous, the Tuberculosis Equalization Fund would continue to receive all or nearly all of its requested allocation, peaking in the 1953–55 biennium, when the legislature appropriated $10 million.[91]

Langlie had acted to some degree from humanitarian concerns but even more because investment in tuberculosis control seemed to make good economic sense. Northrop and his colleagues had convinced Langlie that prompt hospitalization of the tuberculous "result[ed] in the saving of tax dollars in the long run" and thus represented the exact type of economic investment that Langlie had championed since his early years as a member of the New Order of Cincinnatus.[92] Such thinking also fit in well with the opinions of other commentators across the country, who encouraged public health officials to stop behaving like "mendicants" and to demonstrate, in the words of the Colorado physician and public health official Florence Sabin, that "good health is good business."[93]

In urging health officials to carry out strategies like those favored by Sabin, commentators such as Metropolitan Life Insurance Company vice president William Shepard argued that public health spending should be distanced from "less tangible" forms of public spending, such as relief expenditures.[94] Tuberculosis workers in Seattle in the post–World War II era believed they had achieved this distinction. The mandatory tuberculosis millage for King County, the generous State Tuberculosis Equalization Fund, the acquisition of the naval hospital, and the successful mass X-ray survey legitimated tuberculosis control in Seattle as an important public health campaign that was crucial for the continued development of the city.

In the late 1940s, just as the city was solidifying the public health portion of its tuberculosis work, a revolutionary change in the medical management of the disease was occurring. After years of supposed cures that never proved effective, new antibiotic agents were demonstrating clear efficacy against *Mycobacterium tuberculosis.* The availability of these drugs further rejuvenated tuberculosis work in Seattle and across the country. Yet effective medical therapy and a "good business" approach to public health did not necessarily provide simple solutions for one large segment of the tuberculous population: those with severe social problems, such as homelessness, unemployment, and alcoholism. In order to explore how such social issues continued to complicate tuberculosis control efforts, we must reenter Firland Sanatorium.

THREE

Still a Social Disease

Tuberculosis Control in the Antibiotic Era

Most histories of tuberculosis control in the United States describe the post–World War II era as a story of the triumph of antibiotic therapy. The effectiveness of the new medications, according to these accounts, led to decreased length of hospitalization and, in turn, to the closing of sanatoriums.[1] Yet far from becoming less important, the sanatorium actually became the focus of antituberculosis efforts in the 1950s, providing what physicians believed was the optimal setting for monitoring the initial progress of patients on drug therapy. The peak capacity of sanatorium beds in the United States, nearly 120,000, was reached in 1954.[2]

Tuberculosis control in Seattle exemplified this trend. By 1950, Firland housed more than twelve hundred patients, who received not only the latest regimen of antibiotics but also sophisticated physiological testing and, if necessary, aggressive surgical interventions. In contrast with the standard historical interpretation, however, the improved medical techniques for treating tuberculosis proved to be no panacea. Firland, like other sanatoriums across the country, continued to have high rates of discharge against medical advice, undercutting its ability to cure patients and prevent the spread of tuberculosis in the community. As the Firland staff began to address these unapproved discharges, they once again had to confront the pervasiveness of their patients' social problems.

STREPTOMYCIN COMES TO SEATTLE

If tuberculosis control had experienced a revival in the early 1940s, the discovery of antibiotics truly began a new era. The first of these agents was streptomycin, discovered in 1944 by the Rutgers University soil microbiologists Selman Waksman and Albert Schatz. As Frank Ryan has described in *The Forgotten Plague,* the apparent ability of the drug to treat tuberculosis seemed almost miraculous. By 1948, clinical trials in the United States and Great Britain—the latter constituting the first randomized control trial in medical history—had confirmed the antibiotic's efficacy.[3] Small supplies of streptomycin became available for use at Firland in 1947, and the drug's impact was enthusiastically noted in the sanatorium's annual report: "It has produced perfectly amazing results in some patients who would have certainly died without it."[4]

Nevertheless, Roberts Davies and many Firland staff remained reserved in their praise for the medication, which required intramuscular injection and often caused severe side effects, such as deafness and problems with balance. In addition, clinicians at Firland and elsewhere quickly realized that tubercle bacilli developed resistance to streptomycin, often within weeks of the initiation of therapy.[5] Thus, while the drug contributed to the arrest of the disease in certain cases, many patients experienced only temporary improvement. As one Firland physician remarked in 1948, "It is not a 'Miracle Drug.' "[6] Physicians also used caution because they did not want patients to expect that they would necessarily receive the new antibiotic, which remained in short supply throughout 1947.

Given the publicity surrounding streptomycin, deciding who would and who would not receive the drug was difficult. Corwin Hinshaw, a Mayo Clinic physician involved in the earliest testing of streptomycin, had experienced enormous pressure when confronted with the duty of rationing the drug.[7] When the drug became available for use at Firland, staff physicians faced similarly difficult decisions. How did Firland ultimately allocate the small amounts of streptomycin among its hundreds of patients? Financial issues may have played a role. Davies estimated in August 1947 that a course of the drug cost $450 and stated that patients and their families had generally been responsible for raising the necessary funding. Yet Davies also noted that the ability to pay for streptomycin did not determine whether it was prescribed. Thanks to donations from the Firland Endowment Fund and local Lions Clubs, roughly $17,500 was available to finance streptomycin therapy for patients who could not afford it.[8]

Firland staff allocated streptomycin using a utilitarian calculus. As Davies explained, "If the life of the patient is in danger, and the case is not a hopeless one, streptomycin is given. If the life of the patient is not in danger, streptomycin is not given."[9] The drug went not to the sickest patients but to the sickest patients most likely to recover. In addition, the drug was generally reserved for those who had "failed" standard therapy. Davies offered as an "ideal indication for the use of Streptomycin" a woman with far-advanced tuberculosis with frequent hemorrhages whose extent of disease and age precluded the use of collapse therapy. Davies noted exceptions to the basic policy, but existing records do not provide details.[10]

By the early 1950s the major issue was no longer the allocation of streptomycin but rather which of several available antibiotics to use. Para-aminosalicylic acid (PAS), which became available in 1949, was an effective oral medication but often caused abdominal pain and nausea. By 1950 Firland was regularly using a combination of PAS and streptomycin. Clinical trials of this regimen, conducted by investigators in Veterans' Administration hospitals and elsewhere, had given impressive results, in large part because the concurrent administration of PAS prevented the development of resistance to streptomycin.[11]

When a new antibiotic of the thiosemicarbazone family, isoniazid, was introduced in 1952, it, like streptomycin five years earlier, was hailed as a "wonder drug."[12] Part of the antibiotic's reputation stemmed from the fact that an early preparation, known as iproniazid, acted as a stimulant. Pictures of formerly gravely ill patients dancing in the halls at Sea View Sanatorium in New York City had led to overly optimistic assessments of the drug's efficacy. Yet such claims were not totally unmerited. Versions of the pill that lacked any stimulant properties also caused greater reduction of disease than the combination of streptomycin and PAS.[13] Isoniazid was also well tolerated and inexpensive.

Despite the drug's glowing reports, Roberts Davies once again urged caution. "There isn't yet any real evidence that it is better than streptomycin," he stated in 1952, "and there is no proof that it is as good."[14] Davies argued that because the new antibiotics were better at preventing the multiplication of tubercle bacilli than at killing them, it was still necessary "for the healing powers within [the body] to rebuild the health."[15] Bed rest, he concluded, was still "the basic remedy for tuberculosis."[16]

Although Davies and his colleagues continued to preach bed rest, the transformation that antibiotics had caused at Firland and other sanatoriums was unmistakable. With the introduction of isoniazid, drug therapy became a routine part of patient care. As reports of resistance to isoniazid rapidly surfaced, most patients received the antibiotic in combination with either streptomycin or PAS. Certain physicians preferred to give patients all three drugs.[17]

The impact of isoniazid on the average length of hospitalization was striking. Even when receiving treatment with streptomycin and PAS, patients had remained at Firland for an average of sixteen months in 1951 and 1952, but by 1954 the mean length of stay had dropped to nine and one-half months. The census of the sanatorium, which had peaked at 1,219 in April 1950, varied between 600 and 700 during 1954.[18] Discharged patients were expected to complete their antibiotic therapy as outpatients. Although the necessary duration of treatment was unknown in the mid-1950s, physicians generally believed that two years of continuous therapy was sufficient to cure uncomplicated cases of tuberculosis. By 1954, even Davies had conceded that the use of bed rest at Firland was on the decline.[19]

Indeed, Cedric Northrop remarked that it was Davies' confidence in outpatient therapy that had made Washington "more active in shortening the period of hospital stay and lengthening the period of postsanatorium drug management than any other state in the Union."[20] While Davies had been an early advocate of outpatient therapy, Northrop's statement was somewhat hyperbolic. In fact, both Davies and Northrop continued to advocate strongly that all Firland patients be hospitalized for at least six months regardless of the rapidity of their recovery. Health officials in cities and states that, unlike Washington, had been either unable or unwilling to obtain enough sanatorium beds were actually much more aggressive in starting early outpatient treatment. By the mid-1950s, officials in many of these locales had even begun to dispense antibiotics to outpatients who had never been hospitalized. Heretical in its questioning of the continued necessity of the sanatorium, this policy rankled Northrop and many of his peers.

Nevertheless, studies from elsewhere in the United States, most notably those performed by Arthur B. Robins and Aaron D. Chaves in New York City, reported reasonably good results for the treatment of unhospitalized tuberculosis patients. For example, according to a 1957 article by Robins and Chaves, 313 (62 percent) of 501 sputum-positive patients had converted to sputum-negative within twenty-four months of treatment; at the same time, none of 134 treated patients whose sputum had initially been negative reverted to positive.[21] Results like these encouraged officials to either close their institutions or convert them into facilities for other groups, such as the mentally retarded. Among the hundreds of sanatoriums that closed in the 1950s were the fabled Trudeau Sanatorium in Saranac Lake and New York City's Otisville Sanatorium.[22]

Not only were antibiotics decreasing the length of hospitalization, but they were also having a major effect on mortality from tuberculosis. In 1948, 31 percent of Firland's "discharges" were deaths; by 1954 this figure had decreased to 6 percent. The combined Seattle and King County death rate from tuberculosis over this six-year period plummeted from 35.1 to 6.2 per 100,000 population. This dramatic decline mirrored the pattern throughout the United States.[23]

The impact of antibiotics on the prevalence of tuberculosis was less impressive. First, although the drugs prevented deaths among persons with advanced disease who otherwise would have died, as many as one-fifth of hospitalized patients became so-called chronics, with persistent but incurable tuberculosis. Second, the number of new cases reported annually dropped much more slowly than the number of deaths. In Seattle and King County, for example, the number of new cases remained steady, between 450 and 500, from 1951 through 1956, falling under 400 only in 1957. This persistently high incidence of tuberculosis was partially an artifact of more aggressive screening efforts, which identified cases that otherwise would have gone undetected. Yet the new cases also represented the reactivation of old dormant areas of tuberculosis that had been acquired when the disease had been more prevalent. Antibiotics could do nothing to prevent such reactivations from occurring.[24]

Nevertheless, the remarkable ability of antibiotics to treat most cases of tuberculosis engendered a great deal of hopefulness among health officials across the country. This optimism would ultimately peak in 1959, when the National Tuberculosis Association and the U.S. Public Health Service cosponsored a conference on tuberculosis at Arden House in Harriman, New York. Noting that, in the words of conference attendee René Dubos, "miracles do not happen very often,"[25] participants called for an all-out campaign against tuberculosis. With the "widespread application of chemotherapy as a public health measure," they concluded, the "elimination of tuberculosis in the United States" had become a distinct possibility.[26]

The success of antibiotic therapy greatly enhanced the reputations of sanatoriums like Firland. If a sanatorium stay in the era of Betty MacDonald had been the equivalent of a death sentence, admission to Firland in the 1950s offered an excellent chance of recovery from the once dreaded white plague. Local tuberculosis officials constantly lauded Firland. Cedric Northrop, for example, believed that the institution was among the three best sanatoriums in the country. Compliments came from outsiders as well. A team of four prominent national officials who evaluated Firland in 1957 termed it "one of the most outstanding" institutions in the United States.[27] Patients and other Seattle citizens echoed this assessment. "The care here has been the best," reported one patient. "That goes for the janitor, the food, the nurses, and the doctors. This place is doing wonderful work."[28] A relative of another patient concurred: "Every person connected in any way with the hospital does everything humanly possible to help the patient and keep him happy."[29]

If commentators had good things to say about all aspects of Firland, its medical achievements generated the most pride within the institution. As of 1952, the sanatorium employed seventeen full-time physicians, four in training, and thirty consultants. There were also more than a hundred nurses and two hundred nursing aides on the staff. Firland was one of nearly two dozen hospitals that participated in antibiotic trials sponsored by the U.S. Public Health Service. These trials, conducted throughout the 1950s and 1960s, compared the efficacy of various combinations of the original three antimicrobials and a series of new agents that had subsequently been developed.[30] Basic science research, which had essentially been nonexistent at the original Firland facility, blossomed in the 1950s. One physician who performed particularly notable work was Carroll J. Martin, a pulmonary physiologist. With funding from both the U.S. Public Health Service and the

National Tuberculosis Association, Martin examined complex ventilatory patterns of the lungs in tuberculosis and other respiratory diseases.[31]

Firland's clinical and research activities were enhanced in 1948 when it formally affiliated with the new University of Washington Medical School, which had opened two years earlier. The establishment of the medical school was part of the university's evolution from a regional institution in the 1930s to a "national power" after World War II.[32] By the early 1950s, both medical students and nursing students from the University of Washington Nursing School received part of their clinical training at Firland.

The combination of improved medical therapy, an academic affiliation, and a research and teaching program effectively transformed the institution. Although it retained the name Firland Sanatorium until it closed in 1973, by the 1950s it was commonly referred to as a "tuberculosis hospital." If the word *sanatorium* recalled the mountainous Swiss resorts of Thomas Mann's *Magic Mountain,* the word *hospital* increasingly connoted an institution of "irreproachable scientific reputation."[33]

Firland's new status as a university teaching hospital helped Roberts Davies to attract physicians from the best training programs in the country. In 1952, *Pep,* now renamed *Pep and Courage,* reported that nearly one-third of Firland's medical staff had trained in New York City under the renowned Bellevue Hospital physician J. Burns Amberson.[34] The ability of Firland to attract such individuals represented a major change from Robert Stith's era, when even well-respected sanatoriums often had difficulty filling their medical staffs.

Just as the sanatorium became a tuberculosis hospital, its practitioners also changed the way in which they referred to themselves. No longer "phthisiologists" devoted solely to tuberculosis, they had become "chest physicians," and many supplemented their participation in tuberculosis societies with membership in the American College of Chest Physicians.[35] Given the declining mortality from tuberculosis, the adoption of this new title represented a practical decision by physicians whose field of specialization was suddenly shrinking. Yet the term "chest physician" also reflected the process of professionalization that accompanied the expansion of clinical tuberculology into the scientific study of areas such as lung physiology, asthma, and emphysema. Seattle's chest physicians took great pride in their ability to read the hundreds of thousands of miniature screening chest X-rays that were taken throughout Washington state from the 1940s through the 1960s. "To this day," recalled former Firland physician Richard Greenleaf in 1992, "I don't trust anybody but chest people to read chest X-rays. I don't trust an internist or radiologist."[36]

THE RISE OF THORACIC SURGERY

Nowhere were the advances in chest medicine so apparent as in the expanding use of thoracic surgery. World War II played a major role in the rise of this field, as a generation of surgeons gained experience in treating traumatic injuries to the chest. It was not until the widespread availability of antibiotics, however, that thoracic surgery became commonplace in the treatment of tuberculosis. Once patients were receiving streptomycin and other agents, surgeons no longer feared that manipulation of infected tissue would in fact cause the tuberculosis to spread postoperatively.[37]

The first operative intervention that grew in popularity was thoracoplasty. As noted in chapter 1, thoracoplasty was one of several procedures that phthisiologists were using by the 1920s to collapse persistent lung cavities. Thoracoplasty was by far the most aggressive of these procedures, a major operation that required removal of the rib cage and led to permanent deformities.[38] By the early 1950s, however, thoracoplasties had been supplanted by operations that actually resected portions of diseased lung. Although the surgical removal of disease foci had always carried a high theoretical appeal, physicians had used pulmonary resection sparingly in the preantibiotic era.

Statistics from Firland reveal the evolving nature of surgical intervention for tuberculosis. Whereas 26 percent of patients underwent either thoracoplasty or another type of collapse procedure in 1948, by 1953 this number had decreased to 3 percent. Meanwhile, in this latter year, more than 11 percent (239) of the 2,121 patients cared for at Firland had a pulmonary resection performed by one of the three staff surgeons, Fred Jarvis, Waldo Mills, or Roland Pinkham.[39] As at Firland, physicians at other sanatoriums were also increasingly advocating and performing lung resections.[40] The major role played by surgery in the "conquest" of tuberculosis after World War II has been largely neglected.

Why did certain patients undergo resection? Surgical candidates, explained Firland's assistant medical director George Hames in 1952, were generally those patients who, despite several months of antibiotics, had persistent cavities, masses, or nodules on their chest X-rays. The choice of surgical procedure varied based on the extent of the remaining lesion. Resections ranged from the removal of a small amount of tissue (nodulectomy, or wedge resection) to a lobe (lobectomy) or an entire lung (pneumonectomy). Not surprisingly, mortality rates from these procedures, which generally averaged between 2 and 3 percent overall, were highest among patients undergoing removal of a lung. In 1953, for example, four of fourteen persons (29 percent) undergoing pneumonectomy at Firland died during or shortly after their operation.[41]

Prior to recommending thoracic surgery to patients, physicians presented their cases at Firland's weekly staff conferences. Departing from the more traditional model of medical decision making, in which an individual physician makes therapeutic recommendations to a patient, decisions regarding surgery were determined by a vote of staff doctors attending the conferences: an operation was recommended only if a majority gave their approval. Surgeons performed resections only if patients signed consent forms; at times, patients declined surgery.

There was general agreement about the need to remove certain lesions. For example, Firland physicians routinely approved the removal of isolated cavities from patients who remained sputum-positive despite several months of antibiotic therapy. Many of these cases involved drug-resistant bacteria. Other scenarios, however, generated avid debate. Typically, these involved individuals whose X-rays revealed persistent infiltrates despite negative sputum samples. (If such infiltrates were cavitary, the cases were termed "open negatives.") Some physicians favored giving these patients additional bed rest and antibiotics. Others disagreed, however, arguing that prolonged courses of antibiotic therapy were unlikely to lead to cure.[42] These Firland staff members, once again using a military metaphor, were likely to advocate a "resectional attack" on these persistent lesions.[43]

In one 1953 case, for example, a patient whose sputum had been negative for six months had a persistent nodule in the right-lower-lung field. "There was considerable argument," wrote the patient's physician, "about whether the lesion had resolved to the point where surgery was not necessary."[44] Ultimately, the physicians approved a "nodulectomy," by a slim margin of eleven to nine. In another case from the same year, a segmental resection was performed over the objection of one physician, who believed the patient's X-ray demonstrated continued improvement.[45]

These discussions reveal the great authority of the chest radiograph in determining what degree of "disease" was present. Long past the days in which phthisiologists decried X-rays as a poor substitute for the physical examination, clinicians at Firland relied heavily on radiographic findings to ascertain the initial extent of disease and to monitor the healing process. Not surprisingly, therefore, treatment decisions often hinged on what the X-rays revealed.

The power of the chest radiograph became particularly apparent in the case of an entity known as a "tuberculoma," which bore some relationship to the residual nodules described above. Although physicians at Firland generally did not use the term, their colleagues around the country actively debated how to assess and manage this entity. Nineteenth-century pathologists had been the first to identify tuberculomas, defining them as a "gross mass of tuberculous tissue resembling a tumor."[46] The diagnosis of tuberculoma was rarely made during life, nor would the ability to make such a diagnosis change the management of such cases.

With the advent of the chest X-ray, however, physicians began to identify round opacities that correlated with tuberculomas found on pathological examination. Indeed, the radiologic image itself had gradually begun to define the disease. One author, for example, defined tuberculoma of the lung as "a rounded, homogeneous radiographic opacity."[47] There was considerable disagreement as to why such lesions formed, with various commentators claiming they represented cavities, residual areas of dead tissue, or fusion of multiple adjacent areas of active disease.

Despite the growing interest in tuberculomas and what they signified clinically, an X-ray finding of a tuberculoma in someone with known tuberculosis made little difference in the preantibiotic era. Such patients continued to receive the standard treatment of bed rest and fresh air. With the advent of antibiotics, however, tuberculomas attracted growing attention, in part because the residual nodules that at times remained after drug therapy resembled tuberculomas.[48] As with the residual nodules, many commentators began to advocate the surgical extirpation of tuberculomas. In retrospect, it was probably the new ability to resect such lesions that transformed the tuberculoma from a "traditionally benign condition" to "an omnipresent threat" or "time-bomb" requiring excision.[49] In this sense, tuberculoma had become both a radiologically and a surgically constructed disease.[50]

Ultimately, a series of studies vindicated those who had discouraged the resection of tuberculomas or persistent infiltrates. Work by researchers affiliated with both the Veterans' Administration and the Public Health Service demonstrated that resection of residual lesions—including cavities with negative sputum—was unnecessary.[51] Once these results had been disseminated, rates of surgery across the United States dropped. At Firland, for example, less than 7 percent (74) of the 1,187 patients cared for in 1960 received a resection, down from 11 percent seven years earlier.[52] While the overall numbers of resections declined, the debate over the proper indications for these operations grew increasingly intense. As we will see, the most controversial cases generally involved Skid Road alcoholics.

DISCHARGES AGAINST MEDICAL ADVICE

Although the new medical therapies available beginning in the late 1940s had markedly improved the ability of physicians to cure tuberculosis, problems persisted. Most notably, many patients continued to leave sanatoriums against medical advice. At Firland, for example, 47 percent of all discharges (excluding deaths) in 1948 left prior to approved discharge. By 1951 so-called irregular discharges had declined but still totaled 37 percent.[53]

It was not until the 1940s, however, that discharges against medical advice became an issue of major concern among tuberculosis workers nationwide. A large number of articles with titles like "Why Do Patients Go AWOL?" and "Irregular Discharge: The Problem of Hospitalization of the Tuberculous" began to appear.[54] While the issue received some coverage in the lay press, the bulk of the discussion about such discharges occurred at tuberculosis conferences and in medical journals. A patient who left against advice, according to a typical article in the Washington Tuberculosis Association's *Health Pilot,* was a "double menace—to the community through spread of infection—and to himself, because such action almost invariably results in a deterioration of his condition."[55]

What led to the sudden rise of interest in a problem that had existed since public sanatoriums first opened in the early twentieth century? First, World War II had focused attention on the irregular discharge problem among tuberculous veterans—both those who had served in World War I and those who had been diagnosed with the disease during more recent hostilities. Two of the seminal articles on discharges against medical advice, written by Louis I. Dublin and William B. Tollen, specifically examined populations of veterans. In 1943 Dublin reported the astounding fact that up to 58 percent of cases left Veterans' Administration hospitals without consent or authorization; only 36 percent of tuberculous veterans demonstrated any improvement whatsoever. Moreover, much like the "rounders" of the Hermann Biggs era, veterans came and went among inpatient facilities as they pleased. One patient had twenty-four separate admissions.[56]

Dublin's interest in this area stemmed from his long experience doing actuarial work on tuberculosis. As a statistician for the Metropolitan Life Insurance Company, which had organized the Framingham tuberculosis demonstration project (1916–23), Dublin had become a national expert on funding care for the tuberculous. Given this background, it is hardly surprising that he chose to emphasize how much of the Veterans' Administration's roughly $40 million annual allocation for tuberculosis was being squandered by patients unwilling to remain hospitalized.

Similar considerations applied at the local level. As Cedric Northrop and his counterparts elsewhere trumpeted tuberculosis control as both efficient and "good business," their apparent willingness to allow partially treated patients to leave facilities early seemed to be nothing if not a poor investment. This was particularly true in locations, such as Seattle, where funding increases for tuberculosis control had recently been procured. Whereas Robert Stith's disciplinary discharges might have made sense when there were waiting-list patients to fill vacated beds, it was not logical to maintain such a lax standard when the city could finally hospitalize all of its tuberculous citizens. Ensuring that all people with tuberculosis received proper treatment, therefore, became a type of quid pro quo of the health department and its patients to the city and state. The community had a responsibility to hospitalize and care for the tuberculous, wrote one Seattle commentator, but "the control program can be defeated in large part unless each patient with active tuberculosis can undergo the long-drawn-out process of regaining his health."[57]

In one sense, this growing concern with irregular discharges seems paradoxical. Curative antibiotics and surgery had led to a major decline in the average length of stay at tuberculosis sanatoriums. Nevertheless, as noted above, Firland physicians continued to believe that at least six months of hospitalization was still necessary. This mandatory stay served both medical and social purposes. It ensured that doctors had both prescribed the correct medications and imparted the necessary program of "health instruction, moral guidance, and occupational training" that they believed was an essential part of therapy for tuberculosis.[58] As Roberts Davies noted in 1952, only eighteen of the 1,808 Firland patients who had received "apparently proper treatment" during the previous year had died.[59] It thus remained crucial, he believed, to institute a comprehensive therapeutic regimen in the sanatorium.

Spurred by Davies' concern, discharges against medical advice became a preoccupation among Firland staff. In 1950, for the first time, the issue appeared in Firland's annual report. Davies himself continued to criticize patients who left against advice. "Almost all of these people," he wrote, "show poor judgment that is as reckless and may be as fatal as the judgment of a careless driver who tries to beat a train to a crossing."[60] Others also evinced a growing interest in the subject, most notably a group of University of Washington students writing their master's theses and doctoral dissertations. In what became a sort of cottage industry, students in the 1950s trekked out to the Department of Health clinic and Firland, where they conducted a series of projects that examined numerous aspects of the care of tuberculosis patients. A typical thesis title was "A Study of Sixty-Four Tuberculous Patients with Emphasis on Their Social Problems."[61]

Two studies that looked specifically at the issue of discharges against medical advice were those of Barbara Dike and Evelyn Noakes Hadaway, master's degree students in the schools of nursing and social work, respectively. Dike reviewed the charts of ninety-four patients (fifty-four men and forty women) who had left Firland against advice during the first half of 1950; Hadaway examined the records of fifty-four patients (thirty-two men and twenty-two women) who had irregular discharges in 1952. As anticipated, both authors found that such discharges comprised roughly one-third of all discharges and that between 25 and 50 percent of the patients in question had previously left a sanatorium against advice.[62] Although many irregularly discharged patients "left only a little sooner than the medical staff would have advised,"[63] others still had significant disease; 55 percent of the men in Hadaway's study had active tuberculosis when they left Firland.[64]

Dike and Hadaway also studied the demographics of persons discharged against medical advice. Although neither explicitly compared her sample with the larger sanatorium population, irregular discharges appeared to represent a cross section of those hospitalized. Among the men, for example, there were laborers, students, and unemployed persons as well as one accountant. Seventeen of the forty women that Dike studied were housewives, while sixteen of the twenty-two women in Hadaway's study were classified as such. Those who worked outside of the home included waitresses and factory workers. The ages of irregularly discharged patients ranged from six to seventy-one.[65]

Both Dike and Hadaway examined the racial composition of patients who left against advice, finding that between 85 and 90 percent were white. This total actually represented a higher percentage than the general sanatorium population in the early 1950s, which averaged about 80 percent white, 7 percent Negro, 4 percent Oriental, and 4 percent either American Indian or Eskimo. The fact that whites represented a disproportionately high percentage of irregular discharges, noted Hadaway, "dispels the cliché that minority races are troublesome in this respect."[66]

What was more notable than these slight racial disparities, however, was Dike's finding that "the factor of alcoholism stood out as a prominent indication of faulty adjustment."[67] Indeed, despite the long association of tuberculosis, alcoholism, and uncooperativeness, most of the newer studies did not explicitly address the contribution of alcohol to discharges against advice. Yet Dike and Hadaway reported that 36 and 50 percent of their irregularly discharged patients, respectively, carried the diagnosis of alcoholism.[68] The vast majority of these patients were males.

What explanations for discharges against medical advice did the medical charts offer? Obtaining data consistent with other studies from across the country, Dike found that twenty-one of the ninety-four patients (22 percent) had reported "home or family" problems, and thirty (32 percent) had expressed dissatisfaction with aspects of their care at Firland. These findings applied almost equally to both sexes. The remaining forty-three patients (46 percent) had given miscellaneous reasons or no specific explanation for their premature departure.[69] Hadaway also reviewed the summaries of interviews that social workers had conducted with patients at some point during their hospitalization. She reported that patients' major concerns had included financial problems, child care or domestic issues, sanatorium adjustment, and the appropriateness of their therapeutic regimen.[70]

Given these findings, Dike and Hadaway reached a similar conclusion: in order to decrease the number of irregular discharges, Firland staff needed to understand the problems that hospitalized patients experienced. Patients, Dike wrote, were "people with feelings and the rights to have attitudes of their own."[71] Sanatorium care had been set up, remarked Hadaway, "without sufficient understanding . . . that attitudes toward recovery and discharge are complex and laden with conflicts about the resumption of mature responsibilities in the normal workaday world."[72] It was only through individualized case studies, she concluded, that patients' emotions and behaviors could truly be understood and addressed.

Such concerns were hardly new among sanatorium staff members. In fact, the lay and medical literature contained numerous articles that discussed the emotional characteristics of the tuberculous, often positing a relation between the disease and "neurotic" personalities or other specific psychological characteristics.[73] By the mid-1940s, however, authors had specifically begun to emphasize the importance of helping all patients adjust to the emotional tribulations of prolonged hospitalization. Many of these studies encouraged the use of formal psychological testing.[74]

Dike's and Hadaway's recommendations fell on fertile soil. Roberts Davies and Firland business manager Frank Fells had already commissioned two University of Washington researchers, Catherine Vavra and Edith Rainboth, to conduct a study examining patients' attitudes toward the care they received at Firland Sanatorium. The study, completed in 1955, received national attention.[75] While the researchers genuinely sought to improve the quality of hospitalization at Firland, their ultimate goal—strongly shared by Davies and Fells—was to decrease the number of irregular discharges: "The challenge of reducing the discharges against medical advice, the number of reactivations and resulting readmissions is the basic reason for making this study. . . . It is assumed that a patient who is satisfied with his progress and care, is reassured about his family's needs, and is adequately informed about the disease is less inclined to leave the hospital against medical advice."[76]

Tabulating questionnaire results from 857 Firland patients, Vavra and Rainboth found that the majority were pleased with their care. Yet a high percentage of those hospitalized registered various complaints, particularly a perceived lack of communication with medical and nursing staff. For example, 25 percent of patients believed that their doctors "were not really interested in them"; 43 percent perceived a similar lack of interest on the part of nurses. As one patient reported, "Good care . . . indifferent attitude . . . they feel we are a pair of lungs in bed with absolutely no feelings whatsoever."[77] Forty-four percent of patients stated that they did not have adequate private discussions with their physicians, leading one to state that "the motto around here is 'ignorance is bliss.' "[78]

These findings were consistent with the observations of Columbia University sociologist Julius A. Roth, who conducted studies of several sanatoriums in the 1950s and 1960s. Roth discovered that most of the conflicts that arose in such institutions stemmed from patients' frustrations with the often arbitrary "timetables" used by physicians in prescribing therapies and assessing recovery. While patients grasped for reliable guideposts with which to assess their progress, staff members preferred not to discuss such matters unless pressed.[79]

Davies and his colleagues felt "humbled" by the results of Vavra and Rainboth's study. Quoting Robert Burns, Davies thanked the authors for the " 'giftie' gie us tae see oorsels as ithers see us."[80] Davies' response was typical of his receptive attitude toward patients' concerns. After the "new" Firland had opened in 1947, Davies had liberalized a number of the rigid rules that had characterized the Stith era, including the ban on smoking and the segregation of male and female patients. He had also expanded entertainment offerings at the sanatorium, which included a bowling league, concerts, movies, and visits from celebrities, such as Bob Feller, the star pitcher of the Cleveland Indians.[81] Finally, Davies had been particularly receptive to requests made by the Patients' Council, an organization begun by patients in 1948 to promote their concerns.[82]

Responding to a preliminary version of the Vavra and Rainboth study, Davies and his colleagues had already begun to make the types of changes recommended in the final 1955 version. For example, Firland inaugurated formal "patient interview conferences," moved physicians' offices onto the actual wards, and "gradually eliminated" nurses and attendants "who showed little interest in their patients."[83] In addition, Firland became one of the earliest sanatoriums to hire psychiatrists or psychologists to address patients' emotional problems.[84]

The growing role of therapists in tuberculosis sanatoriums in part reflected the rising status of psychiatry and psychology. Both of these professions had achieved a growing legitimacy during World War II as their members helped medical doctors evaluate patients for conditions such as shell shock. Consultation-liaison psychiatry, which specifically emphasized the evaluation and counseling of patients under the care of other physicians, was also becoming a recognized subspecialty within psychiatry.[85]

The man who became Firland's part-time staff psychiatrist in 1949 was not a psychiatrist at all. Thomas H. Holmes was actually an internist who had received additional training in psychosomatic medicine at Cornell University Medical School in New York City. At the University of Washington, however, Holmes served on the faculty of the Department of Psychiatry and began to do psychiatric consultations on sanatorium patients shortly after arriving in Seattle in 1949. At times, Firland's new enthusiasm for addressing emotional concerns led to what might be termed a "psychiatricization" of all elements of patients' lives. As one student noted in her master's thesis: "The doctors' records showed evidence of emotional problems in the past in such areas as general illness patterns, fainting patterns, miscarriages and menstrual difficulties, alcoholism, pregnancy while not married, and past and present marital difficulty. Prenatal and family problems were also seen including psychosis and illness, accidental deaths and poor relationships."[86] Holmes, however, remained modest in his expectations, providing diagnostic assistance and counseling for patients he was asked to evaluate.

By hiring Holmes and attempting to increase sensitivity among its staff members, Firland had taken several steps toward improving communication in the sanatorium. Yet such interventions did little to address the financial, employment, and family issues that seemed to underlie much of the discontent of patients. Davies and his colleagues next turned toward the "treatment" of these social problems.

READDRESSING SOCIAL CONCERNS

Firland's efforts to deal with its patients' social problems were part of a broader resurgence of interest in social issues that characterized postwar tuberculosis control. Many tuberculosis workers between 1945 and 1960 struggled to reintroduce an Oslerian Progressive Era conceptualization of the disease as "a social problem with medical aspects."[87]

This new emphasis was embodied by the French-born Rockefeller Institute microbiologist and philosopher René Dubos. Dubos, whose first wife had died from tuberculosis, had performed some important laboratory work on the disease, but his major contribution was to conceptualize tuberculosis as an interaction of bacillus, man, and environment. In *The White Plague*, coauthored with his second wife, Jean, and published in 1952, Dubos characterized tuberculosis as a "social disease" that presented problems that "transcend the conventional medical approach."[88] Reviewing the history of tuberculosis, Dubos described how the disease had historically thrived in the setting of poor social and environmental conditions. Tuberculosis had declined in recent years, he believed, due to a combination of public health measures and improvement in basic living conditions. Thus, Dubos argued, the solution to the problem of tuberculosis was not a vaccine or stronger medications but better housing, jobs, and nutrition—in other words, "solving the social problem of tuberculosis."[89]

Epidemiological data appeared to back up Dubos's claims. As of 1950, tuberculosis was still the leading killer of persons between the ages of fifteen and thirty in the United States. Such individuals often became tuberculous shortly after exposure to someone who was infectious. Yet tuberculosis was increasingly becoming a disease of those forty-five and older, particularly males, whose tuberculosis resulted from reactivation of dormant lesions acquired in childhood. The noted Johns Hopkins University epidemiologist Wade Frost had predicted this demographic shift in the tuberculous population in a seminal 1937 article.[90]

Moreover, although the new antibiotics had led to marked declines in overall mortality from tuberculosis in the United States, death rates among the poor, minorities, and the homeless remained three to five times that of the general population. In 1948, for example, mortality for white males and white females was 33.3 and 15.4 per 100,000 population, respectively. For nonwhites, these figures rose to 92.1 and 65.4 per 100,000 population.[91]

As a result of the changing demographic patterns of tuberculosis, attention shifted in part from preventing the transmission of infection to addressing the possible factors—such as poverty or homelessness—that lowered the ability of infected persons to resist breakdown of their dormant lesions.[92] Accordingly, the relation of poor housing to tuberculosis, which had received little attention since World War I, once again became the focus of meetings and articles. Similarly, numerous pieces appeared in the medical literature with titles such as "The Increase in Tuberculosis Proportionate Mortality among Nonwhite Young Adults" and "Anti-Poverty-Anti-TB." The authors of these articles called for increased attention to the continued high rates of tuberculosis among poor and minority populations.[93]

The increased emphasis on social issues was also apparent at the National Tuberculosis Association, which in the 1940s organized new committees on rehabilitation, Spanish-speaking people with tuberculosis, and social and economic problems. By 1953, the latter group had been replaced by a Committee on Social Research designed to study issues like public assistance, housing, irregular discharges, and "public attitudes toward tuberculosis and persons who have had it."[94] Meanwhile, the Tuberculosis Control Division of the U.S. Public Health Service called not only for better drugs but also for continued attention to the "after care and rehabilitation of the patient" and "protection of the families of the tuberculous against economic distress."[95]

This growing attention to social issues at the national level appeared to fit well with the efforts of Firland staff to address the social problems that they believed were contributing to discharges against medical advice. After all, promising discharged tuberculosis patients jobs or economic assistance might discourage them from leaving the sanatorium early. Yet, at the same time, the two agendas were at odds. Dubos' call for fundamental social change necessarily conflicted with a concern for social problems that basically emanated from a more limited medical goal: the need to ensure compliance with antibiotic therapy.

This conflict became apparent in 1948, when Firland hired Louise Shaffrath to head a new Department of Social Service. Once again, the interest of government and sanatorium officials had been sparked by the King County Anti-Tuberculosis League, which had begun a demonstration project of social services at the Department of Health clinic and Firland in 1944. By 1950 Firland employed four social workers who could "discuss with the patient some of the fears and worries arising from illness and hospitalization."[96] Yet while this inclination to emphasize patients' psychological problems was growing increasingly popular within social work circles,[97] Firland's social workers generally spent most of their time assisting patients with financial and family matters. One of these activities was an appraisal of the financial status of all persons admitted to Firland. It was this assessment, informally known as the "means test," that determined whether or not patients would contribute to the cost of their hospitalization. Those persons with adequate "means" were expected to fund at least a portion of their care.

Although many private tuberculosis patients in Seattle were hospitalized at either Laurel Beach or Riverton sanatoriums, Firland also housed some middle-class persons, including physicians, nurses, and bankers. For the most part, however, patients came from poor or working-class families whose wage earners worked on the assembly lines at Boeing or for other local manufacturers. Because of the generous funding allotted for tuberculosis control in Seattle and Washington, Firland patients actually paid very little toward their care. According to one 1950 study of ninety-one patients, 86 percent were admitted for free, 8 percent planned to pay, and 6 percent had some outside coverage.[98] Money from the King County 0.6 mill tax levy and the State Tuberculosis Equalization Fund covered those who were unable to pay. In addition, the "quite liberal and flexible" King County Welfare Department continued to provide patients' families with assistance in the form of food, shelter, utilities, and clothing.[99]

Yet despite the relatively generous assistance available to Firland patients, financial troubles figured prominently among the "family" problems that so often led to discharges against medical advice. Unless patients had no dependents, hospitalization meant the loss of either a wage earner or a caretaker. Admission social work evaluations contained numerous examples of tenuous family circumstances. For example, admission of a woman with two children meant that "the husband's earnings would be stretched to the utmost to meet his new budget due to illness." In another case, admission of a married male left his wife and new baby in an "unpleasant housing project" without a source of income.[100] As much as ever, social problems remained paramount when addressing tuberculosis.

Yet both the ability and inclination of Firland's social workers to address such concerns remained limited in scope. Although Davies, Northrop, and their colleagues remained sympathetic to the value of social work, to some extent they continued to regard it as a "frill."[101] What ultimately cemented the place of the Department of Social Service at Firland was the belief of Davies and the Board of Managers that it was "instrumental in reducing the number of discharges against medical advice."[102] Or, in the words of Louise Shaffrath, that it "assisted patients with personal and family problems which may be interfering with medical treatment and 'taking the cure.'"[103]

Perhaps the best example of the ambiguous status of efforts to address patients' social problems was a statement made in 1956 by Denver tuberculosis specialist Gardner Middlebrook, who termed the need to administer isoniazid regularly for many months a "serious psychosocial problem."[104] At first glance, this assertion appears to be an explicit acknowledgement of the need to view tuberculosis and its treatment as more than just a medical matter. Yet Middlebrook's words actually framed social concerns entirely within the context of the limited goal of completing antibiotic therapy. In fact, irregular discharges and noncompliance with antibiotics often reflected the presence of numerous psychosocial problems that would most likely persist even if the patient's tuberculosis was cured. Nevertheless, the message remained clear: the primary reason for addressing the social problems of Firland patients was to facilitate the completion of antibiotic and other medical therapy, first within the sanatorium and then at home. Such a philosophy was entirely consistent with the spirit of the Arden House Conference, which, while emphasizing that tuberculosis was both a sociological and biological problem, had principally called for the widespread application of antibiotic therapy.

VOCATIONAL REHABILITATION AT FIRLAND

As with social work, postwar commentators debated whether the goal of vocational rehabilitation was improving patients' lives or merely facilitating a medical cure. Compared with certain areas of the country, relatively little job retraining had been offered at the "old" Firland, despite the widespread belief that patients who returned to strenuous work would experience a reactivation of their tuberculosis. The King County Anti-Tuberculosis League had formed a rehabilitation committee in 1933 but did not begin an actual demonstration project until 1944, when it hired Helen Wilson to provide job counseling to patients hospitalized at Firland and Morningside.

World War II greatly helped to popularize a broad concept of medical rehabilitation. Soldiers returned from overseas not only with medical injuries but also with uncertain vocational plans and emotional problems stemming from their war service. Medical rehabilitation, wrote one physician in 1949, is "a concept of treatment which combines medical, psychological, educational, and sociologic methods to give the disabled maximum independence commensurate with his limitations."[105]

This definition fit well with the philosophy of tuberculosis workers. At a national Conference on Rehabilitation of the Tuberculous held in Washington, D.C., in March 1946, the following statement was adopted: "Rehabilitation in tuberculosis is the restoration of tuberculous persons to the fullest physical, mental, social, vocational, and economic usefulness of which they are capable."[106] In this sense, the attempts of Firland's social workers to assist patients with both emotional and economic matters were part of the rehabilitation process. But vocational issues—such as job retraining—remained at the heart of such efforts.

The best record of vocational rehabilitation at Firland is a 1953 doctoral dissertation by Alma V. Armstrong, who became head of vocational rehabilitation at the sanatorium in 1946. She directed a staff of three counselors, all of whom were funded by the Anti-Tuberculosis League. Armstrong examined vocational counseling given to 1,361 Firland patients, analyzing categories such as previous occupations, extent of education, desired future work, and doctors' recommendations regarding appropriate vocational goals.[107] As a result of these interviews and aptitude testing, patients embarked on a variety of vocational programs. These included studying with public school teachers hired by Firland, enrolling in correspondence courses to learn business skills, and engaging in occupational therapy, which ranged from watch repair to employment in a sheltered machine workshop operated by the Boeing Airplane Company.

The extent to which hospitalized patients at Firland could undergo meaningful job training was limited by the patient's medical condition, the hospital setting, and, increasingly, the declining length of stay. In addition, as rehabilitation workers often reported, fear of hiring former tuberculosis patients remained pervasive, in Seattle as elsewhere. Armstrong and her staff referred patients who required the most ambitious job retraining to the Washington state Division of Vocational Rehabilitation (DVR), which had been established in 1933. The DVR assumed responsibility for placing the discharged patient in a suitable job, often paying the cost of schooling or on-the-job training.[108]

The number of patients who actually qualified for this program appears to have been limited, even after the DVR itself assumed control of vocational rehabilitation at Firland in 1951. During one twelve-month period in 1946 and 1947, for example, vocational counselors at Firland conducted 457 interviews but referred only twenty-three patients to the DVR. Of these twenty-three, only eight had begun training or had qualified for placement as of mid-1947.[109] Many states reported job placement rates comparable to those attained in Washington, but others achieved much greater success. Michigan and Connecticut, for example, surpassed the National Tuberculosis Association's goal that a minimum of 10 percent of the number of new cases annually should receive job placements. Overall, the NTA reported that state vocational rehabilitative agencies had found jobs for 21,690 persons with a history of pulmonary tuberculosis between 1934 and 1947.[110]

What was much harder to determine, of course, was what such job placements accomplished. Did they, in fact, prevent patients with arrested cases of tuberculosis from reactivating? Even if this were so, did the prevention of relapse justify expansion of rehabilitation programs across the country and the maintenance of a rehabilitation staff of twenty persons at the NTA? Historically, the only statistics on the fate of rehabilitated tuberculosis patients had come from the few aftercare programs designed to provide both employment and intensive follow-up for tuberculosis patients.[111] By the late 1940s, however, commentators had begun to call for the establishment of "prognostic terms that have an unequivocal meaning for physician and rehabilitation worker alike."[112]

Such requests for more scientific data highlighted an underlying disagreement as to how rehabilitation should be conceptualized. Advocates often attempted to "medicalize" rehabilitation, urging their colleagues to view it not only as an important postsanatorium intervention but "as an essential part of the *treatment* of the tuberculous."[113] Others preferred to view vocational rehabilitation as one of many potential "psychosocial" interventions that helped patients deal with the multiple problems that tuberculosis engendered.[114]

By the end of the 1950s, the debate as to whether vocational rehabilitation should be considered a medical or a social intervention became more controversial, as certain commentators began to ask why it was considered part of tuberculosis therapy at all. In the *American Review of Tuberculosis and Pulmonary Diseases* in 1958, two rural midwestern physicians, David T. Carr and Ezra V. Bridge, argued that the goal of finding less taxing jobs for the tuberculous was no longer appropriate for three reasons: (1) antibiotic and surgical therapy had made cure without relapse more likely, regardless of occupation; (2) tuberculosis was affecting a much older age group with fewer career concerns; and (3) the percentage of patients who had been manual laborers prior to developing tuberculosis had declined considerably. Carr and Bridge emphasized that they continued to advocate appropriate nonvocational rehabilitation for the tuberculous but nevertheless were questioning "whether the patient who has had tuberculosis needs training for a better job any more than his fellow citizens, who have not been unfortunate enough to contract the disease."[115] Karl H. Pfuetze and Marjorie M. Pyle, of the Chicago State Tuberculosis Sanitarium, disagreed, continuing to see tuberculosis as a social disease that warranted interventions that were not simply medical. Urban patient populations, they stated, still included a large number of relatively young, unskilled individuals who "need[ed] special vocational rehabilitation services . . . to compete in today's labor market and yet avoid a relapse."[116]

While some of the disagreement between the two sets of authors reflected the fact that they treated different populations of patients, the issue was actually much broader. As we have seen, commentators throughout the twentieth century had continued to view tuberculosis as a social disease. Vocational rehabilitation had embodied this philosophy, aiming not only to preserve the results of medical therapy but also to ensure that "the patient has been returned to a normal and adequate social and economic place in the community."[117] Carr and Bridge's contention—that the tuberculous did not, by virtue of their diagnosis, necessarily deserve any more social interventions than anyone else—served notice that tuberculosis would increasingly be treated as a medical disease that happened to affect the poor and disadvantaged preferentially.

A similar debate arose in the 1940s and 1950s when some commentators called for the abolition of the means test and the liberalization of welfare services to the families of the tuberculous. Policies that promoted financial hardship among the tuberculous, according to one critic, were nothing short of "socio-economic malpractice."[118] Although such comments were inspired in part by the public health threat of tuberculosis, they also reflected the Dubosian belief that ignoring the social factors that predisposed persons to tuberculosis was myopic. Advocating special welfare services for tuberculosis patients, New York City tuberculosis worker George J. Nelbach wrote in 1946: "A clear distinction needs to be made between the kind of public assistance given to tuberculous families and that which is given generally to the poor."[119]

As with vocational rehabilitation, however, the claim that patients with tuberculosis required special social—as opposed to medical—services never became a rallying cry among tuberculosis workers, let alone the general public. As of 1954, the families of only 20 percent of patients with active tuberculosis received public assistance; by 1959 only twelve states had abolished the means test.[120] Similarly, by the end of the 1950s, the new "social" emphasis of the National Tuberculosis Association had sputtered. Sydney Jacobs, the chairman of the Committee on Social Research, reported in 1958 that his committee remained underfunded and understaffed and had received only five grant requests over the previous five years. Although a panel discussion on social research at the 1959 NTA meeting was "generally received favorably," committee members noted ruefully that a "paucity of board members and doctors" attended.[121] Indeed, even a document prepared for the panel discussion, while advocating a comprehensive approach to therapy, noted that it was largely the "oldtimers" who continued to see tuberculosis as a "chronic disease" rather than a curable infection.[122]

Although the 1950s have been accurately characterized as a triumphant decade in the control of tuberculosis, health officials during this era remained acutely aware that social problems continued to predispose persons to tuberculosis and to complicate efforts at treatment. Yet only a minority of commentators, such as René Dubos, believed that a broad attack on social inequities was necessary for successful tuberculosis control. Most tuberculosis workers emphasized the narrower goal of designing strategies that encouraged poor patients to remain hospitalized and to take their antibiotics. Yet just when it seemed that the social aspects of tuberculosis no longer made the disease unique, physicians and health officials in Seattle developed two nationally recognized research protocols that sought to emphasize how social problems interfered with both the prevention and treatment of tuberculosis. The first research program, directed by Thomas Holmes, studied tuberculosis as a "psychosomatic" disease that resulted from stressful events in people' lives; the second program focused on the barriers to the successful treatment of tuberculous Skid Road alcoholics. These efforts are examined in chapters 4 and 5, respectively.

FOUR

Beyond the Germ Theory

Tuberculosis and Psychosomatics

Firland Sanatorium initially hired Thomas Holmes as a psychiatric consultant, responsible for the evaluation of patients' emotional problems. Yet Holmes' major legacy at Firland was a series of research studies that linked both the onset and clinical course of tuberculosis with stressful events in patients' lives.

If René Dubos emphasized the connection of tuberculosis with broad social problems such as poverty and malnutrition, Holmes analyzed the relation of the disease to the psychosocial problems of individual patients. In this manner, Holmes, like Dubos, called into question a strict medical model of tuberculosis. Indeed, Holmes' argument that stress "caused" tuberculosis actually challenged the basic epistemological concepts that underlay traditional notions of disease. Although his ideas never gained a prominent foothold in mainstream medical thought, they nevertheless helped many physicians—particularly those at Firland—to view the disease as more than just a biological entity. Before returning to Firland's efforts to ensure that its patients received appropriate medical therapy, it is worth examining the work of a man whose philosophy made such an approach look exceedingly narrow.

THE HISTORY OF PSYCHOSOMATIC MEDICINE

The idea that the emotions influence health and disease dates back to the days of Hippocrates. In the Hippocratic corpus, patients were characterized by four temperaments: sanguine, phlegmatic, choleric, and melancholic. Based on his or her temperament, a patient was likely to develop specific diseases.[1] The association of the emotions and tuberculosis achieved great popularity during the romantic age of the nineteenth century.[2] For example, the renowned physician René Laennec claimed that consumption was "psychogenic," somehow resulting from emotional disturbances. Others referred to the so-called tubercular diathesis, a combination of physical, environmental, and emotional factors that appeared to predispose certain individuals to the disease.[3] Among the most popular notions was the predilection of tuberculosis for frail, impoverished artists. As Susan Sontag has argued, metaphorical images such as the dying bohemian consumptives in *La Bohème* and *La Traviata* served to validate the purported connection of tuberculosis with an individual's emotional state.[4]

Such constructs of disease fell out of favor in the 1870s and 1880s, when scientists discovered that specific microorganisms caused certain diseases. Thus, when Robert Koch demonstrated that tuberculosis was an infectious disease caused by a particular microorganism, interest in any type of mind-body interaction waned. Yet, the introduction of the Von Pirquet skin test in 1907 revealed that tuberculosis often resulted from the activation of dormant infection. Thus, while prevention of the spread of tuberculosis between individuals remained crucial to control efforts, it was also important to understand why, among persons already infected with tuberculosis, some developed the disease while others did not.

One common explanation for this phenomenon drew on the familiar association of tuberculosis with poor living conditions. Poverty, suboptimal housing, and malnutrition, the argument went, lowered resistance to tuberculosis and thus increased the likelihood that those infected with the bacillus would develop clinical tuberculosis. Conversely, healthful living conditions prevented the activation of dormant disease. This understanding of tuberculosis led René Dubos to call for improved housing and nutrition, which he believed would "increase the resistance of man through a proper way of life."[5]

Yet the traditional concept of mind-body interaction provided another possible explanation for the breakdown of previously dormant areas of tuberculous infection: patients' emotional or psychological problems. The 1920s and 1930s proved to be a fertile time for this approach to disease. A new discipline, ultimately known as psychosomatic medicine, took root in the interwar years, emphasizing the connection of emotional factors to the onset of disease.[6] Historians have concluded that this reemergence of mind-body medicine occurred as a result of the growing prominence of Freudian thought, beginning in the second decade of the twentieth century and continuing through the 1930s, and as a reaction to the increasingly mechanistic orientation of early-twentieth-century scientific medicine.[7]

Scholars have broken down psychosomatic research after 1920 into three schools of thought.[8] While these categories and their major proponents overlap considerably, the scheme is nevertheless useful. The first group, the "dynamic," or psychoanalytical, school, was exemplified by a German émigré psychoanalyst named Franz Alexander. Alexander and his followers explored the connection between specific personality types and diseases such as hypertension, heart disease, peptic ulcer, and ulcerative colitis. Alexander's thinking was heavily influenced by Sigmund Freud, and thus he emphasized the role of childhood conflicts and psychological disturbances in producing physical disease.[9]

The second school of psychosomatic thought was the "mechanismic," or psychophysiological, school, which stressed the impact of emotions on the body's physiological processes. This work drew heavily on the concept of homeostasis, which had been introduced by Claude Bernard in the mid-nineteenth century and subsequently expanded upon by Walter Cannon at Harvard University in the second and third decades of the twentieth century.[10] The theory of homeostasis posited that the body remained in delicate physiological balance by making compensatory adjustments to changes in the environment. The manner in which a given individual's physiology responded to a stressor—which might be either physical or psychosocial—determined whether or not disease would result.[11]

The third trend in psychosomatics was the "organismic," or psychobiological, approach. The major figure in psychobiology was Adolf Meyer, the Swiss-born Johns Hopkins neurologist and psychiatrist. Meyer viewed disease as resulting from a complex combination of biological and psychological forces. He illustrated this interaction by a "life chart," which depicted how disease correlated with important emotional events in a given patient's life.[12] Among those who expanded on Meyer's work were George Draper and Helen Flanders Dunbar, both of whom favored a constitutional or holistic approach that viewed disease as reflecting the constitution and character of the individual patient.[13]

Although research into psychosomatics between 1920 and 1945 emphasized the study of noninfectious diseases, some work was carried out in the area of tuberculosis. Most of this research was of the psychoanalytical type, attempting to identify personality types that might be prone to tuberculosis. For example, Jerome Hartz, a psychiatrist at the Phipps Clinic in Philadelphia, claimed that the disease was caused by episodes of anxiety and conflict in dependent personalities; the English psychiatrist Eric Wittkower identified five types of "premorbid" personalities found among the tuberculous.[14]

In the post–World War II period, research into the psychosomatics of tuberculosis accelerated. One explanation for this phenomenon was the changing priorities of the psychiatric profession. Shifting away from the traditional focus on institutions and psychotic illness, both the newly founded National Institute of Mental Health and the growing social psychiatry movement emphasized the importance of studying sources of emotional stress in the community.[15] Meanwhile, the wartime growth of cities like Seattle led commentators to discuss the potentially deleterious ramifications of "tension" and "modern high-speed living." Articles on the connection of stress and disease increasingly appeared in mainstream publications like *Harper's Magazine*.[16]

Tuberculosis itself was back in the news after 1946 because of the discovery of antibiotics and the subsequent decline in mortality rates. Yet it was the early recognition of the limitations of drug therapy that gave the largest boost to psychosomatics.[17] Once sanatoriums invited in psychiatrists, psychologists, and social workers to address the problems of noncompliance and discharges against medical advice, many of them embarked on formal psychosomatic research projects. The goal of such work was not simply the prevention of irregular discharges but also the opportunity to study tuberculosis in the context of the "entire man," particularly his "intellectual, mental, and spiritual spheres."[18] Thomas Holmes chose to do this by examining the relation of stressful life events to the development of tuberculosis.

THOMAS HOLMES

Thomas Holmes' interest in this area had begun during his years at Cornell University Medical School. Born in North Carolina in 1918, Holmes graduated from medical school in 1943 at the age of twenty-five (figure 4.1). During his residency training in internal medicine at Cornell–New York Hospital, he had undertaken a research project under Harold Wolff, a professor of neurology at Cornell and a major figure in psychosomatic medicine. Holmes formally began to work for Wolff in 1947, having been awarded a Hofheimer Research Fellowship in Psychosomatic Medicine. Holmes remained as a Hofheimer fellow until he accepted a faculty position in the Department of Psychiatry at the University of Washington in 1949.

Wolff had received broad training in neurology, studying with such luminaries as Adolf Meyer at Johns Hopkins, Ivan Pavlov in Russia, and Otto Loewi in Austria. Wolff's earliest accomplishment was the elucidation of the vascular mechanism of migraine headaches, work that demonstrated the interaction of temperament and disease.[19] His subsequent research in psychophysiology, which drew heavily on ideas of Claude Bernard and Walter Cannon, investigated how the body, through the mediation of the neural system, responded to stressful situations. Wolff defined stressors broadly to include both personal events, such as divorce or retirement, and ecological or environmental causes, such as the onset of war or living in a poor neighborhood. The body's physiological responses to stress were "protective" and "adaptive," Wolff concluded, although they could produce disease in certain individuals if present to excess.[20]

During Holmes' fellowship, the two men collaborated on a project that ultimately resulted in a book, entitled *The Nose.* Holmes had conceived of the project based on his own long history of various nasal and allergic symptoms.[21] The research demonstrated how stressful emotional events caused predictable physiological responses in the noses of experimental subjects. For example, anxiety resulting from sexual problems or an "officious"

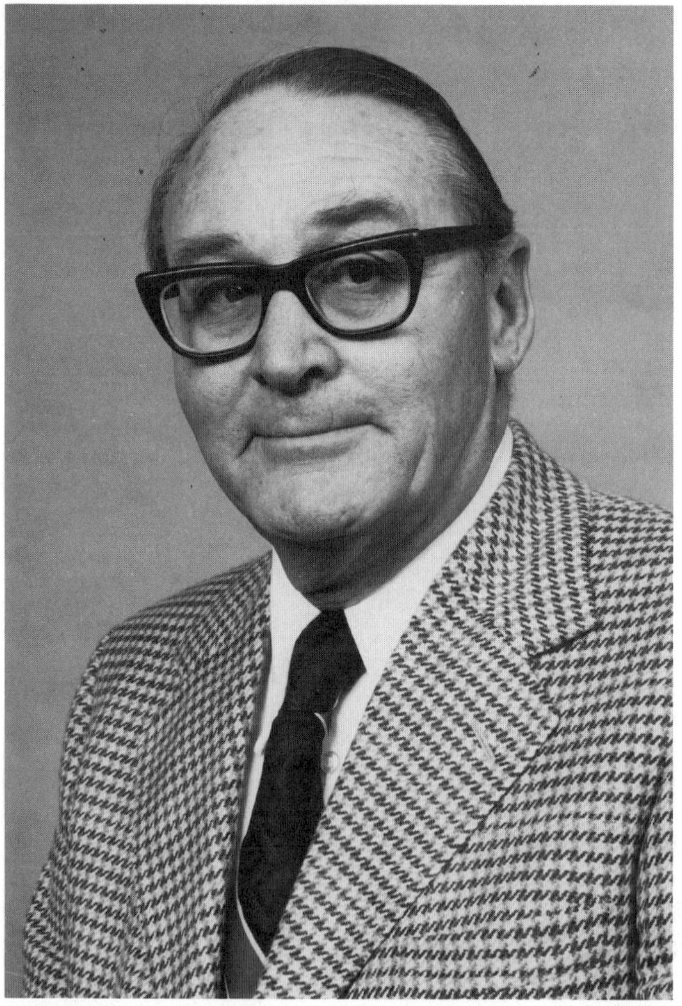

FIGURE 4.1 Thomas H. Holmes, staff psychiatrist, Firland Sanatorium. Courtesy of Marion Amundson.

mother-in-law led to edema of the nasal tissue and to an increase in the number of inflammatory cells present in nasal secretions.[22]

If Wolff and Holmes saw eye to eye on the value of such psychophysiological research, the two men could not have had more different personalities. Wolff was renowned for his punctiliousness, appearing promptly for rounds each morning in a newly starched white coat with a flower in his lapel. Students feared the intense Wolff, and it was said that each year at least one student fainted while presenting a medical case to him. Holmes, in contrast, was quite relaxed, a gentle man who loved to laugh as much as he loved to teach. With both students and colleagues, Holmes was always a provocateur, offering theories that generated a calculated mixture of outrage and intellectual stimulation.[23]

Holmes's distinctive personality became well known shortly after his arrival in Seattle in 1949. Holmes had been offered a faculty position by his Cornell colleague Herbert Ripley, who had just become the head of the Department of Psychiatry at the University of Washington. Holmes had hoped to obtain a joint appointment in psychiatry and internal medicine, but the Department of Medicine did not offer him a position. Holmes' ultimate status—an internist in a department of psychiatry—well symbolized the iconoclastic career path he would pursue in Seattle.[24] Shortly after his arrival in 1949 Holmes began to spend half a day each week as a staff psychiatrist at Firland Sanatorium. Searching for an area of research that would draw on his training with Wolff, Holmes soon decided to use Firland's extensive patient population to study the interaction of stress, resistance, and tuberculosis.

RESEARCH PROJECTS

In his first project, funded by the University of Washington and the U.S. Air Force, Holmes and two colleagues studied how the clinical course of tuberculosis correlated with the excretion of 17-ketosteroids in the urine.[25] Seventeen-ketosteroids were of interest due to the recent work of Hans Selye on the "general adaptation syndrome." Selye, a physician and laboratory researcher at the University of Montreal, had demonstrated how a variety of stressful stimuli produced a standard physiological response in the adrenal glands of experimental animals: the production of a hormone known as glucocorticoid, which was then excreted in the urine as 17-ketosteroids.[26] For researchers in the field, measuring urinary 17-ketosteroids appeared to be a way to quantify the amount of stress someone had experienced.

Holmes and his collaborators studied 109 sanatorium patients in order to understand the relation between 17-ketosteroid levels, the clinical course of tuberculosis, and emotional state. The research team discovered an apparent association between 17-ketosteroids and the extent of tuberculosis (figure 4.2). Persons with normal or high levels of 17-ketosteroids had less severe tuberculosis, and their disease tended to be resolving. In contrast, patients with low 17-ketosteroid excretion tended to have severe exudative tuberculosis and be on the decline clinically. Holmes and his colleagues also examined the emotional state of these patients and found that those with high levels of ketosteroids tended to be anxious and tense, while those with low levels tended to be apathetic or depressed.[27] This latter relationship made sense, given that stress and anxiety caused increased steroid production.

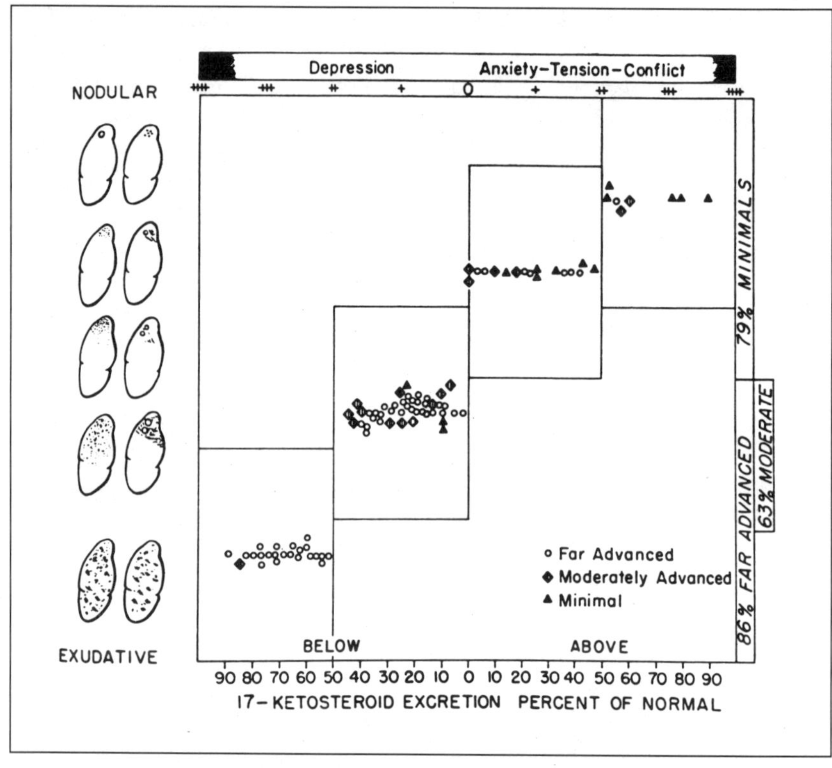

FIGURE 4.2 The relationship of 17-ketosteroid excretion to emotional state and extent and character of disease in pulmonary tuberculosis. Thomas H. Holmes, "Multi-discipline Studies of Tuberculosis," in Phineas J. Sparer, ed., *Personality, Stress, and Tuberculosis* (New York: International Universities Press, 1956), 121, fig. 22.

Holmes and his colleagues drew two major conclusions, although they emphasized that their study was only a "working hypothesis." Because those patients with high 17-ketosteroids were improving clinically, the researchers suggested that this state was "consistent with resistance to tuberculosis." In addition, they inferred that patients' emotional states influenced adrenal gland function and thus the course of the tuberculosis.[28]

The study was flawed in several ways. Like much of the clinical research performed in this era, its uncontrolled and unblinded protocol raised the possibility of numerous types of observer bias. Beyond this, however, was an inherent contradiction. Selye's work had shown that the stress-induced increase in glucocorticoids lowered the levels of immune cells in the blood, thereby promoting the spread of infection. For example, experimental rats normally resistant to tuberculosis became susceptible when exposed to high levels of glucocorticoids.[29] Thus, based on Selye's work, one would have expected that higher levels of 17-ketosteroids would be associated with decreased resistance to tuberculosis and thus more severe disease. Yet in Holmes' study, the patients who fit this category of increased stress and steroid production were the ones who were getting better. Despite this apparent discrepancy, the study was published in 1954 in the prestigious *American Review of Tuberculosis.* The confusion surrounding this issue grew further when the *Seattle Times,* in reviewing Holmes' research, reported that symptoms of fright or anger appeared to be beneficial to tuberculosis patients. At least one Firland patient noted the inherent contradiction between this finding and the standard regimen of bed rest and relaxation.[30]

The 17-ketosteroid study suffered from an additional flaw, one that would continue to plague the work of Holmes and many of his colleagues in the field of psychosomatics:[31] even if one acknowledged that stress was correlated with activation or worsening of tuberculosis, how could one prove that stress or anxiety was the etiology of the medical deterioration? Certainly, one might expect that worsening tuberculosis itself would cause higher levels of stress. The psychosomatics literature often acknowledged this chicken-and-egg dilemma, and later research, by Holmes and others, would try to address this problem by the use of controls and prospective methodology.

In his next series of studies, Holmes supervised the research of Norman Hawkins, a doctoral student in the Department of Sociology at the University of Washington. Hawkins, a World War II veteran, had earned his undergraduate degree at the university in 1949 and had subsequently enrolled in the graduate school. Given his background in sociology, Hawkins' research focused not on physiological mechanisms but rather on the relation between stressful events in patients' lives and the onset of their tuberculosis.

Employing the broad notion of stress favored by Harold Wolff, which included factors such as one's living conditions, Hawkins first examined the ecological characteristics of the 481 Seattle residents diagnosed with tuberculosis in 1952. He found that both the incidence and extent of the disease correlated with where one lived in the city: that is, higher rates of tuberculosis and more severe disease predominated in geographical areas of Seattle that had high percentages of persons who were nonwhite, had lower incomes, and had transient skid row lifestyles. In other words, tuberculosis preferentially affected the "socially marginal."[32]

Yet Hawkins and Holmes were not simply interested in confirming the well-known fact that tuberculosis tended to be a disease of the poor and that such persons tended to have more severe disease. Rather, they wanted to understand why certain persons infected with tuberculosis ultimately developed active disease. The answer, Hawkins postulated, could be found by examining the "emotional and psychological behavior" that resulted from their "social relationships and social interactions."[33]

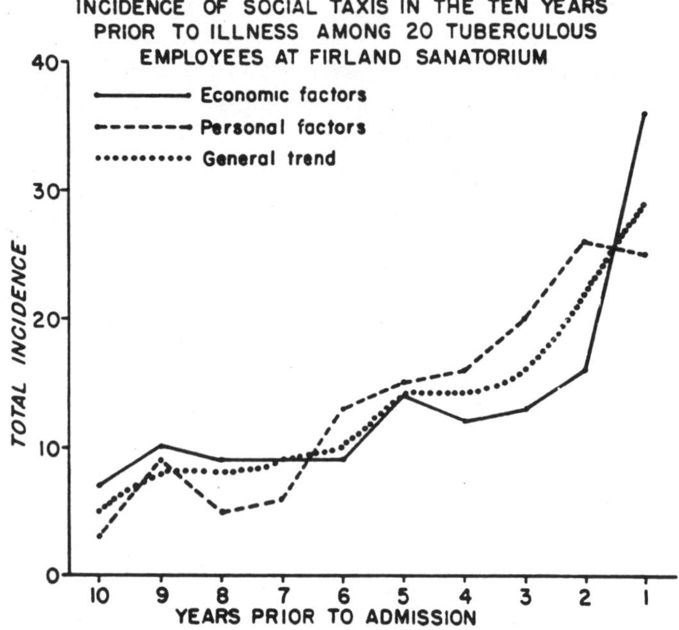

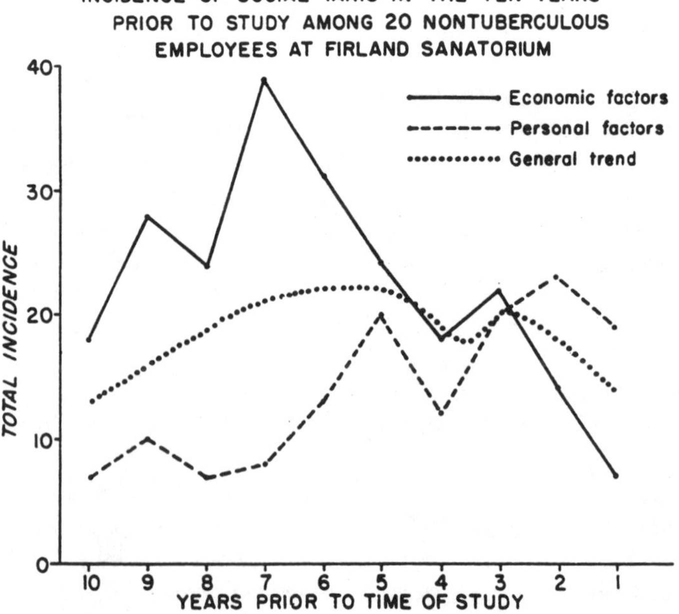

FIGURE 4.3 Social taxis ("disturbing occurrences") among tuberculous employees and control group. Thomas H. Holmes, "Multidiscipline Studies of Tuberculosis," in Phineas J. Sparer, ed., *Personality, Stress, and Tuberculosis* (New York: International Universities Press, 1956), 98, 99, figs. 11 and 10.

Hawkins first tested this theory by conducting interviews with one hundred patients newly admitted to Firland. As this was an exploratory study, no controls were employed. Although the questions covered a broad range of topics, Hawkins gave particular focus to the following subjects: (1) marital break by death, divorce, or separation; (2) irregular sleep or other habits; (3) financial hardship; (4) job dissatisfaction; (5) drug dependence; (6) alcoholism; and (7) disability. Hawkins found very high rates of these problems among the respondents. For example, 71 percent had experienced financial hardship, and 52 percent job dissatisfaction. Thirty-one percent met Hawkins' criteria for alcoholism.[34]

These personal difficulties, Hawkins noted, appeared to cluster in the two years preceding the patient's admission to Firland. This temporal relation, which recalled the life chart of Adolf Meyer, suggested that the "apparently high frequency of disorganizing variables"[35] may have played an etiological role in the activation of the dormant tuberculosis. It was this hypothesis that Hawkins, after adding a control group, subsequently explored.

In this study, which comprised part of Hawkins' doctoral dissertation, he and Holmes compared twenty Firland employees who had become tuberculous between 1949 and 1954 with twenty nontuberculous sanatorium employees matched for multiple variables such as age, sex, race, marital status, income, duration of employment, and, most importantly, the status of their tuberculosis skin test when they began work at the sanatorium.[36] The "previous occurrence of psychosocial stresses" was measured by the use of a form, devised by Hawkins, known as the Schedule of Recent Experience. Examining the same types of variables as in the earlier study, Hawkins and Holmes found that the tuberculous employees reported rising total levels of "disturbing occurrences" during the two years preceding their illness. In contrast, the control subjects, while reporting a high number of such occurrences, demonstrated no such temporal trend (figure 4.3). Moreover, for each of the individual stressors tested, those with tuberculosis were more likely than the controls to have experienced such increases. In the areas of financial hardship, job changes, residential changes, and work stress, the results achieved statistical significance.[37]

As a separate portion of the study, Hawkins and Holmes investigated the psychiatric makeup of their subjects by using the Cornell Medical Index. The index was a questionnaire that measured patients' "level of personal integration" by asking them 195 questions about topics such as the condition of their skin, digestive tract, and nervous system as well as their levels of depression, anxiety, sensitivity, anger, and tension.[38] The results demonstrated that thirteen of the twenty tuberculous persons were "pathologically disturbed" as compared with only five of the nontuberculous individuals. This result was also statistically significant.[39]

In response to the high levels of personality disturbances and the clustering of stressful events among the tuberculous employees, Hawkins and Holmes constructed a scenario that posited an important role for psychosomatic factors in the genesis of tuberculosis. In the first published record of this research, a chapter in a 1956 book entitled *Personality, Stress, and Tuberculosis,* Holmes concluded that since the subjects and controls experienced the same "conditions of infection," it was "reasonable to conclude" that stress determined whether or not an individual developed active disease.[40] By the time Hawkins, Holmes, and Roberts Davies published the study in the *American Review of Tuberculosis and Pulmonary Diseases* the next year, this conclusion had become more tentative. It was "tenable," they wrote, to postulate that psychosocial crisis was one of the precipitant causes of the development of tuberculosis.[41]

This modification may have reflected caution on the part of the *Review*'s editors, but the authors were also well aware of the possible methodological flaws in their work. First, the study was retrospective and thus relied on the ability of the participants to recall stressful events that had occurred months or years in the past. Related to this, Hawkins noted, was the old chicken-and-egg question as to whether stress caused tuberculosis or tuberculosis caused stress. In other words, was it possible that those employees who had become tuberculous had experienced more stressful events because they were developing the disease? Or, alternatively, had the disease process or the "shock of diagnosis" caused them to give the "immediately preceding experiences a heightened emotional tone?"[42]

Holmes' next study attempted to address some of these methodological issues by using a partially prospective design. For this project, James Hart, a University of Washington medical student working under Holmes, looked at sanatorium patients who had "thrown a positive." That is, they had redeveloped positive sputum for *Mycobacterium tuberculosis* after having had negative samples for at least three months. The study, which was conducted in 1957 and 1958, involved twenty-one such patients as well as twenty-four control patients who had not had a recurrence of positive sputum. Once again, efforts were made to find controls who were well matched with respect to both medical and social factors.[43]

Because of the "essential similarity of disease status" and the comparable antibiotic and surgical regimens used within the two groups, Hart concluded that neither the extent of disease nor variations in treatment provided a satisfactory explanation for the conversion to positive sputum. He then compared the "psychosocial histories" of the patients and controls, through the use of interviews, the Cornell Medical Index, and the Suczek and LaForge Interpersonal Check List, an instrument that measured the quantity and type of interpersonal conflicts a subject had experienced.[44]

Hart concluded that those who had developed disease, "when faced with emotional problems and stresses during hospitalization . . . had fewer resources with which to handle problems." This stemmed from their long histories of emotional disturbances, economic problems, unstable lifestyles, and lack of close interpersonal relationships.[45] Because these individuals were less equipped to deal with stressful situations, Hart claimed, their tuberculosis had worsened.

Since this work suffered from the same potentially confounding factors as Hawkins' earlier studies, Hart also added a prospective component. He took a portion of the data from his psychosocial testing and created a new instrument that assigned point totals for various types of emotional disturbances. In September 1957 he analyzed ten of the original control patients and assigned them point scores that reflected their baseline psychological difficulties. Hart predicted that the two patients with particularly high scores would "throw a positive" by September 1958, while the other eight would not. Hart's prediction subsequently came true, as did another prediction that none of the remaining thirteen control patients in the study would undergo sputum conversion.[46]

The final major study in this subject area conducted by Holmes and his colleagues, entitled "Experimental Study of Prognosis," was published in 1961. The researchers employed the Berle Index, an instrument developed by the physician Beatrice B. Berle that identified psychological and social factors characteristic of recovering patients. Thus, a high Berle score suggested that a patient was likely to recover. Not only did the Berle Index look at the patient's perception of issues such as "emotional support from spouse" and "occupational satisfaction," but it also included a psychosocial assessment of the patient by his or her primary physician.

Studying forty-one randomly selected patients, Holmes once again achieved results that confirmed his hypothesis. When twenty-six patients who had achieved medium or high Berle scores (30 to 58) were located five years after testing, none had been classified as "treatment failures." In contrast, five of the fifteen patients with low Berle scores (16 to 28) were considered treatment failures. The researchers carefully acknowledged that factors other than psychosocial adjustment might have contributed to their findings, noting that failure of treatment also was significantly correlated with male sex, old age, presence of nontuberculous illness, alcoholism, and discharge against medical advice (although not with character and extent of disease). Yet in contrast with most researchers conducting epidemiological studies, Holmes was not particularly concerned with teasing out these variables. The research, he and his colleagues concluded, had demonstrated the "interrelationship of the natural history of disease and the physiologic, psychologic, and sociologic disciplines."[47] While few would have disagreed with this statement, it was much less evident that Holmes' decade of work in psychosomatics had proved that stressful events "caused" tuberculosis.

CONTEXTUALIZING HOLMES' RESEARCH

How did the medical community of the 1950s, accustomed to more "scientific" studies of tuberculosis, view a researcher who advanced psychosomatic theories as to the cause of the disease? On the whole, it appears that Holmes succeeded in convincing his peers that his work was important. For example, he was able to attract funding support from sources such as the U.S. Air Force and the National Institute of Mental Health. Holmes or his students made three presentations at annual meetings of the National Tuberculosis Association (NTA) between 1954 and 1959. As noted above, the *American Review of Tuberculosis* published two of Holmes' Firland studies.

Well-respected physicians of the era took Holmes' research quite seriously. The noted New York City tuberculosis specialist Walsh McDermott, for example, maintained an avid interest in Holmes' work. Kerr White, later of the Rockefeller Foundation, characterized a presentation by Holmes at the 1955 NTA meeting as "magnificent."[48] In a recent interview, White recalled Holmes as a "serious fellow doing serious work."[49]

Yet if many commentators included "emotional strain" in their list of contributing causes to tuberculosis,[50] others questioned both Holmes' methodology and his basic claim of a connection between emotions and disease. Reviewing an early version of Hawkins' and Holmes' work, an Air Force lieutenant colonel noted: "It seems that the psychosocial factors evaluated can be either contributing causes of tuberculosis, direct or indirect effects of the tuberculosis, the effect of other factors which may themselves be contributing causes of tuberculosis, and various combinations of these three. . . . In other words, tuberculosis may give rise to social factors which in themselves then influence the course of the disease."[51] Other critics were more tongue-in-cheek. In a 1953 note to Holmes, Emanuel Wolinsky, a friend and basic scientist involved in drug research, asked whether Holmes was "still fooling around with TB." Wolinsky went on to suggest that Holmes "try to make rabbits neurotic and see the effect on their TB by X-ray."[52]

Holmes' reception at Firland Sanatorium was similarly mixed. As a nationally renowned sanatorium in the forefront of the recent medical and surgical advances in the treatment of tuberculosis, Firland was not the most hospitable place for someone like Holmes, whose theories of disease recalled speculations from a more ignorant, less scientific past. As one former colleague of Holmes recalled, it was not uncommon to hear snickering when he made a presentation at the weekly case conferences.[53]

Yet even if some persons believed that Holmes's work was, as one commentator would later say, "the biggest bunch of baloney I ever heard,"[54] it struck an important chord among certain members of the sanatorium staff. Holmes won frequent praise from his colleagues in his role as consultation psychiatrist at the sanatorium. Both Roberts Davies and Daniel W. Zahn, who succeeded Davies as medical director in November 1954, cited theories about the relation of the emotions, personality, and tuberculosis in their writings.[55] Indeed, four internists who were close associates of Holmes at Firland, including Davies, subsequently enrolled in psychiatry residency programs and became psychiatrists.

Holmes also achieved acclaim for his teaching, an activity that consumed much of his time. His responsibilities included both the supervision of students and residents in the Department of Psychiatry and the sponsorship of a broad range of interdisciplinary social sciences research projects among University of Washington students. Holmes also organized lectures and conferences for University of Washington medical students, who, in turn, honored him with several teaching awards.[56] The conferences usually included interviews of patients, many of whom returned annually to meet with students. Holmes used these conferences to demonstrate the importance of an ongoing physician-patient relationship and to highlight how environmental and psychosocial factors contributed to disease. Among the lectures Holmes gave was a discussion of pain, which emphasized the "perception and analysis of sensation and reaction to sensations as well as the setting in which the sensations occur."[57] This broad understanding of pain anticipated many of the subsequent developments in the field.

It was at the weekly Firland case conferences, however, that Holmes, always the performer, made his most vivid impact. After other staff physicians had extensively detailed the patient's medical history, physical exam, and X-ray findings, Holmes would limn a tale of the patient's illness in the context of his or her larger environment. This portion of a presentation regarding a twenty-nine-year-old black female was typical:

> At this point in her life, the man she later married returned from war service to the small town in Louisiana, and after a month of superficial acquaintanceship, they were married. The marital adjustment was always poor. As she phrased it, "My kids come first. I don't drink and I don't smoke. I feel odd when I go out with him; I feel fine if he goes out without me." She spoke of herself as "not a hot-blooded woman" who preferred church activities. Her husband preferred sports and parties. She resented the fact that he was not a good provider and stated, "My father built a good home for my mother. Here we are packed in; I need my own home." The husband chose Seattle as a place to live, and in 1946 they moved here. The choice was on the basis of

his mother's preference. The patient always resented the separation from her family and stated, "I always keep the fare home available."[58]

Holmes then provided his assessment of why this particular woman had become tuberculous: "It was in this setting of unfulfilled dependency needs, and an increasingly strained marital adjustment in a new and unsympathetic environment, that the patient developed pulmonary tuberculosis."[59] Although Holmes' work had grown out of Harold Wolff's emphasis on psychophysiology, much of what Holmes stressed in presentations like these was reminiscent of the holistic, organismic approach to psychosomatic medicine that sought to understand disease in the context of an individual's "life chart." Disease did not simply result from the invasion of bacteria or viruses into the body but rather represented an "adaptation to crisis in one's cultural experience."[60] As Holmes wrote of Firland tuberculosis patients: "These patients, when compared with the cultural norms, were in many ways marginal people at the time of onset of tuberculosis. They started life with an unfavorable social status and grew up in an environment that was for them crippling. They were, in essence, strangers attempting to find a place for themselves in the contemporary American scene."[61]

EPISTEMOLOGICAL ISSUES

What, then, was the relevance of Thomas Holmes' work to the field of tuberculosis in the 1950s? Was Holmes' basic hypothesis regarding tuberculosis—that it was caused by stressful events in the setting of preexisting psychosocial disturbances—a fringe belief of little importance? Or did such a construct actually provide a useful antidote to more reductionist understandings of disease?

Some of Holmes' statements highlight the radical nature of many of his theories. Among his more incendiary assertions were that congestive heart failure had nothing to do with the heart, that antibiotic therapy had not affected the incidence of tuberculosis, and that "germs" did not exist.[62] At first glance, such pointedly outrageous claims about the origin of disease call into question Holmes' credibility. Had he chosen to pursue research in psychosomatic medicine simply because it provided the best forum for a born showman to espouse controversial ideas?

This does not appear to have been the case. Holmes was a notorious provocateur, willing to use such broadsides to challenge his audience. In more sober moments, he readily acknowledged that infection with the tubercle bacillus was a necessary prerequisite for tuberculosis. As Holmes himself suggested, his more outrageous statements were designed to encourage his colleagues to "realize that there is more than one point of view in the science of medicine."[63] In other words, understanding tuberculosis, even in an era of successful antibiotic therapy, required knowledge of social and psychological issues.

Yet Holmes' goal was not simply to foster the consideration of a broader perspective of tuberculosis. Throughout his years at Firland, he was a serious apostle of psychosomatic medicine. For example, Holmes distributed to his students and colleagues a list of roughly twenty diseases along with the fundamental psychological "attitude" that predisposed persons to each disease.[64] Thus, according to Holmes, someone who developed a duodenal ulcer "felt deprived of what is due him, and wants to get even." A diabetic, on the other hand, was "starving in the midst of plenty . . . surrounded by things that have meaning to him but are unavailable." In 1954, Holmes reported that he had "found the answer" for the attitude specific to tuberculosis. Persons who became tuberculous, he claimed, were those who felt "overwhelmed by circumstances . . . despite a valiant effort."[65] The combination of this underlying emotional state and superimposed stressful events, Holmes believed, was much more relevant to understanding who developed tuberculosis than was exposure to the "causative" microorganism. Holmes' work on tuberculosis, his student and later colleague Norman Hawkins concluded, "raise[d] a serious question whether contagion is even an important issue."[66]

Holmes' de-emphasis of the importance of the tubercle bacillus in the spread of tuberculosis was part of a larger epistemological trend in the 1950s that sought to move "beyond the germ theory" in understanding health and disease.[67] Perhaps the most radical proponent of reconceptualizing tuberculosis was Phineas J. Sparer, a professor of psychiatry at the University of Tennessee College of Medicine. Sparer's work expanded on ideas originally suggested in the 1940s and 1950s by Minnesota tuberculosis specialist J. Arthur Myers. Myers had argued that a person with a positive tuberculin test should not be viewed as immune to future disease but rather as a case of tuberculosis that was at risk of reactivating, particularly in the setting of poor living conditions.[68]

In the introductory chapter to *Personality, Stress, and Tuberculosis,* Sparer argued that tuberculosis at the turn of the twentieth century had been epidemic. Its ubiquity resulted from the fact that it was an infectious disease whose spread throughout the entire population was enhanced by poor environmental conditions. A positive tuberculin skin test in this setting was good, signifying immunity. Yet by the 1950s, according to Sparer, tuberculosis had become nonepidemic, limited to small pockets of the community. Agreeing with Myers, Sparer claimed that in the nonepidemic setting, a positive tuberculin test no longer signified protective immunity "but actually disease."[69] Sparer then took Myers' argument one step further. What determined whose skin tests became positive (and thus who was "diseased") in this nonepidemic era, Sparer stated, were psychosomatic factors such as one's personality. "Nonepidemic tuberculosis," he concluded, "is a psychosomatic disease. It is psychophysiologically determined, though still infectious."[70]

In retrospect, Sparer's reasoning seems faulty. One could easily reverse his argument, suggesting that since nearly everyone had a positive skin test in the epidemic era, psychosomatic factors were of particular importance, determining which of these infected persons came down with the disease. In the nonepidemic era, in contrast, infection became the most important factor, since only the small number of individuals exposed to the bacillus could actually develop the disease. Despite these criticisms, it is clear that Sparer had developed a radical new epistemology of tuberculosis, one that stressed the "doctrine of multiple etiology."[71] While Thomas Holmes did not appear to share Sparer's notion of a positive skin test as "disease," he nevertheless agreed with his colleague's attempt to view tuberculosis as considerably more complex than simply a mycobacterial infection.

Although Holmes developed an innovative theory as to why tuberculosis occurred, he offered relatively few recommendations regarding either its prevention or its treatment. This omission is perhaps not surprising if one considers the deep roots of the psychosocial issues identified by Holmes. Addressing these types of problems obviously required a much more intensive effort than simply encouraging people to cough into a handkerchief or to have an annual chest X-ray.

Of course, one potential strategy for reducing stressful events was to advocate social reform measures, such as improved jobs, housing, and nutrition for the poor. As discussed earlier, certain commentators in the early 1950s had once again begun to promote such interventions in order to improve the resistance of persons with dormant tuberculosis. Holmes, however, never openly recommended such major social changes. This decision reflected the fact that Holmes ultimately emphasized the psychological—as opposed to the social—aspects of the "psychosocial" problems he had identified. To paraphrase one of Holmes' students, patients came down with tuberculosis not because of their problems but because of the way they handled their problems.[72]

Not surprisingly, therefore, the preventive and therapeutic suggestions made by Holmes and his students largely addressed psychological and emotional issues. It was essential to educate patients about their "fears, anxieties, and misperceptions," thereby enabling them to anticipate—and adjust to—stressful circumstances.[73] For example, a patient might avoid additional disruptive events during otherwise stressful periods.[74] This emphasis on examining and modifying personal habits through education—rather than altering the living environment—reflected both the triumph of the "new public health" movement and the growing influence of Freudian psychotherapeutics after World War II.[75]

Part of Holmes' reluctance to intervene more directly into the lives of patients may also have reflected the deterministic leanings of some, including Holmes, who explained social problems through "structuralist" or "environmentalist" theories.[76] In 1965, for example, Holmes was taken to task by an audience in his home state of North Carolina for implying that because illegitimacy was endemic among African Americans, it was unnecessary to confront the issue. "Some of us," wrote one correspondent to Holmes, "understood you to say that Negroes have no morals, that illegitimacy is to them a way of life."[77] Although Holmes' comments most likely reflected the racist stereotypes of his southern upbringing, they probably also bespoke a deterministic streak within his philosophical outlook that came close to "blaming the victim."[78]

Holmes remained on the staff of Firland until 1961, at which point he began to drift away from the study of tuberculosis. Given the major impact that antibiotics were having on mortality from tuberculosis, his attempt to promote a psychosocial model of the disease had occurred at an unpropitious time. Yet while Holmes' work never gained broad acceptance in the medical community, he was able to convince a number of colleagues across the country to view tuberculosis from a broader perspective.

During the 1960s and 1970s, Holmes turned his interest to the relation of stressful situations, which he now termed "life events," to disease in general. In conjunction with a student named Richard Rahe, Holmes developed the Social Readjustment Rating Scale, a numerical instrument that predicted the onset of illness based on an individual's recent life events, such as divorce or loss of one's job. The scale, which received acclaim internationally, has served as the cornerstone for modern mind-body research.[79] As a result of this work, Holmes became increasingly associated with the discipline of psychosomatic medicine and even served as the president of the American Psychosomatic Society.

Before Holmes turned his attention away from tuberculosis, however, he became involved in one additional project at Firland: studying the experiences of Skid Road alcoholics at the sanatorium. Most of his work in this area was actually of a supervisory nature. Beginning in the late 1950s, Holmes became a mentor to Joan K. Jackson, a graduate student and later a sociologist who was conducting research on the Skid Road. In one sense, Skid Road alcoholics were the ideal subjects for Holmes to study. If, as he often stated, "sick people have more disease than anybody,"[80] then the sickest patients at Firland Sanatorium were certainly the Skid Road alcoholics. With particularly high rates of medical, social, and psychological disturbances, these individuals caused disciplinary problems at Firland and left the sanatorium against medical advice more often than any other group of patients. The need to ensure compliance among Skid Road alcoholics would remain the major preoccupation of the Firland staff until the institution closed in 1973.

FIVE

Vagrants as Patients

The Skid Road Alcoholic at Firland Sanatorium

The growing interest in the tuberculous alcoholic occurred at a time in which traditional conceptualizations of alcoholism were being questioned. Following the repeal of Prohibition in 1933, both the medical profession and the public had begun to define alcoholism as a medical disease rather than a moral or behavioral weakness. Implicit in this evolving definition was the notion that, in contrast with the traditional stereotype, alcoholism affected all social classes — not only skid row "bums." Yet it was this latter population that caused the most concern among tuberculosis workers in Seattle and across the United States. In an era of declining morbidity and mortality from tuberculosis, skid row alcoholics continued to have high rates of disease and were often noncompliant with therapeutic interventions. The complex social problems of the skid row population reinforced the notion that a strictly medical approach to tuberculosis was unlikely to succeed.

Although the relation between alcoholism and tuberculosis raised concern in many urban areas, the country's most ambitious attempt to address tuberculosis on skid row occurred in Seattle. Given that the city consistently attracted large numbers of transients seeking work on the West Coast,[1] it is not surprising that Seattle tuberculosis workers decided to tackle this problem most directly. By the late 1950s, sociologist Joan K. Jackson and several colleagues in the city had organized a highly praised program of clinical research and rehabilitative services that focused on alcoholic patients at Firland Sanatorium. Eventually, many Firland staff members began to refer to "tuberculosis-alcoholism." By constructing the two conditions as a single condition, they hoped to create a disease entity whose etiology was at once medical and social. That is, in order to understand and treat tuberculosis-alcoholism, caregivers needed to look beyond issues of infection and addiction to factors such as the Skid Road culture, the emotional and psychological problems of its inhabitants, and stereotypes about alcoholics both at the sanatorium and in society more broadly.[2]

The efforts of Jackson and others interested in tuberculosis-alcoholism proved to be far from straightforward. Although they succeeded in demonstrating that the traditional sanatorium regimen for tuberculosis was inadequate for Skid Road alcoholics, their intensive focus on this population inadvertently led to the stereotyping of such people as necessarily "recalcitrant." In addition, the increased interest in alcoholism refocused attention on the familiar question of whether it was essential or even appropriate to treat social problems in a facility designed to cure tuberculosis.

ALCOHOLISM BECOMES MEDICALIZED

If the repeal of Prohibition connoted a growing acceptance of alcohol, public drunkenness remained unacceptable to most Americans in the 1930s and 1940s. The alcoholic actress Frances Farmer, home in Seattle in 1945 after a brief hospitalization in a mental institution, related a confrontation with her mother after Farmer returned, drunk, from a local bar:

> "Where did you get the liquor?" she screamed.
>
> "You're nuts," I screamed back. "You're a crazy goddamned old woman and I don't know what you are talking about."
>
> "Don't you lie to me! The whole neighborhood saw you staggering down the street. Now, where did you get it?"
>
> "I don't know what you are talking about."
>
> She moved quickly across the room and I felt her hand slap hard across my cheek.
>
> "Don't lie to me!" she shrieked and slapped me again.
>
> I put out my hand to ward off another blow.
>
> "You rotten tramp! You filthy whore! Where did you get it?"[3]

Indeed, the repeal of Prohibition hardly had changed the generally hostile manner in which Americans viewed alcoholics. Alcoholism retained its associations with weak-willed, irresponsible, and immoral behavior. Yet the 1930s witnessed renewed debates concerning both the etiology of alcoholism and the proper way to address the problem. "Dry" groups across the country continued to advocate legal measures to limit public accessibility to alcohol, a substance they viewed as an absolute evil. Their opponents, ranging from moderationists to unabashed "wets," agreed that excessive use of alcohol—that is, alcoholism—was the problem, not the liquor itself. Efforts to control alcoholism, according to this construct, needed to focus not on the use of alcohol but on its misuse. By the mid-1940s, this emphasis on alcoholism had triumphed.[4]

Central to the evolving concept of alcoholism was its orientation toward the person drinking the alcohol. Rejecting the traditional moralistic approach that viewed excessive drinkers as sinful, those advocating the new alcoholism portrayed such individuals as sick. That is, alcoholism became reconfigured as a disease, one that, ideally, would be researched and discussed with the same scientific dispassion as diabetes or heart disease.[5] While various commentators defined alcoholism somewhat differently, the fundamental characteristic of the disease was a "loss of control" that the alcoholic was powerless to counteract. Thus, as one researcher wrote: "Alcoholism is generally considered as a sickness characterized (a) by emotional and social maladjustment, (b) by compulsive dependence on alcohol, (c) by drinking which is motivated not by taste sensations or fun or sociability but by the need to enable the drinker to go on facing life, and (d) by resulting damage to the life of the drinker which is obvious to all who perceive him."[6]

The three major organizations that addressed the issue of alcoholism in the 1930s and 1940s adopted this type of definition. The first group was Alcoholics Anonymous (A.A.), a self-help group begun by white-collar, middle-class drinkers in 1935, which recruited alcoholics who had "reached bottom." Through confessional speeches, a "buddy" system, and a twelve-step recovery program, A.A. used an evangelical approach to encourage total abstinence through peer support.[7]

The second organization was the Research Council on Problems of Alcohol, a group of scientists who believed that scientific research into alcoholism would provide objective data to guide preventive efforts. In 1940 the council launched the *Quarterly Journal of Studies on Alcohol*, based at Yale University. Within four years, Yale faculty interested in alcoholism had begun an educational program, the Summer School of Alcohol Studies, and had opened the Yale Plan clinics for the prevention and treatment of alcoholism.[8] The guiding light of what eventually became the Yale Center of Alcohol Studies was Elvin Jellinek, a physiologist who popularized the notion that alcoholism was a medical disease characterized by "phases of inebriety," which culminated in alcohol addiction and loss of control of one's life.[9] Although Jellinek strongly encouraged the medicalization of alcoholism, he and his colleagues at Yale viewed the condition as resulting from a complex interaction of medical, social, and psychological factors, all of which needed to be addressed in order to prevent and treat the disease.[10]

The third group that became involved in alcoholism in the 1940s was a voluntary agency known as the National Council on Alcoholism (NCA). Founded in 1944 by Marty Mann, a recovering alcoholic, the NCA had a three-part statement of purpose: (1) alcoholism is a disease, and the alcoholic is a sick person; (2) the alcoholic can be helped and is worth helping; (3) alcoholism is a public health problem and therefore a public responsibility. Mann, who had also recovered from tuberculosis, consciously used the model of the National Tuberculosis Association (NTA) in structuring the NCA's educational and preventive efforts.[11]

Recent scholarship has convincingly demonstrated that the concept of alcoholism as a medical disease was not invented in the 1930s and 1940s but dated back at least as far as the late eighteenth century. In addition, commentators such as Harry G. Levine and Robin Room have argued that the medicalization of alcoholism was a social construct particular to a capitalist society worried about "loss of control."[12] Alcoholism historian Ronald Roizen has also shown how the decision by the Research Council on Problems of Alcohol to pursue research on alcoholism resulted more from financial than from purely "scientific" factors.[13]

Nevertheless, it is clear that the general public during the 1940s increasingly viewed alcoholism as a medical condition. A 1947 survey reported that 36 percent of adults thought alcoholism was a disease, up from only 6 percent in 1943. The medical community also responded, albeit slowly. In 1956 the American Medical Association passed a resolution urging general hospitals to admit patients with the "disease" of alcoholism.[14] The American Hospital Association issued a similar statement in 1957.

As alcoholism was transformed from a sin to a medical condition, commentators also began to define it as a public health issue. While the secrecy that shrouded alcoholism made estimates of its prevalence difficult, sources in the 1950s estimated that there were between 4.5 and 5 million alcoholics in the United States, a figure that represented roughly 5 percent of the adult population. As early as 1944, the U.S. Public Health Service labeled alcoholism the country's fourth largest public health problem.[15] In 1948 the *Health Commentator* of the Washington State Department of Health noted that "alcoholism is becoming a larger public health problem than venereal disease, and the alcoholic is less understood, more incapacitated, and has less opportunity for treatment."[16]

As had been the case since the frontier era, Seattle citizens were concerned about the amount of drinking that took place in the city. A walk through the Skid Road on any afternoon seemed to provide ample proof that alcoholism was rampant in Seattle. Available statistics, moreover, corroborated this perception. The estimated rate of alcoholism in Seattle in the mid-1950s, one of every twelve adults, was considerably higher than the national average of one of every twenty-one adults. By the end of the decade, moreover, the Washington state Health Department reported that Seattle had the "dubious distinction" of having the highest death rate for male alcoholics of any large city in the nation.[17]

Such figures, in part, reflected Seattle's location on the West Coast. Both during and after World War II, the rapidly industrializing West had served as a magnet for men and women looking for jobs either in the aircraft, shipbuilding, or logging industries or on railroads or farms. Many of these individuals were rootless and transient and settled in the various skid rows located in towns along the West Coast. Rates of alcoholism were often high among this population. Indeed, University of Washington sociologist Calvin F. Schmid claimed that it was the migration of "winos" to Seattle and other cities that had caused much of the 88 percent rise in alcoholism in Washington state between 1940 to 1955.[18] Yet if many western cities housed large numbers of transient alcoholics, Seattle, according to Joan Jackson, was "somewhat unique." The city was often the final destination for migrant alcoholics who populated the West Coast: "Perhaps, after several moves, [the alcoholic] lands in Seattle. There is no place else to go. Some may go to Alaska, where they realize they are hopeless. So they come back to Seattle, where there are more agencies to help them and the climate is milder."[19]

Jackson and others who became involved in the study of alcoholism in the 1950s were careful to stress that alcoholism was pervasive among all social classes. The Skid Road population, she estimated, comprised perhaps 10 percent of all alcoholics in Seattle. Nevertheless, it was the common perception of Seattle as the repository of West Coast Skid Road alcoholics that led to such great scrutiny of this population by city officials. As Jackson and others in Seattle began to devote increasing study to the "unholy alliance" between alcoholism and tuberculosis,[20] it is not surprising that they too chose to focus on the Skid Road.

Jackson's interest in this area came about largely through chance. A native Canadian, she had studied sociology and anthropology at McGill University in Montreal before enrolling in the graduate sociology program at the University of Washington in 1951 (figure 5.1). Jackson initially hoped to research mental illness but soon found herself sidetracked into the area of alcoholism. When beginning work on her dissertation, she had obtained funding, through Washington state's Initiative 171, to work on a Department of Psychiatry project looking at alcoholism at the Seattle Veterans' Administration Hospital. Ultimately, Jackson was hired by the department to continue her alcoholism research. Although she had initially collaborated with other physicians in the Department of Psychiatry, Jackson soon began to work with Thomas Holmes. Holmes was pleased to mentor the bright young sociologist whose interest in the behavioral aspects of alcoholism seemed an excellent match for his own research pursuits.

There was some precedent for Jackson's studies of the Skid Road population. In the early 1940s, the Seattle Police Department was averaging roughly thirty thousand arrests annually for public drunkenness. Noting that "recurrent arrests and jailings are of no avail in controlling the problem or in helping the alcoholic to recover," the department had opened a Rehabilitation Project for chronic alcoholics in 1948.[21] While the project, colloquially known as the "police farm," had been established for the purpose of reha-

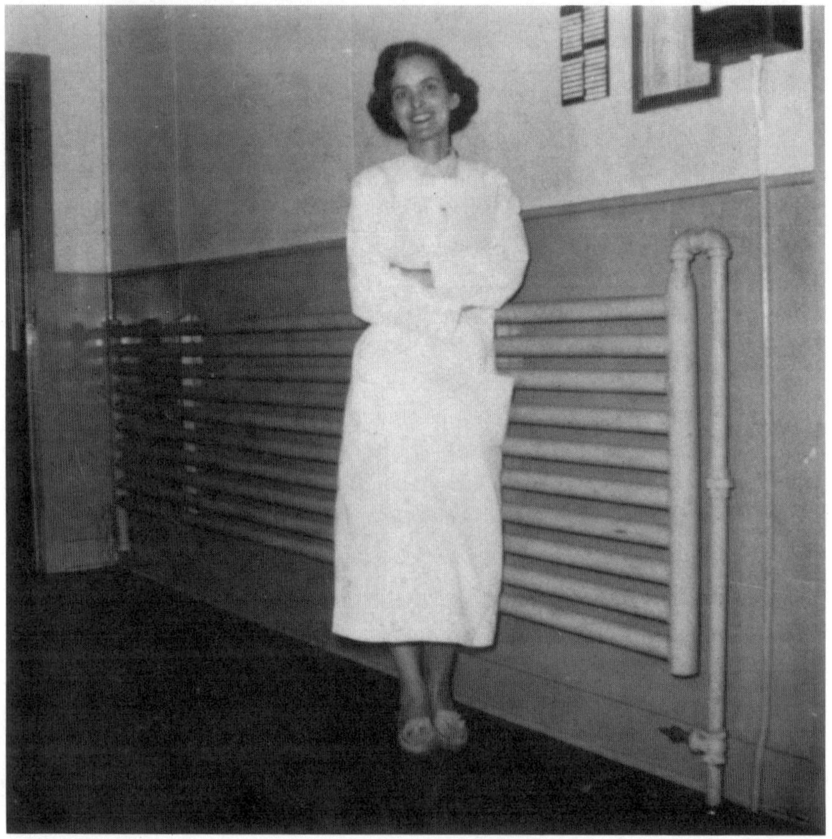

FIGURE 5.1 Joan K. Jackson, medical sociologist, Firland Sanatorium. Courtesy of Joan and Stanley Jackson.

bilitation rather than research, it was, nevertheless, another example of the attention that Skid Road alcoholics received from city officials in Seattle.

Jackson's first project, in which she collaborated with a fellow graduate student, Ralph Connor, was entitled "The Skid Road Alcoholic." In this paper, published by *Quarterly Journal of Studies on Alcohol* in 1953, Jackson and Connor used interviews with Skid Road alcoholics to gain "insight into the motivations and behavior of this type of alcoholic."[22] The findings of the study formed the basis for much of Jackson's later work. To understand the Skid Road alcoholic, the authors concluded, it was essential to understand the Skid Road culture, whose norms had little in common with those of the rest of society. Despite the apparent disorder perceived by the casual observer, the Skid Road was not without its structure. "Group definitions of behavior," wrote Jackson and Connor, provided an informal framework that guided the lives of many Skid Road inhabitants. Various rituals, for example, determined how liquor was to be shared, when and where panhandling was acceptable, and how one should respond to offers of assistance from mission workers and other community agencies. Yet even as they described the "typical" Skid Road alcoholic, the authors also discouraged the use of stereotypes. Not only did many nonalcoholics live on the Skid Road, they noted, but alcoholics themselves could be subdivided into distinctive groups such as "bums," "winos," and "lushes."[23]

Jackson and Connor also spent a good deal of time describing the rehabilitation options available to alcoholics. Although the structured existence the researchers had uncovered on the Skid Road suggested a fierce sense of independence among alcoholics, this was an "illusion." The Skid Road alcoholic, Jackson and Connor argued, had strong "dependency needs," a fact that became evident in settings, such as hospitals, away from the Skid Road. Yet the authors remained optimistic about the ability of Alcoholics Anonymous, which had extended its original focus to include the prototypical "down-and-out" drunk, to rehabilitate Skid Road alcoholics. A.A. was potentially effective, they wrote, "because it manipulates patterns of behavior [the alcoholic] already possesses toward a new end, sobriety."[24]

Because nonwhites made up only 6 percent of Seattle's population in 1950, Jackson and Connor's subjects were, for the most part, white men. Yet even in cities whose poor sections housed relatively high percentages of blacks, Asians, and Native Americans, social scientists researching alcoholism and skid row generally focused on whites. If minorities were often excluded from such studies, so too were women. Well into the 1950s, alcoholism among women, even among women living on skid row, was ignored.[25]

Jackson and Connor's research was hardly the first study to examine migrant urban workers. Numerous sociological works published earlier in the century, such as Alice W. Solenberger's *One Thousand Homeless Men* and Nels Anderson's *The Hobo,* had described the lives of itinerant and homeless men in various cities across the country. Popular writers in the post–World War II era often romanticized the hobo, citing both the freedom of his lifestyle and his constant search for honest work.[26] Yet the characteristics of those persons who populated the run-down portions of cities like Seattle had changed since the turn of the century. Howard M. Bahr has written that skid rows after the depression housed fewer migratory casual workers and more of the permanently unemployed, many of whom were acquiescent and apolitical. The condition of skid rows had also deteriorated. Seattle's Skid Road, for example, no longer included portions of the city's respectable business district but rather was restricted to the "smelly 'hash house,' the pawn shop, the second-hand stores . . . , the cheap hotel, and the dingy beer parlor."[27]

Jackson and Connor's work was important not only because it examined this changing skid row but also because it embodied the new perception that skid row alcoholics had a disease. Jackson quickly became well known in Skid Road settings like Pioneer Square, ultimately earning the moniker of the "alcoholic lady" from the area's denizens. Yet when she returned her attention to Seattle's Skid Road alcoholics, her studies occurred at a venue—Firland Sanatorium—located some distance from their usual habitat.

THE SKID ROAD ALCOHOLIC AT FIRLAND

The long relationship that existed between alcoholism and the skid row also existed between alcoholism and tuberculosis. Yet the exact connection between the two conditions was often unclear. For example, alcohol had once been used as a therapy for tuberculosis. In the mid-nineteenth century, for instance, New York physician Austin Flint had "dispatched some of his [tuberculosis] patients to the mountains with their trunks filled with alcohol."[28] Although some physicians at the turn of the century continued to use liquor as a "stimulant" for the tuberculous, by the turn of the century alcoholism was increasingly viewed as "the most active cooperator of the deadly tubercle bacillus."[29] "It was formerly thought," William Osler wrote, "that alcohol was in some way antagonistic to tuberculous disease, but observations of late years indicate that the reverse is the case and that chronic drinkers are more liable both to acute and pulmonary tuberculosis."[30]

As of the mid-1950s, few health officials disputed the role that alcoholism played in producing high rates of tuberculosis—especially in skid row areas. Among one representative group, homeless men in Minneapolis, roughly 70 percent of whom were alcoholics, the incidence of tuberculosis was fifty-five times higher than that of the general population.[31] Not surprisingly, the association of tuberculosis and the skid row received particular attention in the West. For example, while his estimate was almost certainly too high, the West Coast representative of the National Council on Alcoholism claimed that 70 percent of all tuberculosis patients in the region were alcoholics. Data from Seattle told a similar story. Of 510 jailed alcoholics X-rayed in the city in 1951, 88, or 17 percent, had active tuberculosis. Reviewing these statistics, Cedric Northrop concluded that "the chronic alcoholic who drifts from his regular environment and tries to find obscurity on skid row is particularly prone to tuberculosis."[32] Throughout the 1950s and 1960s, tuberculosis control programs in Seattle and elsewhere placed a strong emphasis on screening skid row alcoholic populations.[33]

Although physicians may have agreed that the overuse of alcohol predisposed people to tuberculosis, the mechanism by which this occurred remained unclear. Some believed that alcohol itself was toxic, but others countered that it produced baleful effects because those who drank had "poor dwellings and bad nourishment."[34] Such an etiologic puzzle was a natural for Thomas Holmes. When Joan Jackson had completed her initial work on Skid Road alcoholics, Holmes suggested that she continue her research at Firland Sanatorium. Firland offered several advantages. First, Holmes and Hawkins had already begun to examine the link between stress, living conditions, and tuberculosis among patients at the sanatorium. Second, because Firland housed a large number of Skid Road alcoholics for relatively long periods of time, it could facilitate research being carried out on an extremely mobile population. Finally, Dike's and Hadaway's studies of irregular discharges at Firland had singled out as a particular problem those patients, mostly males, whom doctors had labeled as alcoholic. For example, 74 percent of the men in Hadaway's study had alcoholism listed as "part of their medical diagnosis." The authors had employed loose definitions of alcoholism. According to Dike, alcoholics were patients who displayed "evidence of an unusual amount of alcohol consumption ranging from excessive drinking to diagnosed alcoholism."[35]

Of greater concern than the actual percentage of alcoholic patients who left against medical advice was the impact of such discharges on both the patients and the community. Two findings in Dike's study had been most worrisome. She had found that 55 percent of irregularly discharged alcoholic patients had sputum positive for *Mycobacterium tuberculosis*, compared with only 32 percent of nonalcoholics. In addition, Dike discovered that it was exceedingly difficult to follow up alcoholics after discharge. While forty-eight (80 percent) of the sixty nonalcoholics could be found at their specified addresses, this was true for only six (18 percent) of the thirty-four alcoholics. The remaining alcoholic patients had either been admitted to jail or a mental institution, had been readmitted to Firland, or had died. Eleven (32 percent) of the thirty-four had altogether disappeared.[36]

The implication of these findings to the Firland staff was clear. If irregularly discharged patients were "very likely to be readmitted later with more disease" and apt to "infect others with their disease" prior to readmission,[37] these concerns applied most dramatically to alcoholics. Accordingly, ensuring compliance with both inpatient and outpatient antibiotic therapy was particularly crucial for alcoholic patients.

To be sure, at the beginning of the 1950s, there were few data to prove this assertion. Firland had just begun to prescribe antibiotics, and it was not until the introduction of isoniazid in 1952 that outpatient drug treatment became routine. Moreover, as noted earlier, the sanatorium had only recently begun to aggressively hospitalize and treat Seattle's tuberculous alcoholics, many of whom had been refused admission during the Robert Stith era.

Nevertheless, since Firland had recently begun to expand its programs of psychological counseling, social services, and vocational rehabilitation in order to decrease the rate of irregular discharges, organizing specific strategies for the alcoholic population at the sanatorium seemed entirely logical. Ultimately, Firland staff went further, articulating an entity they termed "tuberculosis-alcoholism." By constructing the problem of tuberculosis among alcoholics as a specific "disease" in its own right, they sought to emphasize the unique social and psychological issues that continually confounded therapeutic efforts in this population. Joan Jackson had high hopes for this new emphasis on tuberculosis-alcoholism. "We believe," she wrote in 1957, "that the more we come to understand the alcoholic tuberculous patient and the staff's interaction with him, the fewer management problems we will have and, consequently, shorter hospitalizations, fewer irregular discharges, and fewer readmissions."[38]

The availability of funding greatly facilitated Jackson's research at Firland. Taking advantage of the growing interest in both alcoholism and behaviorism, Holmes, Jackson, and their colleagues were able to obtain substantial funding support from agencies as diverse as the National Institute of Mental Health (NIMH), the U.S. Public Health Service, the Boeing Research Fund, and, as noted above, Washington State. By 1962, researchers at Firland had produced fifty-one publications and manuscripts "pertaining to treatment for tuberculosis-alcoholism."[39]

Jackson was not the first researcher to study the Skid Road patient at Firland. When she arrived at the sanatorium in 1953, Norman Hawkins had already undertaken an investigation of the medical charts of 153 patients admitted to Firland from twelve Skid Road flophouses. Hawkins chose to omit from his study the two female admissions, although he included twenty-three nonwhites, including ten Native Americans and seven African Americans. The data revealed the typical characteristics of a skid row population: the mean age was 56.5 years; 149 (97 percent) of the men were unattached—single, separated, divorced, or widowed; 120 (77 percent) were either unskilled or semiskilled laborers; 119 (77 percent) were natives of the United States, although only 12 had been born in Washington state; and 67 (43 percent) had been referred from jail. Most notably, Hawkins found that physicians had classified 72 (47 percent) of the men as alcoholics.[40]

What was unclear from Hawkins' work was how the diagnosis of alcoholism had been assigned. Although the condition was now technically a "disease," physicians at Firland had little or no experience with making a formal diagnosis of alcoholism. Therefore, Jackson began her research at the sanatorium by employing a new diagnostic instrument to study alcoholism among newly admitted patients. She administered the Jellinek Drinking Questionnaire, which had been developed by the Yale specialist, to one hundred white male patients aged twenty-five to fifty-five who lived in one of five Skid Road census tracts. She supplemented the questionnaire with interviews.[41] The following case study, which was typical, bore more than a passing resemblance to the presentations of Jackson's mentor, Thomas Holmes:

> The patient involved was a tiny man of about 55. He had been a Skid Road alcoholic from the age of 19. He had lost his mother at age 2 and his father at age 4. His brother had been killed when he was 11. His childhood was spent in an orphanage, which he left at 12 when he was sent to live with a farmer who wanted cheap and pliable labor. He ran away from the farmer at 15. From that time onward he never remained in the same place for more than two or three months at a time, unless he was in jail. He never had a close friend. Of the last three years before he came into the hospital, he had been in jail steadily for two years. The last year had been spent in a mission, trying to remain sober. . . . He entered the hospital from the City Jail having been arrested for drunkenness.[42]

Jackson discovered, to her surprise, that the staff generally underestimated the amount of alcoholism among Skid Road patients. In contrast to Hawkins' estimate of 47 percent, she found that eighty-five of these hundred patients "were alcoholics at the time of admission or had a history of alcoholism in the past."[43] This statistic suggested that roughly 40 percent of all adult male patients at the sanatorium were alcoholics, a figure that corresponded with estimates made at other municipal sanatoriums across the country.[44]

Jackson next turned to the issue of stress, examining the "illness chains" and "social adjustment" of Skid Road tuberculous alcoholics. In findings consistent with those of Hawkins and Holmes, she concluded that such persons became tuberculous "in a setting of extreme social disarticulation and interpersonal isolation,"[45] often exacerbated, curiously, by recent attempts to stop drinking and renounce the Skid Road lifestyle. In addition, Jackson found that alcoholic patients with more advanced tuberculosis on admission tended to be "solitary and belligerent drinkers" with the most evidence of psychological disturbance. These findings, Jackson noted, supported Holmes' theories on the relationship of emotional stress and the onset of tuberculosis.[46]

Yet these patterns were limited neither to Skid Road alcoholics nor to tuberculosis. When Jackson next studied a group of middle-class alcoholics at Firland, she also found an association of antecedent "personal disequilibrium" with the development of tuberculosis. But what proved most interesting to Jackson was the reaction of Firland physicians and nurses to their middle-class alcoholic patients—or, rather, their lack of reaction. "The middle-class alcoholic," she wrote, "is not usually defined as an alcoholic by the staff."[47] This occurred, Jackson believed, because staff members, who largely came from the same social class as the middle-class alcoholic, were "handicapped in their evaluation of his illness by his similarities to them."[48] Thus, although Seattle was home to the Shadel Sanitarium, one of the foremost hospitals in the country for the aversion treatment of middle-class alcoholics, the public still believed that excessive drinking did not occur in this population.[49]

Jackson's studies of middle-class alcoholics at Firland led her to reevaluate her research protocol. While she had originally emphasized the collection of "objective" data about the past lives of tuberculous alcoholics, she now turned to an examination of the staff-patient interactions that occurred during the actual period of hospitalization. Jackson found that just as preconceived cultural assumptions precluded the staff from making the diagnosis of alcoholism among middle-class patients, stereotypes about Skid Roaders determined whether or not such persons were characterized as alcoholic.

In short, Jackson argued, Firland staff generally gave the diagnosis of alcoholism to those patients who caused management or compliance problems at the sanatorium. "If the patients were misbehaving," she wrote, "it was because they were alcoholics."[50] "It is unfortunate," Jackson later commented, "that the awareness of the problem of alcoholism as a complication in the treatment of tuberculosis arose from the study of 'recalcitrant' patients. Partly as a result of the origins of our concerns, 'alcoholic' and 'recalcitrant' have come to be used as synonyms."[51] Thus, she concluded, the diagnosis of "alcoholism" not only was limited to the Skid Road population but continued to carry its familiar stigma.

If Firland staff were guilty of conflating misbehavior and alcoholism during the period of hospitalization, they did give patients the benefit of the doubt at the time of admission. A review of charts reveals that physicians often withheld the diagnosis of alcoholism from Skid Road patients unless the patients volunteered suggestive information. Once a patient was caught drinking in the sanatorium, however, the doctors generally added the diagnosis of "chronic alcoholism" to the patient's chart.

There was an important corollary to Jackson's findings. If staff members diagnosed alcoholism only in "problem patients," they were disregarding the issue among other Skid Roaders who had not caused disturbances at the sanatorium. Such a response was hardly surprising. Despite the increased calls for a medicalized approach to alcoholism, Firland was first and foremost a tuberculosis sanatorium. "When the alcoholic tuberculosis patient is admitted to the sanatorium," Jackson wrote, "the major concern of the staff is with his tuberculosis. . . . It is assumed that as long as he is not drinking, he is not suffering from alcoholism."[52]

Yet, she argued, it was myopic to ignore how the preexisting culture of Skid Road alcoholics necessarily made their adjustment to sanatorium routine more problematic. Drawing on her earlier work, Jackson stressed the importance of the "illusion of independence and self-sufficiency" on the Skid Road. It was alcohol, moreover, that served as "the basis for membership in a well-integrated sub-society which has its own way of life, its own values, its own view of the world and of the individual's place in it."[53]

Admission to Firland, Jackson claimed, was thus traumatic for Skid Road alcoholics in two ways. First, by restricting mobility and encouraging dependence, hospitalization threatened their usual "adaptive techniques." Second, by ignoring the crucial role that alcohol played in these people's lives, the staff actually promoted recidivism. Although most Skid Road alcoholics abstained from alcohol during the early portion of their stay, the sanatorium was full of both Skid Road denizens and the liquor they managed to smuggle onto the premises. Once the sober alcoholics reestablished relationships with their former cronies, many simply resumed their old pattern of drinking. This, in turn, led to increasing conflicts with the staff and, as we shall see, internment on the locked ward.[54] The final outcome, Jackson concluded, was that alcoholics, having reasserted their independence and rejoined their traditional cultural group, became more likely to leave the sanatorium against advice. This occurred with the Skid Road patient described earlier:

> His one point of pride and self-respect revolved around his health and his ability to work and be self-supporting. His illness left him feeling frightened and helpless. . . . The idea of a lengthy hospitalization mobilized fears about being confined, and reactivated feelings engendered during his long jail experiences. . . . On admission he was a veritable volcano. The staff speedily became impatient with him. . . . The more sterness [*sic*] brought to bear, the higher he blew, calling them policemen, not nurses, etc.[55]

Further miscommunication and tensions between this patient and the staff ensued, Jackson explained, culminating when he left the sanatorium without permission and got drunk.

Once again using language reminiscent of Thomas Holmes, Jackson analogized Skid Road alcoholics admitted to Firland to immigrants who "find themselves in a land among people whose ways are different than theirs."[56] Because it focused only on tuberculosis and ignored alcoholism and its derivative problems, the sanatorium viewed its "immigrant" population too narrowly. This conclusion, however, was not intended to exonerate Firland's Skid Road alcoholics from any responsibility for this situation. Too often, as a group of Jackson's colleagues noted, such individuals fostered an "anti-hospital, anti-treatment sub-culture within the institution." In addition, many of the patients indicated that they were not interested in any form of alcoholism treatment, occupational therapy, or vocational rehabilitation while in the sanatorium.[57] After all, as Elmer Bendiner wrote in his 1961 book, *The Bowery Man,* many men had specifically gravitated to run-down urban areas like Seattle's Skid Road in search of "the sweet delights of hopelessness" and "a place where no one requires anything of them."[58]

RECTIFYING THE SITUATION

What could Firland do to address the situation of the Skid Road alcoholic? The first step, Jackson believed, was to regard alcoholism "as any other illness." Just as the staff treated diabetes in a diabetic, treatment of alcoholism had to begin "at the same time as treatment for tuberculosis and parallel it throughout the hospital stay."[59] Whether or not there was evidence of active drinking did not matter.

Implementation of such an intervention, wrote Jackson and Firland physician Emily B. Fergus in the *American Review of Tuberculosis and Pulmonary Diseases,* required staff members "to equip themselves with considerably greater knowledge about alcoholism and about the agencies experienced in treating alcoholism."[60] Accordingly, Jackson made staff education one of her primary goals at Firland. Working with Thomas Holmes and Norman Hawkins, Jackson gave formal presentations to groups at the sanatorium and held informal discussions with individual staff members. In these venues, she informed her colleagues about her research findings and taught them how to anticipate—and thus prevent—conflicts with alcoholics. On the locked ward itself, Jackson encouraged the use of "milieu" therapy, which was designed to make the ward a conducive environment for the treatment of alcoholism.[61] Essential to the establishment of a successful milieu was the provision of emotional support, particularly to nurses, whose years of contact with Skid Road denizens had engendered significant frustration and, at times, outright hostility. Reminding Firland staff members how tuberculosis patients were stigmatized at the turn of the century, Jackson urged her co-workers not to do the same to tuberculous alcoholics in the 1950s.

Assistance from sympathetic University of Washington and Firland colleagues greatly aided Jackson's efforts. For example, Edith Heinemann, a University of Washington nursing educator, urged student nurses working at the sanatorium to adopt a tolerant attitude toward alcoholic patients. Medical students at the university received formal instruction in alcoholism and in later years participated in A.A. meetings and "alcoholism tours" of the Skid Road.[62] Several of the nurses, who as a group spent much more time with the Skid Roaders than did physicians, developed close relationships with their patients and specifically asked to work on the locked ward. A few Firland physicians, such as Fergus, Archibald Ruprecht, and Marcelle Dunning, took a special interest in alcoholism; Dunning held group therapy sessions for Skid Road patients on her ward. Most helpful, however, was the encouragement provided by Thomas F. Sheehy Jr., who became medical director at Firland in 1956 after Daniel Zahn unexpectedly suffered a fatal heart attack. Sheehy, a Temple University Medical School graduate who had served in Korea, had trained in chest medicine in Detroit prior to joining the

Firland staff in 1950.[63] Perceiving the issue of alcoholism to be central to the control of tuberculosis, he was extremely supportive of the efforts of Jackson, Holmes, and Hawkins.

Although Jackson encouraged physicians and nurses at Firland to identify and begin treatment of alcoholism at the time of admission, she warned against the expectation of immediate results. Skid Road alcoholics, she explained, had often been drinking for more than twenty years. Several months of sobriety in a supportive setting was not likely to cure their alcoholism. Rather, the proper goal of the sanatorium stay was "building the necessary foundations for ultimate recovery."[64]

Central to such a strategy, Jackson argued, was encouraging patients to join Alcoholics Anonymous. An A.A. chapter at Firland had actually been founded in 1950, but it was not until the mid-1950s that the group achieved wide attention at the sanatorium. Numerous articles, written either by outside A.A. members like "Francis from Worcester" or by Firland participants, began appearing in the patients' magazine, which had been renamed *Firland Magazine* in 1955. These pieces urged alcoholic patients to acknowledge their drinking problem and to attend the weekly sanatorium A.A. meeting.[65] The importance of A.A. was also emphasized by Norman Hawkins, whom Firland hired in 1956 as a sociologic consultant and a special counselor for alcoholic patients. Indeed, by the end of the decade, the issue of alcoholism had gained great prominence in the hallways and corridors of the sanatorium. The pages of *Firland* contained many articles, written by Sheehy and others, on the interaction of tuberculosis and alcoholism. It should be noted that Firland—in contrast with other facilities involved in the treatment of alcoholism—did not emphasize the use of either sedatives or disulfiram therapy.[66]

Jackson's work with Skid Road alcoholic patients at Firland earned numerous plaudits. Documents from the National Tuberculosis Association termed her research "bold" and "the most significant of its kind in the country."[67] Jackson delivered talks on tuberculosis-alcoholism to groups across the United States and was appointed to numerous local and national organizations interested in the two diseases. In turn, tuberculosis officials across the country emulated Seattle's efforts, establishing or expanding screening and treatment programs that specifically focused on skid row populations.[68]

Although Jackson's work stressed the period of hospitalization, she was careful not to ignore the discharged tuberculous Skid Road alcoholic. After all, if recovery from alcoholism was to be a gradual process, it was necessary to continue "treatment" in the postsanatorium period. Following discharge, former patients who had attended A.A. meetings at Firland often joined one of the many chapters of the organization that had formed in Seattle by the late 1950s. Yet while A.A. offered the best chance at "curing" skid row alcoholics, Jackson and others also believed that public health agencies in the city had a responsibility to establish facilities to encourage both the prevention and treatment of alcoholism.

As evidenced by the police farm, the country's first college-level seminar on alcoholism, and the establishment of the Studio Club, a halfway house for women alcoholics, there was a great deal of interest in alcoholism in postwar Seattle.[69] Yet both voluntary and government agencies in the city and in the state of Washington proved slow to organize. Not until 1958 did the local chapter of the National Council on Alcoholism, with the assistance of a donation from the Boeing Employees' United Good Neighbor Fund, open an information and referral center in downtown Seattle.[70] As of 1956, Washington was one of only sixteen states that had not established an official program either to study the issue of alcoholism or to provide educational or rehabilitative services to the community. While the state Department of Health finally opened an alcoholism clinic in Seattle in 1959, the Seattle–King County Health Department did not become formally involved until 1963, when it assumed control of the state clinic.[71]

Seattle's traditionally ambivalent attitude toward its Skid Road population accounted for the slow response of its official agencies. As Norman Clark has argued, the city's old "antisaloon" mentality lingered well after alcoholism became an acceptable topic of discussion and regulations on selling liquor were liberalized. The most common public reaction to drunkenness, according to a 1951 poll conducted by the Washington Public Opinion Laboratory, was still one of "disgust." An equal number of poll respondents continued to believe that alcoholics were "weak-willed" rather than "sick."[72]

The persistently negative perception of Skid Road alcoholics was typified by one Firland patient, who, on learning of his upcoming transfer to a predominantly alcoholic ward, feared he would be regarded "just like all these other bums."[73] When Archibald Ruprecht, having left Firland, was named the first director of the state alcoholism clinic in 1959, his fellow physicians treated him with disdain. Ruprecht recalled how one of these physicians verbally attacked him on learning that the clinic had moved into a medical building in Seattle's exclusive First Hill district.[74]

Sensing the slow mobilization of alcoholism work in the city, the King County Anti-Tuberculosis League stepped in to fill the void, popularizing the issue through its newsletter, *Health Notes*, conferences, and a university extension program. Given its role in organizing the vocational rehabilitation program at Firland, the league's involvement in alcoholism was quite logical. "Alcoholism," as one commentator wrote in 1957, "is certainly a rehabilitation problem."[75]

This fact was vividly demonstrated by the King County league's study of "marginally employable" tuberculosis patients, which was completed in 1958. Working with numerous community agencies, such as the state Division of Vocational Rehabilitation, Seattle Goodwill Industries, and the Salvation Army, the league studied thirty-six male patients discharged from Firland who were over age forty and had little education and few job skills. The vast majority of the men lived on the Skid Road and were alcoholics. Although these patients had all received approved discharges, and thus did not represent the worst recidivists, the study's findings were nevertheless bleak. All thirty-six men, reported the league's Honoria Hughes and Clayton Knowles, had appeared at the Department of Public Assistance (formerly the Department of Welfare) within six months of discharge. Moreover, thirty-three of the thirty-six men had "made no progress toward employment" whatsoever.[76]

Despite these results, Hughes and Knowles stressed that rehabilitation of these "hard core" patients was essential in order to prevent further illness, dependence, and disability. The best way to accomplish this, according to Victor I. Howery, a study consultant and dean of the University of Washington School of Social Work, was through a multidisciplinary approach to the problem involving a large number of community organizations. It was necessary, he stated in typically voluntaristic language, to "nourish the patient vocationally, medically, socially, psychologically, and spiritually," thereby enabling him to "pick up the other end of the log and make his contribution."[77]

In sum, Seattle's approach to the issue of tuberculosis-alcoholism in the 1950s was twofold. First, as Jackson had emphasized, it was necessary to view alcoholism as a medical disease and address it openly at Firland. Second, although alcoholics had a "disease," they required more than strictly medical therapy. They also needed social and psychological assistance from groups such as A.A., welfare agencies, the Division of Vocational Rehabilitation, and missions located on the Skid Road. Ideally, these interventions would begin in the sanatorium, which would serve as a "transitional community" or a "therapeutic community" for the recovering patient.[78]

The patient charts document numerous attempts to ease Skid Road alcoholics into life outside the sanatorium. One man, for example, did extensive work in the Firland Exchange Store in preparation for a job in a florist shop after discharge. Many of the alcoholic patients at Firland worked in the Boeing sheltered workshop.[79] In a letter to *Firland Magazine,* one patient detailed his successful attempt at rehabilitation. The staff, he wrote, "understood from the beginning that I was an alcoholic and that alcoholism had undermined my health." During his stay, the patient had joined A.A. and, with the help of the vocational rehabilitation department, was in the process of qualifying for barber school. "I feel that this sojourn at Firland," he concluded, "has changed my life and God will go with me when I have to meet the problems of my future life."[80]

Yet, as with all Firland programs designed to deal with the social and psychological aspects of tuberculosis, this broad attempt to restore the alcoholic patient "to his fullest possible degree of health and usefulness"[81] potentially conflicted with the sanatorium's primary goal: treating tuberculosis and preventing its spread in the community. While it stood to reason that curing alcoholism among Skid Road patients would help antituberculosis efforts, was the treatment of alcoholism and its attendant social problems actually necessary?

Numerous commentators across the country answered yes to this question. The rationale they offered was most often a practical one: control of alcoholism was a prerequisite for effective tuberculosis control. "It is a very rare case indeed," noted Dan Morse, medical director of a sanatorium in Peoria, Illinois, "where a true alcoholic recovers from tuberculosis unless he stops all drinking, and it is almost unheard of for anyone who has an arrested case of tuberculosis, and who goes back to being a chronic alcoholic, to remain well."[82] Similar sentiments were expressed by Pauline Miller of the U.S. Public Health Service. Failure to treat alcoholism, she wrote in 1951, caused "admittedly large sums of money and effort in tuberculosis control [to be] wasted."[83] Such a construct led some to propose broad solutions. "Some authorities believe," reported Philadelphia tuberculosis specialist Donald J. Ottenberg in 1956, that "it is impossible to control tuberculosis on skid row without controlling skid row itself."[84] Discussions about the impact of alcoholism on the future of tuberculosis control were commonplace at National Tuberculosis Association meetings in the late 1950s, and NTA officials cultivated relationships with representatives from both A.A. and the National Council on Alcoholism.[85]

Not surprisingly, many tuberculosis workers in Seattle shared the belief that it was necessary to arrest both the tuberculosis and the alcoholism of the patient. Although Joan Jackson attempted to maintain the neutral stance of a sociologist when performing research at Firland, her work had convinced her of the inherent conflict between a patient's completion of tuberculosis therapy and the Skid Road culture. "As long as the patient suffers from alcoholism," she remarked, "we know we haven't cured him of tuberculosis."[86] Jackson frequently noted that she had never seen an A.A. member of one year's sobriety admitted to Firland.[87]

Yet the alcoholism work among Firland's Skid Road patients signified more than just a prudent strategy for improving tuberculosis control. While curing a patient's tuberculosis was essential, the treatment of tuberculosis-alcoholism offered the possibility of actually bettering the lives of those with both conditions. This philosophy recalled the words of the medical historian and social activist Henry Sigerist, who, in the 1930s, had described both tuberculosis and alcoholism as social diseases caused by poverty. In the case of alcoholism, it was "poor living conditions, a sense of oppression, and a lack of educational and recreational activities [that] drove men to drink."[88] To cure tuberculosis and alcoholism, Sigerist believed, one needed to improve patients' social and economic circumstances. Firland would most explicitly take up Sigerist's challenge in the early 1960s, when Ronald Fagan, who had himself been an alcoholic on Skid Road, opened a special ward for the detoxification and rehabilitation of Skid Road alcoholics.

It should come as little surprise that Firland Sanatorium played a major role in developing the notion of tuberculosis-alcoholism in the 1950s. Given Seattle's long history of addressing the issue of alcoholism on the Skid Road, the new entity of tuberculosis-alcoholism became yet another problem that the city proved willing to tackle. The alcoholism program ultimately established at Firland represented a particularly vivid example of how physicians and other health workers in the city continued to view tuberculosis as both a medical and a social disease.

Yet if enthusiasm existed at the sanatorium for the treatment of alcoholism, few believed that a high percentage of Skid Roaders would actually achieve full rehabilitation. Moreover, given the perceived infectious threat that these men represented, tuberculosis workers in Seattle were unwilling to await the outcome of the efforts of Jackson and the Anti-Tuberculosis League. Thus, even as Firland staff broadly addressed the sociomedical problems of tuberculous Skid Road alcoholics, they worked with local officials to accelerate public health measures specifically aimed at controlling this population. Seattle first forcibly isolated tuberculosis patients in 1949; by the mid-1950s, the city's locked ward had become a model for health departments across the country.

SIX

Temporarily Detained

The Triumph of Coercion

Throughout the postwar era, Seattle physicians tried numerous strategies to ensure that so-called recalcitrant tuberculous alcoholics completed their medical therapy. For example, Skid Road alcoholic patients at Firland received prophylactic lung surgery because of their presumed unreliability and were arbitrarily hospitalized for a minimum of twelve months, regardless of their medical condition. Yet it was the use of formal public health interventions—quarantine and involuntary detention on a locked ward—that most clearly embodied Firland's new use of coercion. Although Cedric Northrop and others had carefully designed these policies to apply to uncooperative patients who posed an immediate threat to the public's health, Firland ultimately employed quarantine and detention for a much broader purpose: to maintain order at the sanatorium. As a result, by the beginning of the 1960s, nearly half of all Skid Road alcoholics at Firland spent at least two weeks of their hospitalization behind a locked door.

Although many tuberculosis divisions across the country accelerated their use of forcible detention in the 1950s and 1960s, it was Seattle—as well as other West Coast cities—that most vigorously implemented a strong-arm approach. This aggressive use of coercion to physically restrict tuberculosis patients represented a significant departure from past practice. Nevertheless, relatively few commentators, either in Seattle or elsewhere, raised objections. This chapter and the one that follows examine the development and implementation of aggressive public health measures designed to control tuberculosis among a population of vagrants with complex social problems.

HISTORY OF QUARANTINE

The policies of public health isolation used in tuberculosis control in Seattle had a long historical lineage. The Bible discusses the confinement of lepers; European cities in the Middle Ages developed the concept of "quarantine," in which officials delayed the landing of ships suspected of carrying victims of bubonic plague or other contagious diseases. The term *quarantine* has since come to mean "the making of a boundary to separate the contaminating from the uncontaminated."[1]

Municipal officials aggressively used quarantine to combat diseases such as cholera well before late-nineteenth-century investigators proved that germs caused disease. But the knowledge that infectious diseases were caused by specific microorganisms transmitted from person to person gave new impetus to the practice of quarantine. The scientific legitimation of the germ theory enabled health officials to solidify their authority to determine the appropriate boundaries between the well and the "diseased." Beginning in the early twentieth century, state laws routinely granted health departments the power to quarantine individuals (generally children) with infectious diseases—such as diphtheria, scarlet fever, or smallpox—either at home or in isolation hospitals.[2]

While officials have implemented such measures with the purpose of preventing the spread of infection, such interventions have often been imposed on "the bodies of those who were least able to protest."[3] On the one hand, this policy made sense, since infectious diseases preferentially affected the poor. The use of quarantine and other compulsory public health measures, however, has also reflected a tendency to stigmatize and punish those groups that become associated with particular diseases.

There are numerous historical examples of this process. For example, health officials incarcerated more than thirty thousand prostitutes in federally funded institutions during World War I in an effort to prevent the spread of venereal disease. Allan Brandt has termed this event "the most concerted attack on civil liberties in the name of public health in American history."[4] Similarly, a surge of nativist beliefs at the end of the nineteenth century led to the arbitrary use of quarantine against Jewish and Chinese persons blamed for the spread of cholera, bubonic plague, and other infectious diseases.[5]

As did health officials selecting persons for quarantine, administrators involved in the day-to-day implementation of enforced isolation enjoyed broad authority. The history of mental hospitals, for example, is replete with accounts of how isolation cells, physical restraints, and other punishments were used to promote discipline.[6] Erving Goffman has termed asylums, mental hospitals, and prisons "total institutions," arguing that such facilities, whatever their underlying purpose, ultimately emphasize the "bureaucratic organization of whole blocks of people."[7]

It was not until the late nineteenth century, when the contagiousness of tuberculosis became widely accepted, that forcible isolation of those with the disease appeared logical. The most aggressive early attempt to segregate tuberculosis patients occurred in New York City in 1903, when Hermann Biggs opened a detention facility at Riverside Hospital on North Brother Island. In her 1994 book, *Living in the Shadow of Death,* Sheila Rothman argues that Riverside, while designed for public health purposes, actually served as a repository for the "fractious and intractable" rounders that so frustrated Biggs and other health officers. Ultimately, Rothman concludes, patients were hospitalized at Riverside not only because of their disease but also for the purpose of controlling populations of poor immigrants, vagrants, and alcoholics.[8]

Although writers across the country continued to decry the "careless consumptive," most health departments did not aggressively quarantine patients after 1920.[9] In Seattle, as elsewhere, officials were reluctant to hold certain patients against their will when there were others willing to fill sanatorium beds. In addition, because tuberculosis was a chronic disease for which no curative treatment existed, the long duration of quarantine that was required made it both expensive and difficult to administer. In contrast, health officials quarantined persons with short-term diseases, such as cholera or influenza, for days or weeks at most.

After World War II, however, health officials dramatically altered their strategy, greatly emphasizing the role of detention. Seattle well exemplified this change in philosophy. In 1948, Washington State instituted a formal quarantine policy for tuberculosis patients; by the next year, Firland had established a locked ward. The timing of these developments was not accidental. By the late 1940s, Cedric Northrop had achieved his original goals of increasing tuberculosis funding and the number of sanatorium beds. As he and his colleagues subsequently turned their attention to the issue of discharges against medical advice, a growing interest in coercive measures, aimed largely at Skid Road alcoholics, accompanied ongoing attempts to improve conditions within the sanatorium. It should be noted that the introduction of quarantine and detention in Seattle antedated the routine use of antibiotics, which did not occur until the early 1950s. However, the subsequent availability of potentially curative drugs greatly promoted the use of more aggressive public health policies.

Northrop believed that the first step in strengthening the public health approach to tuberculosis was to clarify existing quarantine regulations. Building on a 1903 state law that empowered health officials to restrain infectious persons, Northrop drafted two regulations enabling local health officers to quarantine any persons with active tuberculosis who were "uncooperative" and "refused to observe the [necessary] precautions to prevent the spread of the disease."[10] The Seattle–King County health officer generally sent such persons to Firland, where they would remain on quarantine until one of four conditions was met: "(1) the patient's pulmonary disease is considered to be 'apparently arrested' (National Tuberculosis Association Classification—1940); (2) the patient agrees to accept routine sanatorium care; (3) the patient

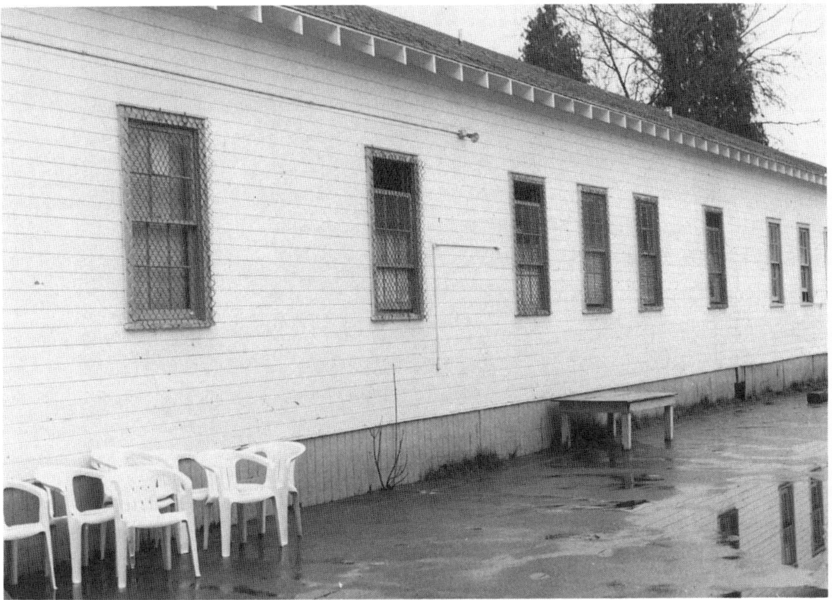

FIGURE 6.1 Heavily screened windows on the outside of Firland Sanatorium's locked ward. Photograph by author, 1993.

dies; (4) other arrangements for adequate isolation are made, which . . . protect the public from the spread of his infection."[11]

King County prosecutors aided Northrop in drafting the regulations, which were subsequently approved by the state Board of Health. The regulations did not define what constituted an "uncooperative" patient or what were the proper "precautions" to prevent the spread of tuberculosis. Like the vast majority of similar ordinances enacted throughout the twentieth century, they gave the public health official great latitude in judging what types of behavior potentially threatened the health of the community.

Although Northrop used the term "uncooperative" when preparing his regulations, health officials most commonly referred to tuberculosis patients who disregarded treatment recommendations as "recalcitrant."[12] The label *recalcitrant,* which is defined by *Webster's Third New International Dictionary* as "obstinately defiant of authority or restraint," strongly implied that those in authority should be fully empowered to determine appropriate behavior. As we shall see, the use of the term *recalcitrant* itself fostered stigmatization and punishment of Skid Road alcoholics, who not only represented a public health threat but also challenged the rules and regulations of Firland Sanatorium.

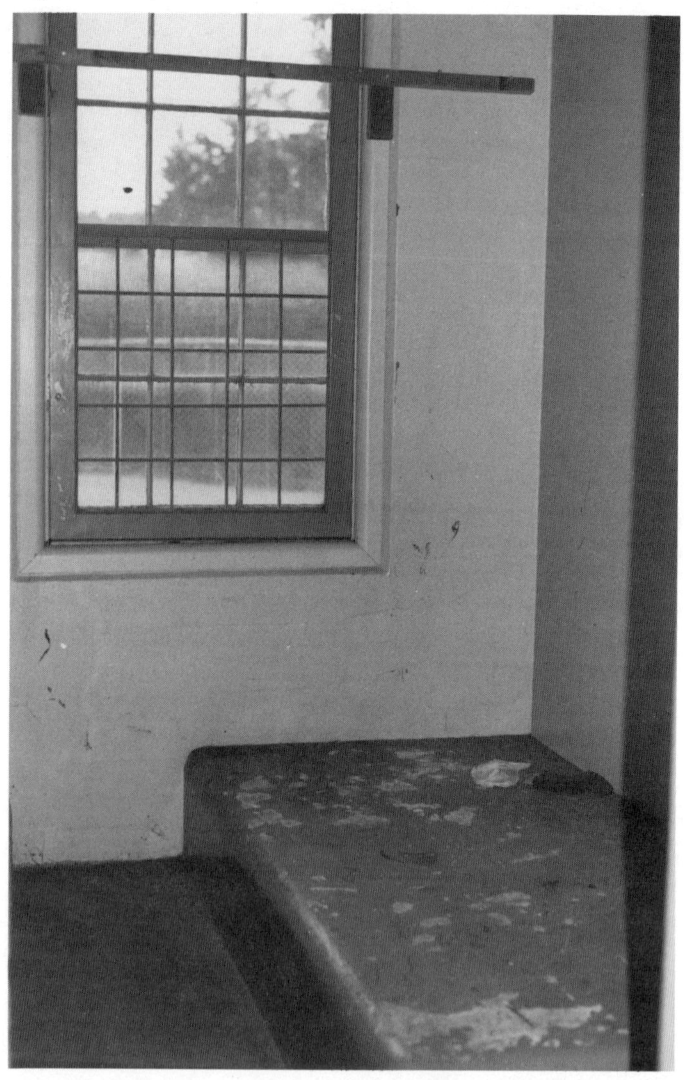

FIGURE 6.2 One of the locked cells used for acutely inebriated tuberculosis patients at Firland Sanatorium. A thin mattress was placed on the concrete slab. Photograph by author, 1993.

Northrop and Firland staff decided to establish a locked ward only after early efforts at quarantine had not prevented unapproved discharges. Known as Ward Six and located in the old naval brig, the unit was opened in June 1949. Its designation as Ward Six had unintended irony. In his short story "Ward Number Six," Anton Chekhov had darkly depicted life within a rusty, rotting hut that housed five Russian lunatics. As the story progressed, the patients' physician, Dr. Ragin, gradually became insane and was himself hospitalized in the hut. Ward Number Six, Chekhov wrote, had the "melancholy, doomed air peculiar to hospital and prison buildings."[13]

Firland's Ward Six bore little resemblance to Chekhov's fictional hospital. It was furnished much like the rest of the sanatorium, with beds for twenty-seven patients, a nursing station, and a common area. Nevertheless, the primary purpose of the ward was involuntary detention, and it was equipped with both locked doors and heavily screened windows (figure 6.1). Included on the ward were seven locked cells, which contained only concrete slabs covered by thin mattresses. Patients admitted to Ward Six (most of whom were intoxicated) spent the first twenty-four hours in one of these cells for purposes of sobering up or delousing (figure 6.2).[14]

Firland staff originally planned to use Ward Six sparingly. "If coercion is needed frequently," Medical Director Roberts Davies wrote, "it is a sure sign that something is wrong, either in the sanatorium or in the administration of the public health part of the program."[15] In fact, the early use of Ward Six was limited. Northrop observed in December 1949 that the locked ward housed only a handful of male patients. No beds had been allotted for women.[16]

"OVERTREATMENT" OF PATIENTS

As Firland began to implement its policies of quarantine and detention, the staff also used another, less formal strategy as a means to ensure that its recalcitrant patients completed their medical treatment. Physicians who favored this approach, termed "overtreatment" by some commentators, recommended additional inpatient medical therapy for patients who they presumed were unlikely to be compliant after discharge from the sanatorium. "It is believed," wrote Firland physician Michael A. Linell in 1956, "that the recalcitrant and frequently alcoholic tuberculous patient definitely requires over-treatment by comparison with the responsible patient."[17] Such over-treatment took two forms: (1) prophylactic surgery to remove foci of pulmonary tuberculosis that would potentially reactivate; and (2) a mandatory sanatorium stay of at least one year regardless of the patient's medical condition.

Many tuberculosis specialists in the 1950s were attracted by the notion of using a surgical procedure as a possible medical solution for noncompliant patients with multiple social problems. Such an idea was not entirely new. As early as 1931, one California physician had proposed "radical" treatment with thoracoplasty for "indigent consumptives" with cavities.[18] Nevertheless, broad advocacy of surgical extirpation of pulmonary lesions in alcoholic or mentally ill patients did not occur until the widespread growth of lung resection in the early 1950s. As we have seen, the debate about performing such surgery in sputum-negative patients with residual foci of disease had generated a great deal of controversy. Yet those physicians who argued that surgery was unnecessary in such cases did so with the assumption that such patients would be compliant with prolonged antibiotic therapy after discharge. Given the presumed unreliability of Skid Road alcoholics, a potential surgical "cure" for tuberculosis became an enticing possibility for this population.[19]

The Firland medical charts from the 1950s document numerous instances in which physicians cited patient unreliability as justification for surgical resections on sputum-negative Skid Road alcoholics. In 1953, for example, the medical staff voted to perform a partial right-upper-lobe excision on a man in his mid-fifties, since there was "no significant disease elsewhere and . . . he is an alcoholic and unreliable as to drug therapy on the outside."[20] So, too, doctors performed a limited resection on another man with diagnoses of both chronic alcoholism and psychopathic personality, providing the following explanation: "The vote of the Section was 5–1 that this patient should have the right-sided surgery as originally voted with the strong feeling that this patient, inspite [*sic*] of multiple promises on his part, will fail to continue on antibiotic therapy and that he will return to his alcoholism and be positive shortly after discharge."[21]

Not all alcoholics at Firland received operations if persistent foci of tuberculosis remained after antibiotic therapy. Staff physicians did not recommend surgery lightly and often decided to forgo an operation with the hope that more conservative management might work. In 1957, for example, the possibility of surgery was considered in a middle-aged man "in view of the patient's unreliability and therefore the question of whether he would take drugs as an out patient." While five physicians ultimately favored surgery for "sociologic reasons," eight others felt that removal of the left upper lobe was "a little more drastic than the present situation called for."[22] An operation was not recommended. It should also be noted that Firland staff honored the decisions of those alcoholic patients who refused surgery.

That physicians at Firland and other sanatoriums included patients' social characteristics when making ostensibly medical decisions is not surprising. As Paul Starr, John Burnham, and others have argued, the authority of the American medical profession probably reached its zenith in the 1950s. Firland's casual and unembarrassed consideration of "sociologic reasons" well demonstrates the ability of physicians in the 1950s to subtly infuse their medical recommendations with value judgments about patients' lives.[23]

Race also influenced clinical decision making at Firland. Although the majority of alcoholics who received operations at Firland were white, the long association of alcoholism with northwest Native American and Eskimo populations appears to have promoted surgery among patients with these racial backgrounds. In summarizing the case conference of a Native American woman in her twenties, a physician wrote that "some of the people thought [the caseous mass] should be resected, since she is an undependable, alcoholic, young Indian female."[24] In a 1992 interview, Firland surgeon Waldo Mills recalled an old saying at the sanatorium: if a patient was an "Indian, alcoholic, school teacher, and divorced, they were sure to get a resection."[25] Such a philosophy was hardly limited to Firland or Seattle. Articles in major medical publications ranging from the *New England Journal of Medicine* to the *American Review of Respiratory Disease* unequivocally supported using racial or ethnic characteristics when evaluating tuberculosis patients for surgery. Nor did objections to the use of race or ethnicity appear in correspondence to these journals.[26]

Yet if Firland's surgery policy for Skid Road alcoholics, and Native Americans in particular, appears to have been coercive, it is important to remember the context in which physicians made clinical decisions. The Firland staff was intimately familiar with its alcoholic patients, many of whom had multiple stays in the sanatorium over a period of several years. Having witnessed repeated failed attempts by these alcoholics to control their tuberculosis, a recommendation advising surgical removal of a lung lesion represented a complex mixture of compulsion and paternalism that took into account both the disease process and the specific patient in question.

The interaction of these factors can be seen in the case of a white male alcoholic in his mid-forties who had formerly worked in the printing industry. The patient's twenty-month hospitalization during 1952 and 1953 was punctuated with frequent elopements from the sanatorium and episodes of drunkenness. In an effort to address this behavior and the issue of postdischarge planning, the patient met with both a vocational rehabilitation counselor and Thomas Holmes. Holmes, after evaluating the patient's life history and his recent existence on the Skid Road, concluded that the feelings of "alienation and rejection" that resulted from his "mixed psycho-neurosis" were unlikely to be treatable. As a result, Holmes concluded that the patient was "a good candidate for long term, unstable tuberculosis."[27]

Given this bleak assessment of the overall prognosis, the staff's ultimate recommendation of a partial left-upper-lobe resection clearly took into account both the disease and the patient. In this sense, Firland continued to view tuberculosis as a social disease. At the same time, however, the solution proposed for resolving the complex social problems of Skid Road alcoholic patients was once again largely medical. Having vividly witnessed the "sociologic reasons" that perennially predisposed such patients to noncompliance, the Firland staff was more than willing to try for a surgical solution.

A similar calculus informed the second type of overtreatment prescribed for Skid Road alcoholics: twelve months of mandatory inpatient therapy, even for those persons who had small lesions that rapidly responded to medications. That is, the presumption of postdischarge noncompliance among alcoholics—in contrast with other patients—led Firland staff to recommend that alcoholics receive a more extensive proportion of their antibiotic therapy while in a supervised hospital setting. The sanatorium never formally codified the one-year rule, although it was mentioned frequently in correspondence, articles, and medical records beginning in 1954.[28] A typical discussion took place in the chart of a fifty-eight-year-old Skid Road alcoholic. "He is being maintained in the hospital," wrote one physician, "mainly because we doubt that he would take his drugs on the outside and would like to have him on them for at least one year."[29] In the case of a fifty-seven-year-old alcoholic with three previous hospitalizations at Firland, physicians decided to keep him for fifteen months despite repeatedly negative sputum samples. They had declined to discharge him at the twelve-month mark, as "it was a little early for him to face the outside world."[30]

That the one-year rule went into effect in 1954 was no coincidence. Although effective antibiotics had been available since the late 1940s, only with the introduction of isoniazid in 1952 did the use of drugs—either INH (isoniazid) and streptomycin, INH and PAS (para-aminosalicylic acid), or all three agents—become routine. Physicians generally recommended approximately two years of continuous treatment. Such prolonged therapy, it was assumed, would be curative; shorter courses of antibiotics might cause patients to relapse. It was important, moreover, that patients received continuous treatment, as erratic use of the drugs appeared to promote resistance.[31] As early as 1953, preliminary data from Firland and elsewhere appeared to confirm the value of prolonged antibiotic therapy.[32] Given these findings, confining alcoholic patients for at least one year of supervised inpatient chemotherapy seemed reasonable.

As concerned with timetables as other patients, alcoholics hospitalized at Firland were well aware of the new rule and apprehensive about it. A 1956 article in *Firland Magazine* suggested that alcoholics were reluctant to go to A.A. meetings at the sanatorium because they would automatically be placed on the "one-year list." "We question the legality of a quarantine for alcolism [*sic*]," stated one patient, "that is given to some patients, and they ar [*sic*] held for a peariod [*sic*] of a year, regardless of the state of their health."[33] Although the policy was relaxed to some degree, extended inpatient treatment of alcoholic patients continued even after doctors in the 1960s decided to shorten the total duration of antibiotic therapy for tuberculosis to as little as eighteen months. Describing a middle-aged patient in 1970, a Firland physician wrote: "Noted in the record is a fairly definite history of chronic alcoholism, residence at the Gospel Mission, and unemployment. Preference is extended for at least one year's chemotherapy at Firland."[34] Thus, as of

1965, alcoholics remained hospitalized at Firland for an average of 259 days, compared with 163 days for nonalcoholic patients.[35]

Overtreatment may have made theoretical sense for patients deemed unreliable, but implementation of the policy proved problematic. While Firland's extensive efforts to improve sanatorium life and address patients' problems had helped to lower its irregular discharge rate from 37 percent in 1951 to 15 percent in 1955,[36] keeping alcoholic patients hospitalized for a minimum of one year of continuous treatment represented a major challenge for sanatorium staff. Seeking to put some teeth in its attempts to carry out this policy, Firland increasingly turned to the strategies of quarantine and detention that Northrop had set in place in the late 1940s.

QUARANTINE AND DETENTION ON THE RISE

Northrop's 1948 regulations had spelled out a formal plan for quarantining tuberculosis patients in Seattle. Yet several problems arose when health officials began to carry out the policy. For example, one of the four criteria required for the discontinuation of quarantine was that "the patient agrees to accept routine sanatorium care."[37] How was such a standard to be determined, especially for patients who had reneged on similar promises in the past?

An issue that caused particular confusion was the severity of the patient's tuberculosis. Northrop had designed quarantine for cases of "active" tuberculosis until they became "apparently arrested." A case of pulmonary tuberculosis went from active to apparently arrested only after a patient had negative sputum cultures and healed X-ray lesions without a cavity for three months. Thus, tuberculosis remained active long after a patient had become noninfectious.[38] Health officials employed this broad definition of active tuberculosis because they saw healing as a slow process that continued long after the sputum was no longer infectious.

In 1950, however, the National Tuberculosis Association (NTA) issued a revised set of diagnostic guidelines that discouraged use of the "apparently arrested" terminology. According to the new 1950 standard, a patient's tuberculosis became "inactive" after six months of sputum negativity and stable X-rays without cavity.[39] Despite this change in nomenclature, neither Northrop nor the state Department of Health revised the original 1948 regulations. As a result, it was unclear which standard—three months or six months—was to be used in determining whether a patient had active disease and thus could be quarantined.

Further complicating the picture was the language of the actual quarantine orders that appeared in the medical charts. Early versions took the form of individualized letters sent from the Seattle–King County Health Department to specific patients. In contrast with Northrop's regulations, which had used the broad definition of active tuberculosis, these letters justified quarantine due to the patient's infectiousness. For example, a 1949 quarantine letter stated that "this measure has been taken in order to safeguard your best interests as well as to protect the public health, because you are suffering with active tuberculosis of the lungs *with a positive sputum which makes your condition communicable to others.*"[40] Similarly, a 1953 letter informed a patient that he had been placed in quarantine because he had tuberculosis "*in a contagious form.*"[41]

The ambiguous nature of early quarantine orders foreshadowed later tendencies to gloss over the exact language of both public health statutes and institutional rules. As did other patients, Skid Road alcoholics with uncomplicated tuberculosis often developed negative sputum after only two to four weeks of inpatient antibiotic treatment. Thus, once Firland began to keep its Skid Road patients hospitalized for the first twelve months of their two-year therapy, they remained noninfectious for most of their stay. Moreover, those patients showing a good response to antibiotic therapy would often convert from active to inactive tuberculosis during their hospitalization—whether one employed the three-month or the six-month standard. Ignoring, for the moment, the issue of infectiousness and using Northrop's broad definition of active tuberculosis, quarantine still should have been discontinued when a patient's disease became inactive. Yet sticking to the letter of the law threatened the carefully constructed new strategy that mandated at least twelve months of inpatient antibiotic therapy for all Skid Road alcoholics.

Questions about the proper implementation of quarantine policy arose in 1951 in the case of V.O., a transient alcoholic with several past admissions to Firland. Given V.O.'s past uncooperativeness, John Fountain, director of the city's tuberculosis division, had placed the patient on quarantine at the time of his admission in January 1950. V.O. had undergone a lobectomy in October of that year and since that time had maintained both negative sputum cultures and a stationary X-ray. Yet when he eloped from Firland in July 1951, nine months after the operation, the Health Department returned him to the sanatorium still on quarantine.[42]

The realization of this problem led to a meeting between public health and sanatorium officials at which each side blamed the other for the oversight. Fountain claimed that the Firland staff had been remiss in not informing his office of the change in V.O.'s clinical status. Roberts Davies conceded this point but upbraided Fountain for what he perceived as too casual use of the public health power of quarantine. "It is hard for me to conceive," Davies stated, that the Health Department could have considered the patient "a menace to the public health" at the time of his return to Firland, regardless of the technicalities of disease classification.[43] Adding that careless use of quarantine could endanger the entire program, Davies continued: "I therefore feel personally that whenever the institution, re-institution, or release of quarantine is being considered, as in the case of [V.O.], that it is wise to lean over backwards to make sure that the patient is not quarantined or his quarantine re-instituted after a lapse if there is any doubt whatever that he is not actually at the time a menace to the public health.[44]

Cases similar to that of V.O. arose throughout the early 1950s, as health officials balanced their public health concerns with the constraints imposed by the actual language of Northrop's regulations. For example, one Firland physician, noting that a fifty-eight-year-old Firland patient was a severe alcoholic and was unreliable, favored continuing quarantine but admitted that it "made little sense so far as the public health was concerned."[45] Even in cases in which all parties agreed that quarantine was appropriate, errors in its implementation were not uncommon. In one representative case, a Health Department secretary admitted that "Dr. Fountain said to put [L.A.] on quar [*sic*] on admission but we slipped up on sending him a quarantine letter—*unfortunately.*"[46]

As had been the case with initial efforts at quarantine, the early use of the locked ward was inconsistent. Although Ward Six was generally intended for persons who had violated quarantine, no formal policies were drafted prior to its opening in June 1949. Of course, Northrop and Fountain had an idea of the type of patient the ward would house: someone like K.S., the first person detained on Ward Six. A white man in his middle thirties, K.S. was not an alcoholic but was "addicted to narcotics" and displayed "irascible" and "psychopathic" behavior. Carrying the diagnosis of far-advanced bilateral pulmonary tuberculosis with a cavity, he had "been in and out of various hospitals for tuberculosis for the past 9 years."[47] Prior to K.S.'s admission in June 1949, the police had arrested him for assaulting his wife. The King County judge hearing the case, however, agreed to suspend his sentence on the condition that he be sent to Firland and remain there until approved for discharge.

The earliest decisions to detain patients were documented inconsistently in the medical charts. For example, in two of the first sixteen cases, there was no explanation for the patient's transfer to Ward Six. One of the sixteen charts contained a typed sheet of rules that stipulated, among other things, that the detained patient was to be "confined in cell until he is sober."[48] Yet none of the remaining fifteen records discussed any aspects of locked ward policy. The duration of early confinement was quite variable, ranging from two days to six and one-half months, with an average of thirty-five days.

Over time, however, the protocol for quarantine and detention at Firland grew more formalized. It is thus possible to depict schematically the usual manner in which health officials curtailed the activities of tuberculo-

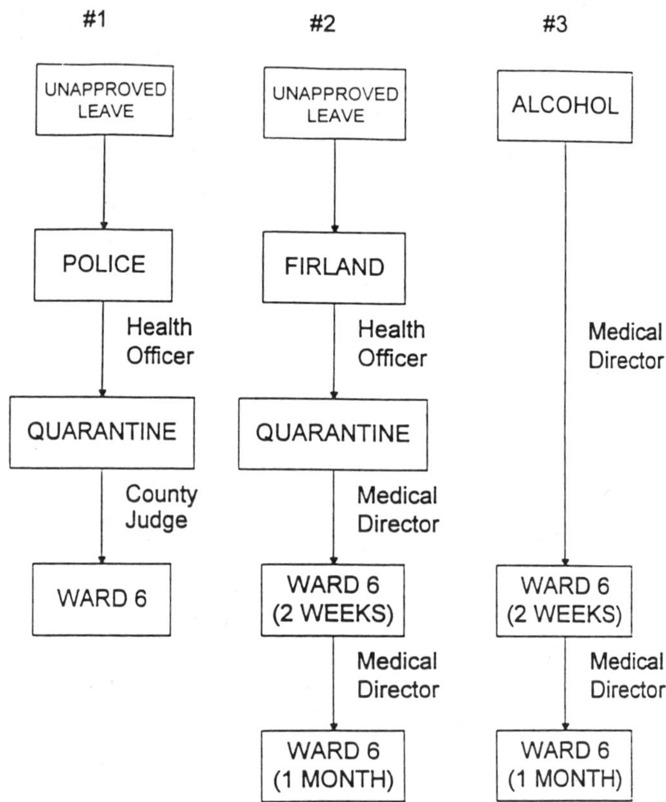

FIGURE 6.3 Three scenarios by which patients were sent to the locked ward at Firland Sanatorium.

sis patients in Seattle in the 1950s and 1960s (figure 6.3). In many instances, King County judges sent to Firland tuberculous persons convicted of crimes ranging from public drunkenness to larceny to forgery. Although jail sentences were suspended in these cases, the judges often sentenced individuals who had committed more serious crimes to serve a specific period of time on Ward Six. K.S., for example, spent the first two and one-half months of his hospitalization on the locked ward. There were two important precedents for this use of hospital facilities for the enforced treatment of alcoholism and related conditions. First, with the growing attempt to medicalize the disease, it had become commonplace for judges to send alcoholics found guilty of crimes to treatment facilities as opposed to jail. In Seattle, for example, some convicted alcoholics qualified for the police farm. Second, there was a long history of involuntary civil commitment of alcoholics to mental institutions—again, ostensibly for therapeutic purposes.[49] Here, given the concurrent diagnosis of tuberculosis, the sanatorium served a similar purpose.

The offenders most often sent to Firland were those arrested for public drunkenness. Although these individuals had technically committed a crime, they were not automatically placed on Ward Six. Rather, they were sent to the unlocked portion of the sanatorium under Health Department quarantine. However, when these individuals, or others on quarantine for different reasons, left the sanatorium without permission, they were deemed to have violated quarantine. In general, persons away from Firland for less than two weeks were termed AWOL, whereas those absent for more than two weeks were considered discharges against medical advice (AMA). Many such patients were eventually found by the police, often when arrested or rearrested for public drunkenness (figure 6.3, scenario 1). When they appeared in court, judges returned the patients to the sanatorium, where they were then detained on the locked ward. As might be expected, AWOL or AMA patients not previously quarantined who were returned to Firland were placed under quarantine in the unlocked portion of the sanatorium.[50]

Not all missing patients arrested for public drunkenness appeared before King County judges. By the early 1950s, the police, who had become quite familiar with Seattle's tuberculous alcoholics, increasingly returned such persons directly to Firland. In addition, other patients who had gone AWOL returned to the sanatorium on their own, often after drinking sprees. Many had overstayed twenty-four- or forty-eight-hour passes approved by the medical director. When these patients returned to Firland, whether unaccompanied or accompanied by police, they too were quarantined and detained. That is, those patients without previous offenses were placed on quarantine, and those already on quarantine were sent to Ward Six.

Since this process took place entirely at the sanatorium, detention occurred in these cases without formal legal process. The medical director, Roberts Davies, sent these patients directly to Ward Six for a length of stay that he and his staff determined (figure 6.3, scenario 2). This ability to detain persons on the locked ward without a judge's ruling derived from the Health Department's letters of quarantine, which stated that patients were to remain "in that section of the Sanatorium designated by the Medical Director."[51]

As Firland increasingly dealt with issues of quarantine and detention within the sanatorium, it also began to use these powers more frequently. By 1952, fully 10 percent of Firland's nearly eleven hundred patients were under a Health Department quarantine order. As the use of quarantine grew and the staff instituted the mandatory one-year hospitalization rule for alcoholics, reliance on the locked ward increased. By the early 1950s, the ward regularly had a census of ten to twenty-five persons.[52]

As anticipated, Ward Six largely housed Skid Road transients. According to a 1953 study, 88 percent of men who had spent time on the ward carried the diagnosis of alcoholism. Various psychiatric diagnoses were also common, such as "constitutional psychopath" and "character disorder."[53] The men ranged in age from twenty to seventy and had held working-class jobs such as logger, cook, sailor, and farm laborer. One-third to one-half were veterans. Reflecting the population of both Seattle and the Skid Road, the locked ward population was overwhelmingly white. Of the first thirty patients placed on Ward Six in 1949, twenty-eight (93.3 percent) were white, one was a "Chinese Indian," and one was African American. The distribution was similar in 1957. Of the seventy-two men detained between January 1 and June 30, sixty-one (85 percent) patients were white, six (8 percent) were Native American, four (6 percent) were black, and one (1 percent) was Japanese. More than half of the men detained in 1957 had had multiple admissions to Firland, and several had logged six or seven separate admissions.

As the number of patients being quarantined and detained rose, Davies and his successors attempted to routinize the use of coercive measures. By 1952, for example, Firland had begun to keep patients on Ward Six for standard periods of time, based on how often they had previously been interned on the ward. A patient's first stay lasted two weeks, the second, one month, and the third, three months. The few patients requiring more than three stays were evaluated at a Ward Six staff conference attended by the medical director.[54] In addition, the Health Department stopped using personalized letters of quarantine and replaced them with two standard forms, which contained spaces for the patient's name. In contrast to the earlier individualized letters of quarantine, these forms made no mention of either positive sputum or contagiousness.

Yet as Firland and the Health Department stopped using infectiousness as the basis for isolation orders, a seemingly paradoxical development was taking place: sanatorium staff had begun to ignore whether forcibly isolated patients even continued to have active disease. As a result, alcoholics who went AWOL or overstayed a pass during the last days or weeks of their mandatory twelve-month hospitalization—a period in which their tuberculosis might likely have become inactive—could be placed on quarantine or sent to the locked ward. Indeed, the staff thought nothing of discharging patients to home directly from Ward Six, a practice that belied the notion that detention was reserved for true public health threats.[55] This new policy was in marked contrast with the earliest efforts at coercion at Firland, when Roberts Davies had urged the Health Department to "lean over backwards" to prevent the abuse of public health powers. Clearly, quarantine and detention at the sanatorium had begun to serve a purpose other than simply preventing the spread of tuberculosis.

MAINTAINING ORDER AT FIRLAND

An understanding of why Firland used the public health powers of quarantine and detention to discipline patients with inactive tuberculosis requires an analysis of its institutional needs. Because the sanatorium housed hundreds of persons in close quarters for long periods of time, the staff saw potential disorder as a persistent problem. Periodic episodes of violence, often instigated by patients with a history of criminality or psychiatric problems, did little to dispel this notion. In 1950, for example, one patient attempted to engineer a mass escape from Firland. Placed in solitary confinement after this episode, he set fire to his mattresses and blankets.[56] Physical altercations, while not frequent, nevertheless left a lasting impression on the staff. "Today when on rounds on the South side of Ward 6," wrote one physician,

> A.C. came to my help when I was being attacked by another patient, D.G. D.G. had already struck me on the jaw once in the corridor and was about to hit me again, when A.C. stepped between us and received the blow that was intended for me. D.G. then lost his control completely and struck A.C. many times both on the face and the body. A.C. retaliated in self defense and, considering his age, made quite a good account of himself.[57]

Most indicative, perhaps, of the overall preoccupation with conduct at Firland was a statement that appeared on all medical charts. In a gesture that would have made Betty MacDonald smile, the discharging physician was asked to evaluate each patient's "attitude and behavior while in sanatorium."

Alcohol particularly disrupted sanatorium routine. A 1947 King County resolution had made the "giving or selling of intoxicating liquors" at Firland a misdemeanor, a fact well publicized to those hospitalized at the sanatorium.[58] Nevertheless, patients who had obtained liquor while on a pass devised numerous methods for getting it past the guards at the sanatorium gate. For example, they frequently tossed bottles over the fence and retrieved them once on the inside. So-called bootlegger patients proved especially adept at smuggling in large quantities of liquor. When the bootleggers returned, loud, raucous drinking parties often followed in the unlocked areas of the sanatorium. Not only were such activities disruptive, but they also led other patients to request early discharge.[59]

The prospect of "utter chaos" strongly influenced the evolution of detention policy at Firland. Missing patients who returned to the sanatorium, many of whom were extremely inebriated, were judged less on the state of their tuberculosis than on their potential for causing additional disorder at the sanatorium. The staff believed that merely allowing such persons, once sober, to return to the regular wards encouraged both elopement and drinking. Conversely, having such persons spend time on the locked ward potentially deterred such disruptive behavior.[60]

Firland used this same justification—the need to maintain order—to send to Ward Six patients caught drinking or selling alcohol at the sanatorium (figure 6.3, scenario 3). Patients sent to the locked ward for drinking or bootlegging need not have previously been on quarantine (although they were subsequently placed on quarantine). Rather, they were sent to the locked ward for having broken the 1947 resolution prohibiting such behavior at the institution. Once again, Firland staff handled these cases without instituting formal legal proceedings.[61] Whether or not the patient had active tuberculosis or was an actual public health threat was irrelevant.

Thus, a patient who had always been compliant with his medical therapy, had never eloped from Firland, and had been noninfectious for three to six months could be sent to Ward Six for drinking. One such patient was P.C., a white cook in his fifties who remained on Ward Six in 1957 despite having negative sputum for eight months and stable X-rays for five months.[62] As demonstrated by the case of M.P., a forty-five-year-old white transient laborer, the quarantine and detention of patients with inactive tuberculosis who were caught drinking continued well into the 1960s. Despite having inactive disease, M.P. "was transferred to the locked ward from Ward Four on 6-29-67, having been drinking on the open ward."[63] Also in 1967, doctors sent an inebriated thirty-two-year-old Native American to Ward Six for the fifth time, although he had more than six months of negative sputum and stable X-rays.[64]

What transpired at Firland beginning in the mid-1950s appears to have represented the confluence of two long-standing historical trends: the broad power of health officials to isolate the "diseased" and the need for institutions to control their inmates.[65] Health officials in Seattle originally established policies of quarantine and detention to protect the community from recalcitrant patients with active tuberculosis. Yet the larger goal turned out to be custodial: to keep Skid Road alcoholics institutionalized, and reasonably well behaved, for twelve months of antibiotic therapy. Once this latter strategy was put into place, it became necessary to define the disruption of institutional order as a public health violation punishable by quarantine and detention. Given the great disciplinary authority of the medical profession in the 1950s and 1960s, it is little wonder that Firland so successfully blended these public health and institutional imperatives in order to achieve control of a disruptive and socially marginal population.[66]

When tuberculosis officials in the early 1950s first began to employ overtreatment and coercive public health measures, they had assumed that ensuring two years of supervised antibiotic therapy would prevent relapses and thus benefit both patients and the community. By the end of the decade, data in the medical literature had provided "substantiation of the belief that long-term, uninterrupted chemotherapy is essential in the treatment of tuberculosis."[67] In 1956, for example, a New York City tuberculosis specialist reported a three-year cumulative relapse rate for patients on antibiotics of only 6.1 percent, compared with 19.1 percent in the preantibiotic era. Another clinical study found that only 8.8 percent of patients with approved discharges who had been treated with multiple drugs, including isoniazid, relapsed within four years. In contrast, a historical control group at the same sanatorium in the 1940s had a relapse rate of 21.2 percent. Reviewing selected studies in 1960, John Crofton of Edinburgh, Scotland, reported a considerably lower relapse rate—only 1 percent—among patients receiving INH, PAS, and streptomycin in various combinations for at least twelve months.[68] While admitting that there was still much uncertainty, an expert panel at the 1959 annual meeting of the National Tuberculosis Association concurred that the overall relapse rate had dropped with chemotherapy and probably totaled somewhat less than 10 percent.[69]

Yet if prolonged drug treatment was leading to fewer relapses in "compliant" populations, what about patients who were less likely to achieve adequate follow-up? Firland itself addressed this question in 1959, compiling data on 669 patients discharged five years earlier. Irregularly discharged patients relapsed at a rate of 29.4 percent, more than double the 13.7 percent figure for those discharged with medical advice.[70] Another "ominous prognostic concomitant" was alcoholism; patients with this diagnosis relapsed 26 percent of the time.[71]

The Firland statistics confirmed the staff's basic presumptions about recalcitrance and also supported the use of overtreatment. Among the same group of 669 patients, relapse rates were lowest for those who had received twenty to twenty-nine months of antibiotic therapy. Moreover, patients who remained in the sanatorium with six to eleven months of negative sputum relapsed only 11 percent of the time. This number fell to 6.4 percent for those with twelve months of negative sputum prior to discharge. Most notable was the improvement in "overtreated" alcoholic patients. One year of supervised drug treatment in the hospital reduced relapses in this population to 10 percent—a rate comparable to that of the general population of tuberculosis patients.[72]

Armed with this evidence that an aggressive public health approach to Skid Road alcoholics and other uncooperative patients was working, the Firland staff increasingly relied on coercion. The proportion of patients on quarantine increased from 10 to 30 percent between 1952 and 1960. Firland enlarged Ward Six in 1954, from twenty-seven beds to fifty-four, and now included six beds for women.[73] As with male patients, women were largely detained for unapproved leaves and drinking at the sanatorium and were at times placed on Ward Six when their tuberculosis had become inactive.

By 1960, Washington state had detained over a thousand patients, more than any other state for which data were available. Although health officials held some of these persons in locked wards at sanatoriums elsewhere in Washington, Firland's Ward Six housed the vast majority. The growing reliance on the ward was demonstrated by a study of 124 male and female alcoholics admitted to Firland during a twelve-month period in 1961 and 1962. Forty-four percent of these patients had at least one stay on Ward Six during their hospitalization.[74] Detention, initially meant for the occasional severely recalcitrant patient, had become a standard part of the management of the Skid Road alcoholic at Firland.

Concurrent with its increased use of quarantine and detention, Firland gradually codified the policies that had evolved during the 1950s. In 1960, Byron F. Francis, Sheehy's successor as medical director, drafted an eighteen-page document, "Policies Covering the Operation of the Detention Ward at Firland Sanatorium," which detailed issues such as visiting hours, smoking privileges, the searching of patients, the locking of individual rooms, and the proper protocol for personnel working on the locked ward. Francis also delineated the admission policy for Ward Six, verifying that intoxication or otherwise belligerent behavior warranted admission to the ward. While the document asserted that the stay on Ward Six was to be "temporary" if a patient "has not been quarantined to the hospital and is not considered a menace to the public health," in practice, as we have seen, such patients were quarantined *post hoc* and generally remained on the locked ward for at least two weeks.[75]

DETENTION ACROSS THE COUNTRY

Seattle's increased use of compulsory public health powers after World War II epitomized developments across the United States. A 1955 survey conducted by the Social Research Committee of the National Tuberculosis Association revealed that since 1948, twenty-two states had passed new legislation pertaining to the isolation of recalcitrant tuberculosis patients. By 1960, thirty-one states and the District of Columbia employed detention as part of their tuberculosis control programs.[76]

Because the NTA did not issue any relevant guidelines until 1959, much variability existed in the use of detention. Although most health departments confined patients in locked hospital wards, three states and three cities employed actual prison facilities.[77] Some states required extensive legal proceedings prior to detention, including the provision of lawyers to potential detainees.[78] Others, however, agreed with the attorney general of Oregon that constitutional guarantees of due process of law did not place limitations on the police power of the state regarding protection of the public's health. At least three other states—New York, Michigan, and Indiana—detained patients for "disorderly conduct" in the sanatorium, although they all required specific court orders permitting such confinement.[79]

Health departments differed widely in defining what degree of disease warranted the use of detention. Cases suitable for forcible isolation ranged from "communicable" in one state to "infectious" and "open" in others.[80] One article describing detention in Ohio referred to "positive sputum" cases in the title but "active" cases in the text, terms that had very different meanings.[81] On the whole, it appears that health officers across the country, as in Seattle, were often less than meticulous in demonstrating that detained persons actually constituted a public health threat. The broad discretion given to local officials was apparent from a statement made by the Virginia health commissioner. It was the role of the health officer, Mack I. Shanholtz claimed, to judge the "degree of infectiousness" and to decide which persons had tuberculosis in a "dangerously communicable" form.[82] Regardless of the terminology used, patients in many states were confined for periods of six to twelve months. Thus, other states also detained persons with both noninfectious and inactive tuberculosis.[83]

Although detention protocols varied considerably, Seattle's overall strategy served as a model for other health departments. Large numbers of people, noted Thomas Sheehy, "come to Firland from all points of the country to observe Ward Six in action."[84] Northrop and Firland staff wrote several articles in major medical journals describing the "practical management of the recalcitrant tuberculosis patient."[85] At NTA meetings, Seattle officials gave advice to colleagues from Wisconsin, Minnesota, Georgia, and other states regarding programs of forcible confinement that they were establishing. Indeed, as Northrop noted somewhat ruefully, he was probably asked more about compulsory isolation than about any other aspect of his work.[86]

While perhaps lacking the passionate commitment of Northrop or California tuberculosis control officer Edward Kupka, the vast majority of tuberculosis workers in the 1950s advocated some use of detention for recalcitrant patients. Most of these recommendations urged health officials to use coercion only after all other possible interventions had failed. Thus, a 1958 editorial in the *Journal of the American Medical Association,* while noting the controversial nature of enforced isolation, agreed that for persistently obstinate patients it was necessary to "resort to available legal measures."[87]

A few commentators in the 1950s, however, decried the use of detention. What patients required, argued Ruth Taylor of the U.S. Public Health Service, was not to be locked up but "more, or better, or different types of help in understanding and accepting medical recommendations."[88] Similarly, the Philadelphia alcoholism specialist Donald J. Ottenberg suggested that forcible isolation might not be necessary if comprehensive treatment programs and facilities existed, "staffed by carefully selected, properly oriented and dedicated doctors, nurses, and other personnel." Locked wards, Ottenberg believed, were, for the most part, "morally unjustifiable and therapeutically unsuccessful."[89] Denver physician Sidney Dressler agreed and frequently warned colleagues at tuberculosis meetings that forcible detention was a "misapplication of police authority" by which health officials treated patients like criminals.[90] This was particularly true in facilities that confined tuberculosis patients alongside criminals. "Now I think it must be very difficult," noted Ottenberg, "to convince those patients that they are there for therapy and not for punishment."[91]

WHY SEATTLE?

Why did Seattle's Firland Sanatorium come to house the country's most aggressive policy of forcible isolation for tuberculosis patients in the 1950s? In order to answer this question, it is necessary to revisit the historical relationship of Seattle, alcoholism, and the Skid Road. Although city officials had long paid particular attention to the high rates of crime and disease on the Skid Road, they often did not adequately distinguish between these two problems. As was exemplified by the quarantining and jailing of prostitutes and other Skid Road denizens for syphilis during World War I, Seattle health officers regularly had difficulty deciding whether vagrants and transients who became sick deserved medical treatment, punishment, or both. And as was demonstrated by the Washington state Supreme Court's 1918 decision, the state's legal and governmental apparatus consistently recognized the scientific authority of these officials to carry out whatever restrictive policies they deemed necessary.

A similar intertwining of politics, punishment, and public health occurred in the case of tuberculosis control. Having once again identified a population of Skid Road alcoholics that was creating both health and legal problems, Seattle responded with its typical mixture of medical treatment and discipline. While this combination of care and coercion of uncooperative tuberculosis patients occurred to some degree throughout the United States after World War II, it was particularly pronounced in Seattle, because the patients in question so clearly raised the same incendiary issues—infectiousness, disobedience, and lawlessness—that had so long been associated with the city's Skid Road alcoholics.

Firland's policies also reflected Seattle's long-standing ambivalence as to whether alcoholism on the Skid Road needed to be cured or controlled. Beginning with the ministrations of the early mission workers through the efforts of the police farm and Alcoholics Anonymous, attempts to rehabilitate and promote abstinence among alcoholics took place throughout the twentieth century. Yet such programs had generally been overshadowed by strategies that restricted the rights and privileges of alcoholics, ranging from passage of Initiative 3 during the Progressive Era to the jailing of alcoholics in the city's "drunk tank" in the 1960s.[92] In 1967, Seattle's legalistic approach to alcoholism would be substantially reinforced by a Washington state Supreme Court ruling. In a case unsuccessfully argued by the Washington chapter of the American Civil Liberties Union, the judges ruled that public drunkenness was still considered to be a crime, even though the underlying problem—alcoholism—had been reclassified as a disease.[93]

There is one additional reason why compulsion came to dominate Seattle's attempts to treat its tuberculous alcoholics. As noted above, Cedric Northrop and other local health officials consistently used the term "recalcitrant" to describe Skid Road alcoholic patients who did not cooperate with sanatorium rules. Even though Northrop probably sincerely wished to employ compulsory measures only as a last resort, the very language he used to justify his policies likely promoted the excessive use of coercion. "At the present time," Northrop wrote in 1949, "we find that the great majority of our recalcitrants are individuals who simply can't think—they are alcoholics, and others whom we technically call 'constitutional psychopathic inferiors.' It is the same type of individual who fills up our jails and penitentiaries."[94] This conflation of criminality, mental inferiority, alcoholism, and recalcitrance helped to cement the notion, among both sanatorium staff and the general public, that alcoholic and psychiatric patients were by definition uncooperative and thus were likely to require some form of forcible isolation in order to complete their antituberculous therapy. As Joan Jackson wrote, "The probability of both renewed drinking and behavior which the staff defines as 'recalcitrant' increases in direct proportion to staff expectations that these behaviors will occur."[95]

Ironically, these stereotypical notions of alcoholism may have been reinforced by the efforts of Jackson and her colleagues to achieve a better understanding of the Skid Road culture. That is, even as she attempted to medicalize alcoholism, Jackson's emphasis on the distinctiveness of Skid Road alcoholics may have perpetuated the tendency to stigmatize these men based on preexisting assumptions and beliefs. As Jackson herself realized in retrospect, her actual charge at Firland was not to achieve a better understanding of alcoholic patients but "to come up with some specific ways of making known alcoholic patients behave the way the staff of the hospital felt patients ought to behave."[96] Thus, when alcoholics misbehaved at the sanatorium, they were punished, in effect, for violating the rules of conduct that Jackson was supposed to have established.

While the criticisms of Taylor, Ottenberg, and Dressler, in retrospect, raised valid concerns about the overuse of detention, their voices constituted a distinct minority. In the years following World War II, tuberculosis officials in the United States, with strong legal backing, pursued aggressive policies aimed at ensuring that recalcitrant patients completed their prescribed antibiotic regimens. More than any other American city, Seattle embodied this approach. Confronted with a population of tuberculous Skid Road alcoholics with a seemingly insurmountable number of sociomedical problems, Seattle "temporarily detained" them until they had received twelve months of supervised, reasonably regular antibiotic therapy. Such a regimen, sanatorium staff believed, was the minimum required to prevent the spread of tuberculosis in the community. By the end of the fifties, earlier plans to use detention only as a last resort had largely been forgotten.

Yet it would be inappropriate to view tuberculosis control among Skid Road vagrants simply as an example of "social control" of a deviant, lower class population. Once again, Firland provides a useful case study. As with its decisions regarding the use of prophylactic lung resection, Firland's policies of forcible isolation grew out of a thorough knowledge of both the Skid Road and alcoholism. By examining day-to-day life at the sanatorium in the 1950s and the 1960s, chapter 7 explores the extensive negotiations and bargaining that characterized quarantine and detention at Firland. Closer scrutiny of what transpired at Firland raises the possibility, at least, that the sanatorium's restrictive policies may have been a somewhat realistic approach to a nearly insoluble problem.

SEVEN

"A Jail in Every Sense of the Word"

Conflict and Negotiation at Firland Sanatorium

Firland Sanatorium's extensive use of coercive strategies did not go unchallenged. For example, in 1957, the Washington state chapter of the American Civil Liberties Union conducted an investigation that corroborated patients' claims that Firland was committing civil liberties violations. Yet even the ACLU ultimately registered faint opposition, at best. Some detained patients attempted to work within the system, bargaining with health officials and physicians to obtain favors. Ironically, such privileges often led to further misbehavior and thus additional punishments. If Firland physicians used the locked ward too liberally, the persistent uncooperativeness of certain patients may have made such an outcome nearly inevitable.

Glimmers of change did not come until the mid-1960s, when evolving notions of due process and legal rights produced some liberalization of existing policies at Firland. Most notably, a local judge held formal hearings at the sanatorium to evaluate complaints lodged by patients regarding detention proceedings. Yet even as confinement policies were being reevaluated, Firland staff grew increasingly reluctant to tackle the complex sociomedical problems of tuberculous Skid Road alcoholics. As tuberculosis in Seattle and the rest of the United States began to decline, so too did the notion that curing the disease entailed anything more than the ingestion of enough pills.

PATIENT PROTESTS

Although patients had periodically complained to the Firland administration about its use of forcible isolation, the years 1956 and 1957 witnessed a "small epidemic of letter-writing."[1] The letter writers constituted only a small percentage of Firland's patient population, but they distributed their missives widely. For example, they sent copies to sanatorium and health department officials, local newspapers, the district attorney's office, Governors Arthur Langlie and Albert Rosellini, U.S. senator Warren Magnuson, and even President Dwight D. Eisenhower.

At times, such letters were almost certainly the work of mentally disturbed individuals. One patient referred to local tuberculosis officer John Fountain as "Gestopo [*sic*] Fountain," terming him a "cheap booking agent for Firland Sanatorium." The sanatorium, he claimed, was "50 percent TB Hospital and 50 percent graft."[2] One woman, a former psychiatric patient at Western State Hospital who believed she did not have tuberculosis, referred to Firland as a "concentration camp" and a "little Russia."[3]

Other letters, however, were written by individuals who had become spokespersons for other patients in the institution. Only some of these people had actually spent time on the locked ward. Among the most vocal were Doris Hilberry and Courtney (Duke) Dugent, who were members of the Patients' Council and often wrote for *Firland Magazine.* Both patients had cooperated with the administration in the past, and Hilberry had written an encomium in memory of Daniel Zahn after his untimely death in 1956.[4] Although Thomas Sheehy, in succeeding Zahn, appears to have continued and formalized strategies already in place at Firland, he was often vilified by Hilberry and Dugent. Sheehy, they wrote to the *Spokane Chronicle* in 1957, "has instituted an administration which has done nothing but destroy patient morale and make people fearful of coming here, which is certainly no help in the fight to curb tuberculosis."[5] "Free-born people," they concluded, "are not accustomed to dictatorship that forces indignaties [*sic*] on them while they are helpless."[6]

If somewhat prone to hyperbole, Hilberry and Dugent offered reasoned arguments against Firland policies. In a letter to Governor Rosellini, for example, Hilberry asked why the health officer was able to quarantine noninfectious patients, thereby preventing them from having home passes. "The patients themselves," she wrote, "would be the first to condemn another who left here illegally if he were contagious, however, contagiousness has nothing to do with the quarantines." Hilberry noted that "people who have had negative sputum for months may be placed under quarantine."[7] Other patients also questioned the manner in which quarantine was employed. According to a group of Firland patients, quarantine at the sanatorium was akin to a "state of parole," which was instituted for "any deviation from a set pattern."[8]

Not surprisingly, patients registered the most objections to Ward Six. One asked why a patient returning from a valid pass after having "one or two drinks" was "treated as an alcoholic" and had a "very good chance of being thrown in jail."[9] To Hilberry, Ward Six was "a jail in every sense of the word; heavily screened windows, locked doors, cells with mattresses on concrite [*sic*] slabs and restrictions that are to be expected in a regular jail."[10] Hilberry, Dugent, and others particularly resented Sheehy's characterization of Ward Six as an "opportunity ward" or "health aid" that "has never been used as a unit for a penalty."[11]

Patients also strongly objected to the lack of formal legal proceedings prior to internment on the locked ward. The doctors, claimed one patient, "may sentence a patient from one day to six months, as they see fit. . . . We want to know by what right, and on what authority this is being done."[12] "There is no *legal* procedure involved," wrote Hilberry and Dugent, "and the patient is not allowed to defend himself in any manner, as he could in a court of law. We feel that if we are lawless enough to go to jail, we'd rather go to town to court, where we would at least have an opportunity to tell our side of the story."[13]

Patient dissatisfaction culminated in 1957 when a sympathetic former Firland employee, Harvey Hurtt, compiled a fifty-one-page report of "patients' grievances," which he sent to Governor Rosellini. Hurtt cited three specific problems: (1) the use of quarantine as punishment; (2) censorship of mail without authorization; and (3) incarceration in punishment quarters without due process. As a result of his efforts, he stated in a follow-up letter to Rosellini, he had been barred from visiting his friends at Firland.[14]

Few if any of these complaints appear to have generated much response from their recipients. Newspapers neither printed the letters nor undertook independent investigations of conditions at Firland. Government officials generally passed the letters on to the local or state health department. Most ultimately wound up on the desk of Cedric Northrop, who, ever the communicator, had volunteered to respond to them.

Although Northrop was generally an open-minded individual and was willing to listen to the complaints of individual recalcitrant patients, he had no patience whatsoever for the type of criticisms contained in these letters. In a memorandum to a colleague, he offered his advice for handling such "crank" letters written by "paranoid persons who are maladjusted in society": "We write them a polite, but firm, answer that the best and surest way to health is to cooperate with the medical staff who [have] their best interest at heart and [are] doing their best to help them. . . . Under no circumstances . . . promise that the 'matter will be given further attention.' That is exactly what these children want—attention."[15]

Yet one organization did pay attention to the letter writers: the Washington state chapter of the American Civil Liberties Union (WCLU). The WCLU had had a rocky history, having been founded in 1931, then disbanding in 1940, and reforming in 1946.[16] The WCLU had initially learned of the Firland situation when Harvey Hurtt, who was a member of the organization, submitted a copy of his report to the group's Civil Liberties Committee. After reviewing the document, the committee designated two of its members, Byron Coney and Arthur Kobler, to investigate Firland. In compiling their report, Coney, an attorney, and Kobler, a psychologist, were assisted by Robert Boland Brooks, an attorney who was at the time the WCLU executive secretary.

The subcommittee's report claimed to have "independently confirmed and enlarged upon most of the facts set out in [Hurtt's] document." The following civil liberties "abuses" existed at Firland: "mis-use of quarantine, opening of patients' mail, the assignment of patients to maximum security wards, and the use of solitary confinement."[17] These findings engendered a great deal of discussion at several meetings of the WCLU Board of Directors in 1957. While noting that the police power in use at Firland was "absolutely essential for the welfare of society," the board members agreed that such authority "is exercised at present without provision of safeguards of due process."[18] Ultimately, in December 1957, a group of WCLU members formally aired its concerns to the administrative staff of Firland.

When Seattle tuberculosis officials largely disregarded the WCLU's recommendations, the libertarians backed down. Quite simply, having identified several legitimate civil liberties violations occurring at the sanatorium, the WCLU dropped the ball. Such an outcome, to be sure, was not surprising. It was not until the 1960s that American courts significantly expanded due process protections, such as providing the accused with a fair trial and with representation by counsel. Moreover, legal rulings limiting the involuntary civil commitment of both prisoners and mental patients did not appear until the early 1970s.[19] Nevertheless, it would be eight years before WCLU members returned to Firland to take action against the exact problems they had first identified in 1957.

There are several other explanations as to why the WCLU did not pursue the Firland matter more zealously. For one, despite the fact that more aggressive detention of tuberculosis patients was occurring throughout the country, both the national ACLU and its local affiliates were focusing on cases involving the protection of free speech. This was certainly true for the WCLU, which was immersed in *Baggett v. Bullitt,* a case that challenged the constitutionality of loyalty oaths at the University of Washington.[20] The Washington ACLU chapter was also undergoing considerable internal turmoil in the late 1950s, including a temporary break with the national chapter and Brooks's stormy resignation as executive secretary in response to Kobler's election to the Board of Directors.[21]

Indeed, this latter event may have been related to the WCLU's 1957 investigation of Firland. In his unpublished history of the WCLU, Mason Morisset suggested that Brooks and Kobler had been at loggerheads ever since Brooks had attempted to insert some of his own ideas into the subcommittee report on Firland. In fact, Brooks had persuaded the Board of Directors to pass several motions urging the WCLU to make somewhat more pointed recommendations to the Firland staff. These included discontinuing the routine use of solitary confinement cells and educating incoming patients about the process of quarantine.[22] Yet, according to Morisset, Brooks had resented being excluded from greater participation in the matter. While Morisset concludes that the Brooks-Kobler affair may ultimately have represented a personality clash, the evidence also suggests that Brooks, once termed "personally and completely devoted to civil liberties"[23] by a WCLU colleague, may actually have feared that a whitewash of the Firland situation was imminent. Brooks's departure from the WCLU in 1958 ensured that the issue would remain on the back burner.

STAFF-PATIENT NEGOTIATIONS

If those patients seeking to reform Firland's use of quarantine and detention made little headway, others relied on a more subtle strategy of bargaining to combat the elaborate rules in operation at the sanatorium. As in the institutions described by Erving Goffman and Julius A. Roth,[24] much of the negotiation between staff and patients at Firland centered on issues of "privileges and punishments." If bad behavior warranted punishment, patients argued, then good behavior should be rewarded. One such reward formally existed within the city's public health regulations. When quarantined patients exhibited medical improvement, "good behavior," and "cooperation with . . . staff physicians," they often qualified for a status of "modified" quarantine that permitted them to have twenty-four- or forty-eight-hour passes.[25] While this new status was granted by the Seattle–King County Health Department, John Fountain relied heavily on the reports of the Firland staff in relaxing the quarantine.

The implementation of modified quarantine provoked considerable contention. Firland physicians often disagreed with patients' claims that their clinical condition and comportment had improved sufficiently to warrant a relaxation of restrictions. Occasionally, the situation resolved itself. When a physician presented one patient with his modified quarantine order in 1957, she found him to be drunk and thus destroyed the letter.[26] Most often, however, intense negotiations occurred between physicians and patients.

This system of give-and-take extended to a whole range of privileges sought by patients. Despite Roberts Davies' efforts to improve sanatorium life, day-to-day existence at Firland was rather mundane. Recovering patients generally felt well and received little therapy aside from daily antibiotics. Seeking and attaining privileges made hospitalization less monotonous. The charts of alcoholic patients are full of letters requesting various favors, in which they express remorse for past indiscretions and promise good behavior in the future. For example, when requesting a typewriter for use on Ward Six, one patient wrote: "I'm quite sure you'll cure my T.B., however this alcoholic problem is much more dangerous to me, and I'll have to be the Dr. there, this is the ground work to it I am laying now, in other words this is my first prescription to myself."[27]

Physicians who acceded to requests for these and other types of favors frequently came to regret these decisions. Of E.N., a forty-five-year-old laborer and "chronic alcoholic," one doctor wrote: "This patient asked for a town leave on 9-20-56 and inasmuch as he had recently become negative, this was granted for twelve hours. He returned from this leave one hour late, quiet, but apparently had done some drinking because he was nauseated during the night. The following morning he dressed quietly and has not been seen since that time."[28] When P.G., a migrant farmworker in his twenties, was sent from Ward Six to the open wards in 1956, his physician offered him a carrot as opposed to a stick. "I had a long discussion with him," the physician wrote, "pointing up to him the reasons for his trouble before and giving him an opportunity to accept medical recommendations at the present time." The doctor added that he had been "fairly liberal" with the patient "and allowed him full bathroom privileges with showers and gave him a recreation pass with the only restriction being that he remain on the Ward at all other times. Two days later, P.G. was noted to have a "strong odor of alcohol on his breath." When questioned, he admitted to drinking. P. G. was subsequently returned to Ward Six.[29] In yet another case, a detained Native American housewife who had previously gone AWOL pleaded for early release to the open ward. "And I *promise* that I'll *never* do such a foolish thing again!" she wrote. Although she kept her word for three months, she eventually escaped from the sanatorium, only to be returned to Ward Six one week later.[30]

The most notorious case in which a patient reneged on a promise to sanatorium staff may have been that of Beatrice Tolbert. In August 1960, Tolbert, a thirty-nine-year-old Firland patient and former nurse, drove into an oncoming car, killing the other vehicle's two passengers, a mother and her three-year-old daughter. Already late from her twenty-four-hour pass and having had three highballs at lunch, Tolbert had a Breathalyzer reading of .210, well over the .150 limit for intoxication. The tragic event received a great deal of coverage in the local newspapers. A prominent headline in the *Seattle Times,* for example, read "Drinking by Patients Big Problem, Says Firland Director." The accident reinforced sanatorium physicians' misgivings about giving privileges to patients who were likely to abuse them.[31]

The news that special favors granted to alcoholics or other quarantined patients had backfired quickly reached other Firland residents via the sanatorium's active gossip network. The Patients' Council was particularly concerned and told the administration that the "discrepancies of a few" should not threaten the entitlements of all patients.[32] Yet even when privileges were not abused, they still remained problematic. The granting of exceptions ran counter to Firland's efforts during the 1950s to codify its quarantine and detention procedures. Introducing arbitrariness into the system, Joan Jackson discovered in her sociological research, led Skid Road alcoholics to conclude that the staff was insincere and weak. This conclusion, in turn, may have encouraged alcoholics to further challenge the system.[33]

Arbitrariness was an even greater problem in the case of punishments. Although regulations prohibiting unapproved discharges and drinking ostensibly applied to all patients, in practice Skid Road alcoholics generally received harsher punishments. Once again, this disparity resulted from the concern about maintaining order at the sanatorium. Skid Road alcoholics who drank at Firland or returned to the sanatorium after a "drunk" tended to be disruptive. In contrast, the "middle-class" alcoholics identified by Jackson usually drank quietly in their rooms. As they rarely "caused a commotion," they were neither quarantined nor detained for drinking.[34] Similarly, Firland staff was also reluctant to lock up non-Skid Road patients who had eloped. "It always poses a difficult problem," wrote Cedric Northrop of an uncooperative King County dentist, "when a professional man has tuberculosis and doesn't cooperate well."[35] Not surprisingly, certain Ward Six patients complained "very bitterly" about "favoritism" and "inconsistency in the rules and regulations."[36]

Skid Road alcoholics themselves were also treated arbitrarily. Although the sanatorium physicians tried to enforce the policy of progressively longer stays on Ward Six, the existing regulations did not address certain situations. For example, what should the staff do about frankly manipulative patients who refused medications or other treatment if they remained on the locked ward?[37] What about patients whose violent behavior posed a threat on the open wards? Should exceptions be made in such cases? Finally, what strategy was to be used for the confinement of patients who remained at Firland for many years and required multiple stays on the ward?

All of these questions arose in the case of D.A., a white unskilled laborer and Skid Road alcoholic who would spend most of the last seventeen years of his life at Firland. D.A., wrote one physician, was "one of the most recalcitrant patients in the history of Firland Sanatorium. His attitude was impossible and his behavior appalling."[38] During a seven-year stay at Firland between 1951 and 1958, D.A. had thirteen admissions to Ward Six. He also threatened a nurse with a bottle on at least one occasion. The situation was further complicated by D.A.'s frequent refusal to take antibiotics when interned on Ward Six. The patient's erratic compliance had led to the development of bacteria resistant to both para-aminosalicylic acid (PAS) and isoniazid (INH), which, in turn, made the possibility of a cure and an approved discharge highly unlikely.

Having long since exhausted the existing confinement protocol, the Ward Six Committee struggled with the question of how to discipline D.A. Ultimately, it decided to make him a "permanent ward sixer," although it continued to give him periodic chances on the open wards in order to get him to take his antibiotics. Elopements and drinking violations routinely followed such trials. Readmitted to Firland in 1959, D.A. once again spent most of his hospitalization on the locked ward until he suffered a stroke and died in 1967 at the age of sixty-six.

A similar pattern of negotiation characterized the three hospitalizations of S.M., a middle-aged machinist and veteran with a "history of heavy drinking," first admitted to Firland in 1964. S.M., who also took his medications sporadically and developed drug-resistant disease, was another patient who defied the rules established to deal with misbehavior. He spent almost none of his three years at Firland on the open wards. In a situation that closely resembled the notorious "revolving door" of alcoholics jailed on public drunkenness charges,[39] S.M. constantly escaped from the locked ward, only to be readmitted there each time he was returned to the sanatorium. A typical sequence occurred in 1965: on August 3, he threatened a Ward Six orderly with cut glass, obtained the orderly's keys, and escaped over the hospital fence; on August 19, he was readmitted, inebriated, to Ward Six; on September 4, he again broke out of the locked ward as the food cart was brought in; on September 9, he once again returned in a state of inebriation.[40]

The fact that Ward Six patients were allowed to "escape" from Firland also bespoke a policy of negotiation. At times, health care personnel, sanatorium guards, and deputies from the county sheriff's office used force to quell disturbances on the wards. Yet Firland was not a prison by design. For the most part, staff was instructed to let potentially violent patients leave the sanatorium, either from the open wards or Ward Six.[41] Given that Firland had established an ambitious program of detention that had easily withstood periodic legal challenges, such a lenient attitude regarding escapes seems paradoxical at first glance. Why go through the trouble of locking up recalcitrant individuals if the mere threat of violence would win them release?

One explanation for this policy is that escapes actually occurred relatively infrequently. Moreover, as we have seen, escapees often returned to Firland within a few days, either accompanied by the police or of their own volition. The fact that many patients willingly returned, despite the likelihood of a period of detention, suggests an unspoken compromise. Patients insisting on occasional drinking sprees would be allowed to "escape" with the presumption that they would return for further hospitalization. Of course, many patients who eloped from Firland never looked back. Yet the frequency of return admissions probably discouraged Cedric Northrop and other government officials from pushing for absolute control over uncooperative patients. Elements of negotiation and compromise would always persist.

At the same time, Firland hardly took its role as protector of the public health lightly. Working in conjunction with the state Liquor Control

Board and the federal Tax Alcohol Unit, many staff members participated in "stings" designed to thwart the smuggling of liquor into the sanatorium. One physician who helped organize such efforts was Walter Miller, a genial Scotsman who arrived at Firland in 1955 and soon took over operation of Ward Six. In one instance, Miller admitted a phony patient with actual Skid Road connections who was supposed to infiltrate a bootlegging ring. The man entered on a Friday, thus delaying until Monday his admission chest X-ray (which would have revealed that he did not have tuberculosis). At other times, Miller and the liquor board received tips from the local Lake City package store, indicating that a Firland patient was making a large purchase. When the patient returned to the sanatorium, sneaking over or under the surrounding fence, Miller and his colleagues would be waiting. Although his extensive training in London and at Cornell University Medical School in New York City had been in chest medicine and not law enforcement, Miller quite enjoyed these stakeouts. He even came in on his days off to participate.[42]

Other sanatoriums outside Washington state also used employees as "detective[s] . . . to find out who is bringing in liquor and who the troublemakers are among the patient population."[43] The conflict of interest that such activities entailed was quite apparent—not only to staff members involved in ambushes but also to those who participated in any aspect of detention. As one Firland physician asked, "How can you ever build up a positive relationship when you send a patient to Ward Six?"[44] The undesirable role of "double agent" was a particularly difficult issue for Firland's nurses, who were actually responsible for much of the day-to-day enforcement of the medical director's detention orders.

HOLDING COURT AT FIRLAND

Firland finally began to reassess its use of quarantine and detention in 1964. The decision to do so stemmed from several ongoing developments, both in society and at the sanatorium itself. Perhaps most important was the major expansion of the rights of the institutionalized, one of many movements during the 1960s that questioned authority and promoted the rights of "oppressed" groups. First, a series of rulings by the U.S. Supreme Court, including *Mapp v. Ohio, Gideon v. Wainwright,* and *Miranda v. Arizona,* incorporated into the due process clause of the Fourteenth Amendment the rights to compulsory process, a speedy trial, and trial by jury. Of even more importance were a series of cases at the state and national level—many of which were litigated by the ACLU—in which courts intervened in the management of prisoners and the mentally ill. These rulings placed significant limits on the methods by which institutions maintained order and, in the case of mental hospitals, circumscribed involuntary commitment policies that deprived persons of their civil liberties.[45]

Changes were also occurring at Firland. Byron F. Francis, the well-respected doyen of Seattle's chest physicians, had taken over for Thomas Sheehy as sanatorium medical director. Sheehy had taken it upon himself to convince his subordinates of the necessity and worthiness of the locked ward. Francis, on the other hand, viewed the ward more as an albatross. By the time he assumed his duties at Firland, Francis was fifty-nine years old and in declining health. He rarely visited Ward Six and preferred to leave the details of its operation to others.

Yet as Francis tried to play down the issue of forcible detention, members of his staff had begun to question the same rules and regulations that certain patients had long criticized. In a letter to Francis in 1964, Sue M. Berger, an alcoholism program assistant, asked whether "patients [are] confined because they really need the kind of care they can only receive on a locked ward, or . . . because we feel the need to punish them?" She was convinced, Berger concluded, "that we are not consistent in the enforcement of our current policies."[46] Both staff and patients, noted other observers, increasingly referred to detention on Ward Six as "punishment," which, in turn, caused growing resentment among persons placed on the ward.[47] As movements promoting social justice for the poor and disadvantaged gained strength in the 1960s, commentators both in Seattle and elsewhere became more outwardly critical of detention policies that treated tuberculous alcoholics "as if they were criminals."[48]

Echoing the objections to mandatory confinement of the mentally ill, the one-year hospitalization rule for alcoholics at Firland also came under attack. "Although it may seem logical," wrote the authors of a 1964 Department of Health study of the state's remaining three sanatoriums, "there is no objective evidence that the twelve months is more successful in preventing readmission than a shorter holding period."[49] Berger agreed, urging Francis to evaluate the utility of the one-year policy. "If adequate data does not show that this policy has significantly reduced relapse rates in 'unreliable' patients, we must be willing to replace it with a better approach."[50] One small study, in fact, had found that twelve of fifteen Skid Road alcoholics discharged from Firland had continued to take their medications.[51]

Meanwhile, certain patients continued to voice their objections to the use of quarantine and detention through letters to sanatorium and government officials. Yet in contrast with the late 1950s, these critics now had a somewhat more effective mouthpiece: *Firland Magazine.* Whereas patient magazines such as *Firland* had traditionally echoed the philosophy of sanatorium administrators, the magazine now periodically printed complaints about hospital policies. "It seems it would be nice to have a 'Doctor-Patient' relationship," wrote one patient in 1962, "rather than a discipline set up." [52]

If *Firland* at times voiced the concerns of patients regarding issues of confinement, more often the magazine treated the subject as a type of standing joke. Its barbs were directed both at the Skid Road characters most likely to be detained and at the staff administrators and physicians who dutifully enforced the system. Readers of the February 1963 edition of *Firland,* for example, were treated to the following poem, entitled "Ward 6":

> No matter what I do "for kicks,"
> I'm always ending up in "6,"
> As anyone can plainly see,
> This must be where I like to be.
> The keys and locks could go — it's true,
> And heavy screens don't help our view.
> But if in "6" I have to stay,
> My friends are with me — anyway.[53]

The locked ward received similar treatment in a *Firland* advice column entitled "San Landers." "Dear San Landers," read one letter, "If you get a twenty-four-hour pass and stay forty-eight will they put you in six if it's the first time?" "Can't answer that one," the purported advisor replied. "Try it and let me know!" [54] *Firland*'s humorous commentary on disciplinary issues included topics other than Ward Six. A photograph in the December 1962 edition, entitled "SAN-did Camera," featured a patient escaping over the Firland fence.[55]

This combination of growing internal criticism of confinement and a changing legal climate led Firland to relax a number of its rules. By the middle to late 1960s, Ward Six patients were allowed out of doors during the day and had permission to work at the Boeing sheltered workshop. The administration redecorated the locked ward and converted a portion of it into a "minimum-security area." Eventually, use of the locked detoxification cells was discontinued.[56] The staff also grew more tolerant of patients who drank on the premises. As long as they remained "orderly," even Skid Road patients "suspected of drinking almost daily" were allowed to remain on unlocked wards. Much of the credit for these reforms belonged to Jonathan Ostrow, a young pulmonologist who joined the Firland staff in 1968 and became its last medical director in 1970.

The most striking change in Firland policy, however, occurred in 1965. Having received requests from Byron Francis for assistance in reviewing Firland's detention procedures, representatives of the WCLU and the civil liberties committee of the Seattle Bar Association devised a solution that provided formal legal redress for sanatorium patients. Beginning in January, a local District Court judge, Robert M. Elston, held monthly sessions at Firland to hear complaints from Ward Six patients. Also attending these meetings was George E. Hames, a longtime Firland physician who served as acting medical director between Francis's retirement in 1965 and the arrival of Jonathan Ostrow. A few patients requested legal assistance prior to these hearings, although lawyers rarely, if ever, attended the actual proceedings.

This innovative solution for addressing questions of commitment and institutionalization appears to have been unprecedented in this era. By the 1970s, once cases involving the rights of prisoners and the mentally ill became commonplace, local magistrates often traveled to and observed the actual institutional setting.[57] Yet it is noteworthy that the precedent for this type of activity took place in a tuberculosis sanatorium.

Not only did Firland permit Ward Six patients to have hearings with Judge Elston after 1965, but it also further formalized the process by which patients were sent to the locked ward. All persons placed on Ward Six received a memorandum that indicated the reason for detention and the duration of confinement and offered patients a hearing with the judge. This memorandum was then placed in the patient's chart. The stated reasons for detention included:

1. Drinking on the wards, or on the premises
2. Possession of alcoholic beverages on the premises
3. Gift or sale of alcoholic beverages to other patients
4. Violation of quarantine, including AWOL
5. Participating in gambling
6. Specific request of the health officer, prosecuting attorney, or court
7. Other causes

In practice, the medical director generally cited numbers 1 or 4.

Many patients indicated on the memorandum that they did not want a hearing with Judge Elston. Interestingly, those who did request hearings often had no complaints about civil liberties issues but rather were dissatisfied with certain aspects of care at Firland. One patient, for example, informed the judge that he had no objections to his confinement on Ward Six but just wanted to see an eye doctor. Others, however, disputed their sentences, such as the patient who wrote the word "lie" on the portion of the memorandum that indicated he had been drinking on the wards.[58]

At times, Judge Elston, or other justices of the peace who came to Firland in later years, sided with patients, indicating that the sanatorium staff had overstepped its bounds. For example, Judge Elston reversed a decision made by the Ward Six Committee to detain "indefinitely" B.V., a farmworker in his fifties, after he left Firland without permission for the second time. Having decided that B.V. was being treated unlike other patients, Elston decreased his internment to one month. To the surprise of no one, B.V. "disappeared" from the sanatorium four weeks after returning to the open portion of Firland and never returned.[59]

Much more commonly, however, Judge Elston agreed with the decisions made by Firland staff, even if such decisions appeared to conflict with accepted practice. One typical example occurred when S.M., the machinist described above, contested the hospital's decision to detain him indefinitely on Ward Six. Although such a punishment was not stipulated in the locked ward policy manual, Judge Elston upheld the sentence in order to "protect the public and also to assure [S.M.'s] own treatment," both of which had proven impossible on an open ward.[60]

A similar situation arose in the case of G.Z., a transient in his late thirties who carried the diagnoses of chronic alcoholism and a character disorder, in addition to tuberculosis. At the time of his second offense in April 1967, he was placed on the locked ward for three months, rather than the usual one month; similarly, for his third offense, he received a six-month stay as opposed to the standard two months. The Ward Six Committee had justified this action "because of his previous history of leaving hospitals AWOL." When G.Z. complained to Judge Elston about the arbitrariness of such treatment, he was informed that Firland "had not acted improperly in confining him to the locked ward."[61]

Judge Elston's presence at the sanatorium, therefore, did not transform the nature of detention at Firland. To be sure, it took much larger offenses as a rule—most notably, frequent elopements—for the staff to employ disciplinary tactics, but such measures continued to be used as they had been in the past. Thus, as late as 1971, one-third of all Firland patients were under quarantine orders, and one-quarter spent time on Ward Six. In addition, the staff still detained persons with inactive disease.[62] Physicians also continued to recommend that certain patients be hospitalized for a minimum of one year because they were chronic alcoholics. The treatment in 1972 of G.B., a former salesman in his mid-forties who was a "regular member of the Skid Road community," differed little from what he might have received in the 1950s. The Ward Six Committee, for example, voted G.B. an indefinite stay on the locked ward. Eventually, the patient received a right-upper-lobe segmental resection. Noting that G.B. was an alcoholic, transient loner without a regular job or family, one physician wrote that "the main indication for surgery here was the adverse social status."[63]

The fact that Judge Elston largely acted as a rubber stamp for Firland's detention policies should come as no surprise. Despite the gesture of ensuring due process protections for the civil commitment of tuberculosis patients, few persons in Seattle were eager to release potentially infectious Skid Road alcoholics from confinement that physicians indicated was necessary. The

Department of Health nearly always won the occasional legal challenges raised by patients. Indeed, in 1967, Firland's policies received formal legal validation when the Washington state legislature passed a law giving health officials the right to indefinitely quarantine people suffering from tuberculosis. Such a quarantine, moreover, could occur without the provision of an attorney or a detention hearing.[64]

If detention policies remained relatively unchanged during Firland's last decade of operation, so too did the demographic composition of those detained. The denizens of Ward Six in the late 1960s continued to be Skid Road transients, many of whom had formerly worked as loggers, cooks, and farm laborers. Although there were a growing number of blacks and Native Americans on the locked ward, some 70 percent of detained men were white.[65]

The racial and social composition of the women placed on Ward Six also remained stable from 1954 until Firland closed in 1973. In contrast with the men, however, detained women were predominantly Native American—67 percent (ten of fifteen) of the total in 1957 and 64 percent (nine of fourteen) in 1964, for example. While a number of these women worked as barmaids on the Skid Road, others came from small towns in western Washington—such as Salkum, Neah Bay, and Pacific Beach—that were home to various Native American tribes. With the closure of all but one of the state's other sanatoriums (Edgecliff, in Spokane), Firland had gradually become responsible for hospitalizing all tuberculosis patients who lived west of the Cascade Mountains.

The women detained on Ward Six were perhaps the most stigmatized patients at Firland. The staff certainly looked down on male Skid Road alcoholics, but in the 1950s alcoholic drinking was seen as "acceptable" male behavior. By contrast, alcoholism among females carried especially strong negative associations: women who drank were often viewed as either masculine or excessively promiscuous.[66] Moreover, the fact that a majority of women requiring detention were Native Americans served to reinforce the stereotype of the Indian as "unreliable, shiftless, demanding, alcoholic, somewhat potentially or actually criminal, [and] unable to form long, intimate relationships."[67]

The hostility shown at times to female Native American patients is demonstrated by the case of N.M., a young alcoholic woman of mixed American Indian and white descent. During her hospitalization in 1954, she attacked an aide and was sent to Ward Six. Even Thomas Holmes, who had been asked to interview N.M. in her "cell" on the locked ward, was thoroughly frustrated by this admittedly difficult patient. "She is at times vindictive and vituperative," Holmes wrote, "show[ing] impulsive outbursts of anger during which time she is completely uncontrollable." Due to her "bizarre and erratic behavior," Holmes recommended that she be managed as a "permanent resident of Ward Six."[68] It is notable that statements in N.M.'s chart consistently equated her ethnic heritage and behavior through the use of expressions such as "This wild young Indian girl" and "This twenty-three-year-old irresponsible Indian girl."

BALANCING COERCION AND REHABILITATION

Despite the evident disdain that certain staff members had for uncooperative patients, such as alcoholic women, Firland in the 1960s did not rely merely on coercive strategies to reach such individuals. As in the previous decade, the sanatorium continued to search for ways to address the social and rehabilitative needs of both its female and male alcoholic patients. By the beginning of the decade, however, Joan Jackson, who had initiated such programs at Firland, had begun to focus on other interests, notably Al-Anon, an organization that addressed the impact of alcoholism on families. Jackson formally ended her relationship with Firland in 1964 when she moved to New Haven, Connecticut. By the early 1960s, Thomas Holmes, too, had left Firland, increasingly emphasizing his research on life change events.

Yet even as Jackson and Holmes loosened their ties to Firland, sanatorium staff inaugurated a second phase of alcoholism work. The first phase, which had included Jackson's research, educational programs regarding alcoholism, and the Anti-Tuberculosis League's vocational rehabilitation project, had been ambitious and well received. Yet, as of 1962, Firland still "failed . . . badly" in treating patients' alcoholism. Alcoholics, staff members conceded, continued to drink at a rate "close to 100 percent" after discharge.[69]

The second phase of Firland's program, which was inaugurated by a National Institute of Mental Health (NIMH) workshop held in Seattle in 1962, sought to establish "an intensive treatment program for tuberculosis-alcoholism and for the social and psychological problems which are correlated so often with this dual illness."[70] This strategy, Jackson explained to the workshop's 170 participants, entailed efforts both within the sanatorium and by community agencies, which were well represented at the conference. As had its earlier efforts, the second phase of Firland's tuberculosis-alcoholism work set the standard for many other sanatoriums and communities attempting to establish similar programs.[71] The involvement of the NIMH at the Seattle workshop, as well as at another tuberculosis-alcoholism conference at Glenn Dale, Maryland, in 1959, paralleled the agency's attempts in the early 1960s to develop community mental health centers that treated drug addiction as a disease rather than a crime.[72]

The man who implemented the hospital phase of this new program, Ronald J. Fagan, was as intriguing an individual as his predecessor, Joan Jackson.

A tall man with a hooked nose and a soft voice, he was, in the words of the noted Seattle journalist Emmett Watson, "the only person I've ever been around who truly embodied the quality of greatness." Fagan had spent much of his youth haunting the speakeasies along First Avenue, drinking "everything from rotgut bootleg whiskey to raw alcohol to fortified wine to canned heat."[73] But in 1947, having traveled the skid rows of the West Coast for most of his thirty-seven years, Fagan had taken offense when Seattle Municipal Court judge John Neergaard referred to him as "a common drunk" and sentenced him to the Seattle Police alcoholism farm.[74] At the police farm, Fagan took a job as a cook and began to turn his life around. Eventually, having stopped drinking, he enrolled at Seattle University and began work as an alcoholism counselor. Fagan obtained his college degree in 1960, graduating magna cum laude. By this time, he had become a nationally recognized authority on treating alcoholism among the same Skid Road population to which he had once belonged.[75] Fagan, according to Watson, treated, counseled, and saved the lives of thousands of alcoholics.

Fagan worked periodically at Firland in the late 1950s and was formally hired in 1961. Fagan's title, special consultant on medical and social problems, was vivid testimony to Firland's persistent attempts to characterize tuberculosis as a social disease.[76] With the goal of creating a "total in-hospital program" to encourage all sanatorium staff to view treatment of alcoholism as part of their primary responsibility, Fagan and several colleagues formalized and accelerated the types of strategies begun by Joan Jackson: systematic in-service staff education on alcoholism, individual and group counseling for alcoholics, and Alcoholics Anonymous meetings. In addition, Fagan established a special ward to "resocialize" a selected group of "socially marginal" alcoholic tuberculosis patients, although he conceded that this goal was realistic for only a small number of individuals."[77]

Because he himself had hit "rock bottom" and spoke their language, Fagan had a great influence on Skid Road alcoholic patients at Firland. It is impossible to know to what extent Fagan's entreaties and his own inspirational history led alcoholics at the sanatorium to pull themselves up by the bootstraps much as he had. Fagan's own data on the percentage of alcoholic patients who had stopped drinking or had become more cooperative with their tuberculosis therapy were inconclusive.[78]

Clearly, however, Fagan's attempts to get Firland staff to intensify its focus on alcoholism were largely unsuccessful. "Apparently," wrote Fagan and coworker Arnold S. Linsky in their 1966 evaluation of the program, "the only members of the Firland staff who were completely committed to the importance of the alcoholism program were the alcoholism program director and [his] staff."[79] There were several explanations for this lack of enthusiasm.

One problem was Fagan himself, who, by his own account, was "viewed as an outsider, with a different background, with different goals and values."[80]

Another impediment was the continued assumption of Firland staff that alcoholism work would result in a "low success ratio, poor patient cooperation, and a . . . lack of appreciation." This opinion, Fagan believed, resulted from the persistent perception of alcoholics as "unacceptable people"—not as persons suffering from a disease.[81] Given the continued stigma surrounding alcoholism, staff members had remained wary of being viewed as "treaters of alcoholics rather than of tuberculosis patients."[82] Such attitudes were hardly limited to Firland. One sanatorium administrator, as quoted by Philadelphia tuberculosis specialist Donald Ottenberg, wrote the following about his own staff's response to alcoholic patients: "Most of the recalcitrant patients, in the opinion of the staff, are just plain bums and the staff is sick and tired of the maudlin sympathy which is sometimes showered upon these people by ill-advised social workers, because they have never seen anything constructive come out of this."[83]

Yet what ultimately thwarted Fagan's program, which was discontinued in December 1964, was the unwillingness of Firland staff to alter its traditionally established routines. Although the Firland administration had been sincere in its efforts to establish an alcoholism treatment program, the institution remained first and foremost a tuberculosis sanatorium. "We set our sights low," recalled staff physician Helen S. Marshall, who began work at Firland in 1949 and ran the locked ward from the early 1960s to 1973. "We could get them over their TB, but I wasn't sure we could do much about their alcoholism."[84] Even Fagan acknowledged that the major goal of his program had been to "return the tuberculosis-alcoholism patient to the community in good physical health with the danger of relapse from tuberculosis held to a minimum."[85]

Among the existing routines that Firland sought to preserve was its use of disciplinary measures. Although Fagan was at times critical of Ward Six, his alcoholism treatment program did not challenge the sanatorium's policies regarding detention. Even patients on Fagan's special ward continued to be sent to Ward Six if they committed infractions. Thus, even though Firland did "considerable soul searching about the extent to which [quarantine and detention] are beneficial with respect to the patient's alcoholism,"[86] the underlying message was clear: Firland physicians would continue to do whatever they believed had the best chance of controlling tuberculosis. In the face of a feared disease that presented a major public health threat, Ron Fagan was unable to use tuberculosis as a wedge either to treat alcoholism or to improve the lives of the "socially marginal."[87]

COERCION IN RETROSPECT

"Prisoner at the bar, you have been accused of the great crime of laboring under pulmonary consumption, and after an impartial trial before a jury of your countrymen, you have been found guilty.... You are a bad and dangerous person, and stand branded in the eyes of your fellow-countrymen with one of the most heinous known offenses."[88] So spoke the judge in *Erehwon,* Samuel Butler's 1872 satire of English society. In Butler's imaginary country of Erehwon ("nowhere" spelled backwards), merely being unfortunate was itself a crime. Hence, the prisoner referred to above, having been diagnosed with tuberculosis, was sentenced to "imprisonment, with hard labor, for the rest of your miserable existence."[89]

Given the coercion of patients that occurred at Firland Sanatorium, it may be tempting to draw an analogy with Butler's Erehwon. Many social historians, in studying the response of health officials and physicians to epidemics and other illnesses among disadvantaged groups, have interpreted such events through a "social control" model.[90] That is, in response to disease outbreaks, society has relied too heavily on strategies that regulate the behaviors of supposedly infectious or dangerous individuals.

Underlying such historical interpretations has been the centrality of the institution. First, health officials have been quick to rely on institutionalization when confronted with infectious diseases among "deviant" populations. Second, those confined have been subject to the ramifications of internment. Specifically, the custodial need to manage the behavior of those detained has regularly become conflated with the medical care that such individuals receive. Such was the case in the Progressive Era mental hospitals and prisons studied by David Rothman, where the need to maintain institutional order ultimately thwarted a series of ambitious therapeutic initiatives designed to help patients and prisoners become productive members of society. "To join assistance to coercion," Rothman concludes, "is to create a tension that cannot persist indefinitely and will be far more likely to be resolved on the side of coercion."[91]

At first glance, the "militant zeal"[92] with which postwar tuberculosis workers at Firland and elsewhere pursued their policies of detention may suggest a similar story. After all, by the 1950s and 1960s, with the discovery of antibiotics and the development of impressive new surgical techniques, the medical profession had reached the pinnacle of its authority. Physicians, as we have seen, casually recommended certain medical procedures based on "sociologic" factors, such as a patient's ethnicity, race, or social circumstances. Meanwhile, public health officials who significantly restricted the activities of presumably infectious persons continued to enjoy broad legal and societal support. The logical outcome of this broad authority in the realms of medicine and public health was the temporary detention of socially deviant, potentially infectious tuberculous skid row alcoholics. As in earlier institutions, the desire to control behavior on the wards of Firland Sanatorium became inextricably intertwined with the actual mission of the facility—preventing the spread of tuberculosis in the community.

That a West Coast city, Seattle, most strikingly came to embody the maxim *Salus populi suprema lex* (The public health is the highest law)[93] should come as no surprise. As with the syphilitic prostitutes jailed in the city during World War I, the presence of stigmatizing medical conditions—tuberculosis and alcoholism—only added to the disrepute with which Seattle already held the largely migrant population that resided on the city's Skid Road. That physicians had recently classified alcoholism as a medical disease requiring rehabilitation mattered little when physicians and nurses in Seattle invoked terms such as "uncooperative" and "recalcitrant" in a manner that confirmed existing stereotypes about Skid Road alcoholics. Ultimately, it proved easier to change the definition of alcoholism than to change long-standing attitudes about Skid Road alcoholics.

Perhaps the most damning feature of Seattle and Washington state's detention policies was their violation of the very guidelines and protections that health officials had carefully designed. When Firland established its program of detention, Medical Director Roberts Davies had warned that overuse of coercion "was a sure sign that something is wrong." Later, he urged his colleagues to "lean over backwards" to prevent the inappropriate use of quarantine. Even before Davies' departure in 1954, however, the cultural forces promoting physician authority, institutional order, and suppression of deviant behavior had begun to foster the overuse of quarantine and detention. Ultimately, Firland was guilty based not on modern standards but its own standards.[94]

Yet to compare Seattle with Erehwon is too simple. In contrast to the earlier tuberculosis workers described by Sheila Rothman, Firland staff members did not lose their hearts as they cured lungs.[95] Although Firland did employ quarantine and detention to discipline Skid Road alcoholics, as confirmed by the Washington Civil Liberties Union in 1957, the sanatorium's motives were not solely punitive. For one thing, by keeping a segment of recalcitrant Skid Road alcoholics hospitalized and properly medicated for up to twelve months, detention most likely contributed to the cures of patients who otherwise would have died. One such patient was K.G., a fifty-year-old farmworker admitted to Firland in 1970 with active pulmonary tuberculosis. K.G. had drunk heavily since age sixteen and continued to do so while at the sanatorium. After nine months at Firland, most of which was spent in the locked ward, the patient was discharged with medical advice and inactive tuberculosis. As of 1986, K.G. was alive and had not relapsed.[96]

Of course, such an anecdote hardly constitutes conclusive evidence. Perhaps, if given the chance, K.G. might have stayed in the unlocked portion of Firland long enough to be treated successfully. Lacking well-controlled studies that examined the outcomes of detained and nondetained patients, it is difficult to prove that forcible confinement was beneficial either to individual patients or as a public health measure. Even with access to much more extensive data, historians and epidemiologists continue to debate whether the dramatic fall in tuberculosis mortality during the twentieth century resulted from improved living conditions, better nutrition, public health campaigns, or the changing virulence of the tubercle bacillus.[97] What is clear, however, is that tuberculosis workers in Seattle strongly believed that their use of forcible isolation contributed significantly to the city's rapidly declining tuberculosis death rate. It was no coincidence, Cedric Northrop and his colleagues argued, that Washington state—which had perhaps the most aggressive program of detention—had experienced the country's largest decrease in tuberculosis mortality between 1946 and 1958.[98]

But even if such a consequentialist argument—that the end (control of tuberculosis) justified the means (detention)—is unsatisfying, there are other reasons to view Firland's coercive policies as more than just punitive. For one thing, Firland staff's advocacy of aggressive surgical treatment, prolonged hospitalization, and involuntary detention was based on intimate knowledge of the lives of Skid Road patients, many of whom remained hospitalized in the sanatorium for years. In contrast with other hospitals and with jail, where Skid Roaders were treated with "indifference at best and often hostility and contempt," even detained alcoholics at Firland "got a pretty good shake,"[99] receiving both close medical attention and the benefits of a therapeutic milieu. Indeed, some Skid Road alcoholics told Firland staff that they preferred the structure of Ward Six to the unlocked portion of the sanatorium, with its constant temptations of liquor and gambling.[100]

In retrospect, Joan Jackson, Ron Fagan, and others at Firland who promoted Alcoholics Anonymous, rehabilitation measures, and the destigmatization of alcoholism were perhaps the strongest advocates these men and women had anywhere in society. Even Cedric Northrop, the redoubtable "policeman of the Northwest," had proposed in 1957 that Washington state convert at least one of its remaining tuberculosis sanatoriums into an "alcoholic research and treatment center."[101] It is true that other municipalities declined to enforce quarantine ordinances for alcoholics with tuberculosis. Yet that decision may have been based on concerns other than civil liberties. At least one physician active in tuberculosis control claimed that New York City officials viewed tuberculosis on skid row as a "self limiting" problem that "should be allowed to contain itself."[102]

Firland staff developed a series of complex strategies for addressing comportment problems within the institution. Even as physicians and nurses implemented an extensive program of coercion, they actively negotiated and bargained with patients, using any number of incentives to improve cooperation and thereby avoid confinement. All too often, such efforts at assistance either backfired or were rejected. Throughout the 1950s and 1960s, a large percentage of Skid Road alcoholics hospitalized at Firland continued to get drunk, go AWOL, or both. Given this reality, staff members increasingly came to view Ward Six as a last-ditch mechanism for providing essential medical treatment to their alcoholic patients and for preventing the spread of tuberculosis in the community.

Yet the strategies used at Firland did not arise only from practical considerations. In the postwar era, paternalism still exerted a strong influence on the decision making of health professionals. Viewed from this perspective, some Firland staff believed that periodic use of the locked ward was an appropriate or even necessary intervention in the lives of many tuberculous Skid Road alcoholics. Joan Jackson, for example, saw the sanatorium's detention policies and its efforts to address the social situation of alcoholics as largely complementary. In a 1992 interview, Jackson recalled that upon discharge from Firland,

> these guys . . . did nothing to maintain a good state of health. Ever. Their whole way of life was such that you knew that as soon as they got out of the hospital they were not going to eat well, they were not going to sleep, they were not going to take their medicine, they were going to mix with a whole bunch of people, they were going to drink from the same bottles as them, they were probably going to get reinfected if they didn't become infectious and infect someone else.[103]

From this standpoint, an authoritarian approach that provided structure and lifesaving medical treatment to the lives of tuberculous Skid Road alcoholics seemed entirely consistent with Firland's overall efforts to understand and rehabilitate a population whose lives outside the sanatorium were in disarray.[104] "The doctors totally took it as a given, as an article of faith," Jackson noted, "that [these patients] would relapse and probably have a drug-resistant strain if they didn't take the drugs well beyond when they were negative."[105] Few could dispute that discharged Skid Road patients—even if still alcoholic and unemployed—left Firland in a considerably better condition than when they were admitted.

This discussion is not meant to suggest that paternalism toward disadvantaged patients justifies the use of coercive measures. As the thirty-year effort to champion patients' rights has demonstrated, the preservation of autonomy is all too important. Nevertheless, the history of Ward Six reminds us that efforts to confront public health epidemics—even in an era that emphasizes the importance of civil liberties—are likely to include measures that place significant limitations on persons deemed to be public health threats. Moreover, some may view such constraints as beneficent or rehabilitative. What remains essential, however, is that coercive components of public health programs not be obscured.

DENOUEMENT

By the middle to late 1960s, debates over the most appropriate strategy for managing tuberculosis-alcoholism had begun to wane. While numerous health workers continued to link tuberculosis control with the multiple social problems of vagrant alcoholics inhabiting American skid rows, this approach was becoming increasingly obsolete.[106] For one thing, skid row was itself changing. Urban renewal projects in the 1960s and 1970s in cities such as Seattle attempted to revitalize skid row neighborhoods, often forcing their residents to relocate.[107] Meanwhile, deinstitutionalization of the mentally ill and worsening poverty led to a diversification of the populations that lived in run-down urban areas. The classic tuberculous skid row alcoholic was becoming less readily identifiable.

Paradoxically, perhaps, the War on Poverty may also have contributed to the declining interest in the links between tuberculosis and alcoholism. By 1965, tuberculosis agencies across the country had instituted a series of new programs "designed to break the cycle of poverty and disease." For example, the Nassau County (New York) Tuberculosis and Health Association participated in health examinations at local Project Head Start centers, and the Nevada Tuberculosis Association received a VISTA grant and participated in the administration of Office of Economic Opportunity programs.[108] While such programs revived the old connection between antituberculosis and antipoverty efforts, they also most likely deflected attention away from the issue of alcoholism. In addition, as poor urban dwellers benefited from various War on Poverty achievements—such as improved medical insurance and community-based social support services—inpatient rehabilitation strategies like those attempted at Firland grew obsolete.[109]

Changes in the field of alcoholism also discouraged continued emphasis on the skid row tuberculous alcoholic. Noting the limited results attained both in inpatient facilities and various "transitional communities,"[110] researchers in the early 1970s began to stress the prevention—as opposed to the treatment—of alcoholism. This public health approach, which gained momentum with the founding of the National Institute on Alcohol Abuse and Alcoholism in 1971, sought to prevent alcohol abuse through the use of educational campaigns. This new perspective drew attention away from the broader "sociological" strategies of Jellinek, Jackson, and Fagan, who had emphasized treatment and rehabilitation of heavy drinkers.[111]

The final element that discouraged a comprehensive treatment strategy for skid row alcoholics resulted from the changing nature of tuberculosis therapy itself. Although Firland continued extended inpatient treatment of Skid Road alcoholics until it closed in 1973, therapeutic trends favored much shorter hospitalizations followed by close outpatient follow-up. No longer did the sanatorium provide sufficient time either for "indoctrination of the patient" or for the "organization of a long-term therapy plan,"[112] both of which had long been components of the social approach to tuberculosis.

While explicit connections between the care of the tuberculous and that of the mentally ill were not often made, it is likely that the trends in the hospitalization of psychiatric patients contributed to growing disenchantment with the sanatorium. Propelled by the discovery of effective antipsychotic medications, legal challenges to traditional civil commitment procedures, reports of the inhumane treatment of inpatients, and growing concerns about costs, critics began to call for the deinstitutionalization of both the mentally ill and the mentally retarded.[113] In their frequent reliance on forcible detention, sanatoriums raised similar questions about the use of excessive coercion, but it was probably a broader dissatisfaction with institutionalization that contributed to the closure of nearly all inpatient tuberculosis facilities by the early 1970s.

Naturally, the demonstration that tuberculosis patients could be successfully treated as outpatients was a requirement for the end of the sanatorium era. While a few tuberculosis specialists had advocated ambulatory treatment of the disease during the 1950s, by the mid-1960s the efficacy of such a strategy could no longer be questioned. The most convincing studies of outpatient therapy had come from Madras, India, where investigators demonstrated that apparent cure rates among a group of patients treated at home were as good as those of a hospitalized control group. Supporters of outpatient therapy in the United States published similar data, often focusing on the treatment of extremely uncooperative patients. For example, an outpatient program of twice-weekly supervised antibiotic treatment begun by John Sbarbaro in Denver, Colorado, in 1965 reported only one relapse among 101 such individuals.[114] Sbarbaro's program was the precursor for the modern tuberculosis control policy known as directly observed therapy (DOT).

By the time Firland closed in 1973, the Seattle–King County Health Department was prepared to treat all its patients predominantly in the outpatient setting. Patients with uncomplicated cases of pulmonary tuberculosis generally received approximately two weeks of inpatient therapy at one of the local hospitals, such as Harborview. They were then managed as out-

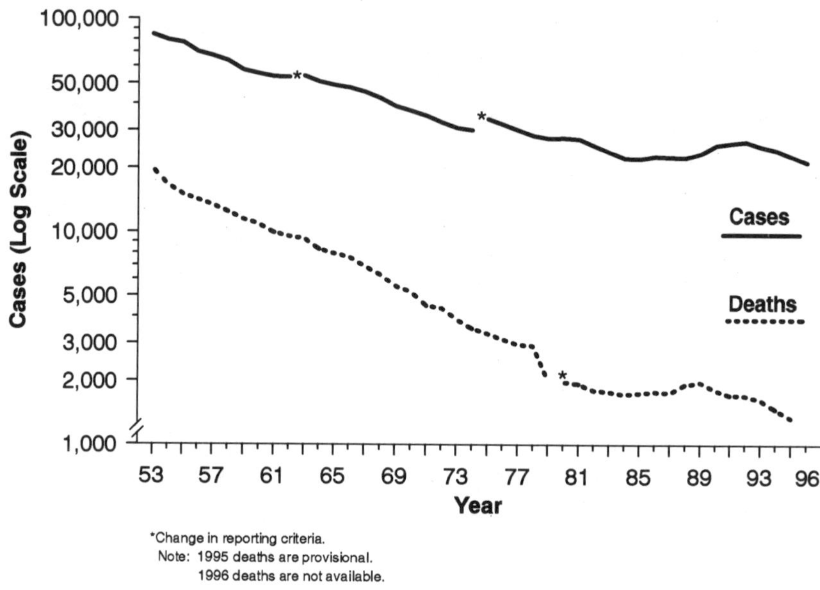

FIGURE 7.1 Tuberculosis morbidity and mortality, United States, 1953–1996. Graph courtesy of the Centers for Disease Control and Prevention, Atlanta, Georgia.

patients, completing eighteen to twenty-four months of antibiotic therapy under the supervision of either the Department of Health or private physicians. In addition, the Health Department had instituted a program similar to that of Sbarbaro for the treatment of potentially noncompliant vagrants and alcoholics. Health workers tracked down these men and women in bars, flophouses, or on the street to ensure that they complied with their medical regimen.[115]

By this time, the incidence of tuberculosis in Seattle had declined markedly. As of 1972, there were only 122 new cases in King County and only 8 deaths attributable to the disease. In contrast, only one-quarter of a century earlier, 619 county residents had been diagnosed with tuberculosis, and 226 people had died.[116] This pattern mirrored the decline of tuberculosis that occurred throughout the United States during the first decades of the antibiotic era. Annual morbidity and mortality rates from the disease, which had totaled 53.0 and 12.4 per 100,000 population, respectively, in 1953, would ultimately decrease to 9.3 and 0.7 per 100,000 by 1985 (figure 7.1).[117] Yet even as Seattle's antituberculosis efforts wound down in the 1960s and 1970s, local health officials, in the spirit of the conference at Arden House, remained steadfast in their attempts to eliminate the disease from the city. Part of the reason for Seattle's persistence stemmed from the fact that the area's two most prominent tuberculosis workers—Cedric Northrop and Honoria Hughes—remained active in the field. Northrop actually had relinquished his position as state tuberculosis control officer in 1959 and had become director of the Seattle–King County Public Health Department's Division of Tuberculosis. In 1962, he began Operation Double Check, which sought to use skin-testing and X-rays to identify all remaining cases of tuberculosis in Seattle and King County over a period of five to seven years.[118]

Hughes remained in charge of the Anti-Tuberculosis League until 1961, when the league's Board of Directors forced her to resign. There were several explanations for this turn of events, but one reason was yet another chapter in the long history of disagreements between the medical profession and the voluntary tuberculosis workers. Physicians in Seattle, using an argument that was becoming increasingly familiar throughout the country, claimed that the National Tuberculosis Association (NTA) and its affiliates devoted too high a percentage of their receipts to administrative costs and educational programs. Funding, these physicians argued, needed to be earmarked for further research into the disease.[119]

By the late 1960s, other critics were suggesting that the league, having accomplished its mission of controlling tuberculosis in King County, should fold. "I proposed that if they believed their job was done," recalled former league board member Harold Laws, "that they should close up shop and quit raising money from the public in order to maintain their staff and offices and so forth."[120] The league eventually decided in 1968 to expand its focus to include all respiratory diseases, an option it had begun to explore as early as 1962. This decision mirrored those made by both the NTA and most other antituberculosis associations across the country. In 1968, for example, the NTA changed its name to the National Tuberculosis and Respiratory Disease Association; it became the American Lung Association in 1972.[121] After 1968, the King County league was known as the Tuberculosis and Respiratory Disease Association of King County. By the late 1960s, league annual reports routinely discussed not only tuberculosis but also asthma, smoking, emphysema, and lung cancer. Eventually, the Tuberculosis and Respiratory Disease Association merged into the Washington Lung Association.

The declining attention to tuberculosis did not occur only within the voluntary sphere. The Seattle–King County Public Health Department's 1971 annual report, commemorating the end of the department's mobile X-ray screening program, featured a picture of a bus bearing the message "Tuberculosis: End of the Line." In January 1973, the department announced that food handlers would no longer be required to have screening chest X-rays prior to obtaining employment.[122]

Even when local agencies attempted to generate interest in tuberculosis, the response was poor. In 1971 a number of groups, including the city and state health departments, the Tuberculosis and Respiratory Disease Association of King County, Firland Sanatorium, the University of Washington, and the King County Medical Society, organized a two-day conference on the treatment and care of tuberculosis patients. Embarrassingly, only forty-five people attended. Meanwhile, that same year, 280 local physicians attended the ninth annual symposium on respiratory diseases held at the University of Washington.[123]

As the number of tuberculosis cases dropped and sanatorium stays shortened, government officials began to question why antituberculosis efforts continued to receive mandatory funding allocations. By 1971, in fact, the state legislature had lowered the annual county property tax earmarked for tuberculosis control from 0.6 mill to 0.125 mill. At the same time, state health officials had accelerated their efforts to close Firland, which had been taken over by the state in 1971.[124] Stressing Firland's almost legendary status in the Seattle community, a few holdouts continued to raise objections. By 1973, however, the decision to close the facility had finally been made. Between October 1 and 31, 1973, the forty remaining Firland patients were either discharged or transferred to Harborview, Providence Hospital, or the local Veterans' Administration Hospital.

Many readers of the *Seattle Times* may have missed the short article on October 30, 1973, that announced that Firland's last patient was to be transferred the next day.[125] In an edition filled with news about the recent resignation of Vice President Spiro Agnew and the escalating Watergate crisis, a story about the closing of Seattle's tuberculosis sanatorium could hardly have been expected to generate much interest. Yet tuberculosis had not disappeared, either from Seattle or from the rest of the country.

EIGHT

An Epidemic Returns

Tuberculosis in the 1990s

Writing in 1952, Cedric Northrop had speculated that thirty years hence a medical student might find a case of tuberculosis as uncommon as a case of typhoid fever.[1] Northrop was nearly correct. Thanks in part to the development of a new antibiotic, rifampin, rates of tuberculosis continued to decline during the 1970s, both in the Seattle–King County region and across the United States. Yet by 1982—the same year to which Northrop referred—the situation had begun to change. The incidence of tuberculosis in New York, Los Angeles, Washington, D.C., and other cities had begun to rise dramatically, once again affecting predominantly poor, disadvantaged populations. By 1992, the media was loudly announcing the "deadly return" of an "old killer" and offering advice on "how we can protect ourselves."[2]

Faced with a potential epidemic of tuberculosis, including worrisome drug-resistant strains of the disease, moribund tuberculosis control programs were revived. Health officials devised and implemented numerous control strategies, most notably directly observed therapy (DOT), a program in which outpatients take their medications under the direct supervision of an outreach worker. Certain health departments are also using forcible detention, although with much less frequency than forty years ago.

As of late 1997, health officials believe that such interventions have "turned the tide"[3] against tuberculosis. Rates of the disease have fallen dramatically, and it has once again disappeared from the front pages of newspapers and magazines. Yet DOT and other modern strategies, while seemingly effective in controlling tuberculosis, have raised many of the same questions that earlier health officials, physicians, and patients confronted. Is tuberculosis an infection, a social disease, or both? Should control efforts among the poor emphasize the amelioration of patients' social problems or merely the ingestion of appropriate antibiotics? How are patients' civil liberties and the public health best balanced? Finally, how should health professionals address the perennial problem of the noncompliant patient? The attempts of tuberculosis workers after World War II to craft appropriate public health strategies and to address both the medical and social problems associated with the disease can shed important light on these modern dilemmas.

THE WHITE PLAGUE RETURNS

The resurgence of tuberculosis occurred earliest (and most dramatically) in New York. The rate of new cases of the disease in the city, which had declined to 17.2 per 100,000 population by 1979, rose steadily thereafter. By 1992, the rate had tripled to 52.0 per 100,000, which translated into 3,811 new cases of the disease.[4] By the mid-1980s, tuberculosis was on the rise throughout much of the United States: between 1985 and 1992, the annual number of new cases increased by 20 percent, from 22,101 to 26,673 (figure 8.1). In Seattle and King County the number of new cases also rose, increasing from 84 in 1984 to 127 by 1992.[5]

Of even more concern than the rising incidence of tuberculosis was a growing inability to treat many cases of the disease. A 1991 study from New York City reported that 19 percent of patients had "multidrug-resistant" tuberculosis that was no longer sensitive to either isoniazid or rifampin. Both Florida and New York experienced outbreaks of multidrug-resistant disease that killed 80 to 90 percent of patients who were concurrently infected with the human immunodeficiency virus (HIV).[6] Such percentages exceeded mortality rates from the preantibiotic era.

Many factors contributed to the return of tuberculosis in the 1980s. First, worsening economic conditions during the decade promoted the spread of the disease, once again demonstrating the historical relation of tuberculosis to poverty. Second, the elaborate public health infrastructure that had once existed to combat the disease had deteriorated. Lacking sanatoriums, sufficient clinic facilities, and screening programs, many cities and states were caught unprepared. Third, immigrants from Third World countries with high rates of tuberculosis brought into the United States large numbers of new cases.[7]

The most important factor promoting the resurgence of tuberculosis in the 1980s, however, was probably the acquired immunodeficiency syndrome (AIDS). Persons whose immune systems had already been weakened by infection with HIV proved particularly likely to develop tuberculosis. In addition, tuberculosis in persons with HIV disease often had atypical manifestations, which complicated efforts at both diagnosis and treatment.[8]

As in the past, commentators were quick to note that a successful tuberculosis control program needed to address the medical aspects of the disease, the public health threat, and the social circumstances of patients. From the medical perspective, physicians employed combinations of sev-

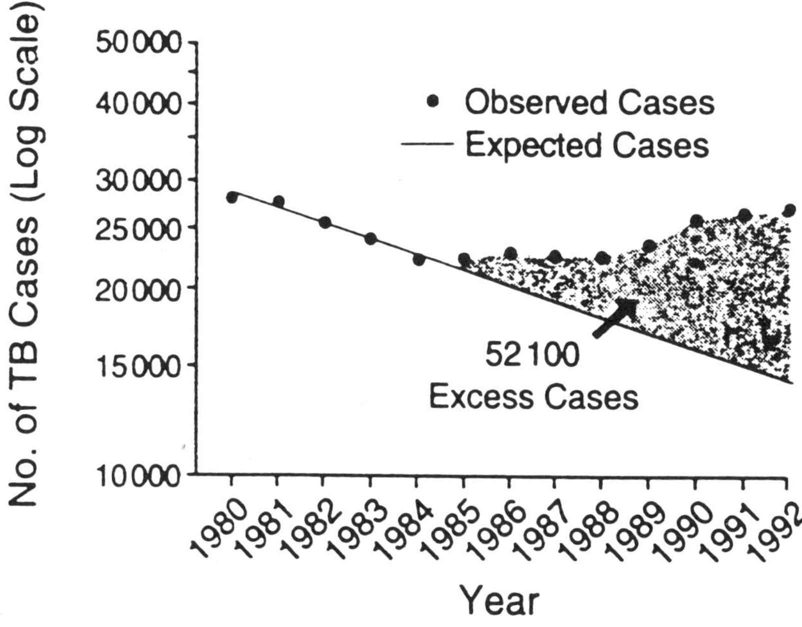

FIGURE 8.1 Observed and excess cases of tuberculosis, United States, 1980–1992. Michael F. Cantwell, Dixie E. Snider Jr., George M. Cauthen, and Ina Onorato, "Epidemiology of Tuberculosis in the United States, 1985 through 1992," *Journal of the American Medical Association* 272 (1994): 536.

eral antibiotics to treat persons with resistant strains. Lung resection, largely abandoned after 1970, returned to the therapeutic armamentarium for the treatment of particularly complex, drug-resistant cases.[9]

Meanwhile, with significant infusions of federal and local dollars, public health officials attempted to rebuild their divisions of tuberculosis and revive screening programs. Most notably, these officials made plans to address the issue of noncompliance with antibiotic regimens. Indeed, it appeared that much of the drug resistance to tuberculosis could be traced to noncompliance, which occurred in up to 90 percent of patients.[10]

The cases that modern health departments confronted were, if anything, even more challenging than those addressed by the Seattle–King County Department of Health twenty-five years earlier. One New York City patient, for example, was a thirty-four-year-old homeless man with schizophrenia who repeatedly failed to take his medications. He had been jailed for spitting at patrons of a laundromat and also denied having contagious tuberculosis. In another case, a thirty-three-year-old New York woman with infectious tuberculosis repeatedly left the hospital against medical advice and continued to visit her healthy children. The woman used numerous aliases, thereby interfering with efforts to track her case. When eventually placed on DOT, she reportedly threw away the medicine in the presence of the person supervising her treatment.[11]

Despite such problems, many health officials in New York and elsewhere quickly stressed that extensive reliance on involuntary isolation was no longer acceptable. Given the earlier legal rulings limiting the civil commitment powers of the state and the more recent efforts of AIDS activists to champion patient autonomy,[12] noncompliant persons with tuberculosis in the 1990s were clearly entitled to full due process prior to detention. In fact, in a 1986 case, a District Court judge in Seattle had ruled that the 1967 Washington state quarantine law did not permit forcible confinement of a non-infectious, noncompliant, alcoholic patient at Harborview Medical Center.[13]

Such considerations led a number of cities and states to update their tuberculosis control statutes. These new regulations stipulate that persons with tuberculosis are entitled to due process protections, including a formal hearing and legal representation. In addition, more coercive measures, such as detention, are not to be employed until "less restrictive alternatives" have been exhausted. Finally, health department regulations permitting the use of forcible confinement must contain safeguards, such as periodic reviews, even for patients who do not request them.[14]

Less restrictive alternatives may include various incentives, such as the provision of subway tokens or food coupons. The foremost strategy, however, is directly observed therapy. Modern DOT is an updated version of the program originally developed in Denver in the 1960s and 1970s.[15] In DOT, tuberculosis patients receive their daily or twice-weekly antibiotics under the eye of an outreach worker. This monitoring may occur either at a tuberculosis clinic, at a patient's home, on the street, or at other community locations. Much of DOT is done on a voluntary basis. The vast majority of patients diagnosed with tuberculosis are offered DOT as a service to assist them with the often difficult task of successfully completing their antibiotic therapy. At the same time, DOT may be mandated for individuals who have demonstrated an inability to adhere to prescribed medications. In the latter case, local health departments may issue an order that requires a given patient to begin DOT. Such supervised therapy is often extremely popular, even among patients obliged to participate. "I definitely needed medical therapy," noted one New York City DOT patient, "but I also definitely needed the attention I was getting. It built my self-confidence. That's what really made me complete therapy."[16]

Although occasional commentators have challenged its widespread acceptance,[17] most medical and public health commentators have endorsed DOT as the standard of care for both compliant and noncompliant persons with tuberculosis. Indeed, treatment completion rates in certain DOT programs exceed 95 percent.[18] In many areas, the success of DOT has made forcible institutionalization of persons with tuberculosis almost obsolete.

Because confinement of tuberculosis patients is now used less frequently, the concerns raised by institutionalization have become somewhat less pressing. Yet health officials remain aware of the need to employ outpatient DOT appropriately. For one thing, DOT, although itself not very coercive, likely derives some of its effectiveness from the threat of future detention. In addition, because earlier calls for universal DOT have been rejected as either unnecessary, too expensive, or a violation of the civil liberties of compliant patients, only a percentage of patients are mandated to have DOT.[19] Officials must continue present efforts to base DOT decisions on actual noncompliance as opposed to preconceived notions about the lifestyles or supposed unreliability of specific disadvantaged groups.

The historical record also reminds us not to obscure the restrictive aspects of DOT. A recent article, seeking to highlight the multiple benefits accrued by poor persons receiving supervised therapy, suggests that the term "DOT" be replaced by "TLC" (tender loving care).[20] Similarly, another author has written, "It should be kept in mind that DOT is a positive intervention, not a punitive one."[21] Such language is reminiscent of Thomas Sheehy's tendency to term Ward Six an "opportunity ward" or "health aid" that was not used for punishment. Having developed a sophisticated system of least restrictive alternatives, health officials should readily acknowledge that public health interventions like DOT have both positive and restrictive elements.

Similar arguments apply to the recent use of detention, which is now being employed by several cities and states, particularly those with high numbers of noncompliant patients.[22] As tuberculosis in the 1990s predominantly affects disadvantaged populations, it is not surprising that those detained in cities such as New York are overwhelmingly minorities, homeless people, and substance users. For example, one study of forty-six patients confined at New York's Goldwater Hospital found that forty-six (100 percent) were minorities, forty-two (91 percent) were substance users, thirty-two (70 percent) had a history of homelessness, and twenty-five (54 percent) were HIV-positive. Given the potential for discrimination against each of these groups, close observation of the selection process remains essential.[23]

Moreover, in New York and elsewhere, modifications of health codes now permit the detention of persistently uncooperative persons until they finish treatment.[24] Although this policy avoids the situation at Firland, where incompletely treated patients often relapsed after discharge, it does allow health officials to detain noninfectious persons for months or even years based solely on predictions of future behavior. Yet there is debate about this policy even within the public health literature. For example, Denver officials recently reported that 90 percent of patients detained for an average of only twenty days successfully completed treatment.[25] In order to justify the continued use of long-term detention, tuberculosis officers must conclusively demonstrate the need for "confinement until cure."

Continued scrutiny of the actual implementation of isolation policies is also essential. Even at facilities that have successfully de-emphasized a punitive approach, there is still a tendency to equate misconduct within the institution with future public health endangerment.[26] Yet such behavioral problems may actually reflect the effects of institutionalization itself.[27] Moreover, despite the extensive discussion of least restrictive alternatives, some jurisdictions continue to commit tuberculous persons under criminal as opposed to civil statutes. As a result, when locked areas are not available in hospitals, sick patients may be confined in prisons. As such a policy crosses the line from restriction to punishment, commentators have urged that health officials and governments establish proper guidelines and facilities that permit the use of civil detention.[28]

RETHINKING TUBERCULOSIS AS A SOCIAL DISEASE

In addition to raising concerns about excessive coercion, the issue of noncompliance has once again underscored the concept of tuberculosis as a social disease. Although vagrant alcoholics now garner less attention, modern health officials have emphasized the predilection of tuberculosis for minorities, substance users, the homeless, and those with HIV disease. The multiple social problems of such individuals both predispose them to tuberculosis and prevent them from successfully completing treatment.[29]

Yet the characterization of tuberculosis as a social disease has changed considerably over time. As Paul Starr has argued, tuberculosis control in the twentieth century has moved "away from the broad advocacy of social reform toward more narrow judgments that could be defended as the exercise of neutral [medical] authority."[30] As early as the second decade of the twentieth century, certain health officials had promoted the practical advantages of such an approach, which Minnesota public health specialist Hibbert W. Hill termed the "new public health." "If 'general environment' be the great factor in tuberculosis," Hill remarked in 1916,

> the hundred million people of these United States must have his or her [*sic*] own individual environment brought up to and kept at some standard-level

designed to maintain each individual in his or her own alleged "state of health."

If, however, the infectiveness of the disease be the great factor, only two hundred thousand people (the actively infectious cases) need this supervision in the United States, and they need it, not for the improvement of their "general environment," but *merely to prevent them from infecting others.* This problem, even numerically, is one five-hundredth of the magnitude of the other.[31]

Despite the growing acceptance of the new public health, efforts to address patients' social problems remained prominent after World War II. As we have seen, tuberculosis control strategies in Seattle included the provision of social services and vocational rehabilitation, research into the culture of the Skid Road, and the inpatient treatment of alcoholism. Many Firland staff members, echoing sanatorium workers earlier in the century, believed that these social interventions themselves were a necessary component of the treatment of tuberculosis. As Joan Jackson and her colleagues contended, a social disease like tuberculosis could never truly be "cured" without also addressing a Skid Road patient's alcoholism and the realities of his life outside the sanatorium. Yet most tuberculosis workers, even in the 1950s and 1960s, did not share this broad vision. Rather, they viewed social interventions essentially as strategies for achieving a more limited medical goal: helping patients to complete their antibiotic therapy.

Today, this narrower approach to tuberculosis control has gained almost universal acceptance. Certainly, modern tuberculosis officials have advocated a series of interventions that seek to improve patients' social circumstances. For example, officials may now attempt to provide homeless patients with housing and to channel those with drug addiction into rehabilitation programs.[32] A few commentators, echoing the philosophy of tuberculosis workers earlier in the century, have argued that control of the disease in the 1990s still requires social change, at least for individual patients.[33] In other words, it is inappropriate to detain noncompliant people with tuberculosis or even to mandate DOT unless they have been provided with a secure residence and access to drug treatment and mental health services. As Ronald Bayer of the Columbia University School of Public Health remarked during hearings on New York City's revised health code in 1993, "It is unfair to threaten with deprivations of liberty" those whose circumstances "make compliance almost impossible."[34]

For the most part, however, modern interventions that take into account patients' social problems, such as providing them with financial incentives, are basically strategies to improve compliance with medical follow-up. The triumph of this philosophy is most apparent in the case of DOT. Health officials designing and implementing DOT programs most certainly address the social circumstances of their patients. Based on often intimate knowledge of patients' living conditions, social networks, and personalities, outreach workers tailor DOT regimens to individual patients. "We're teachers, hand holders, coaches, and a parental influence," noted one DOT supervisor. "We'll do anything we think will work."[35]

Yet DOT, while based on a careful assessment of patients' social problems, does little, if anything, to alter social circumstances. This fact was made clear by John Sbarbaro's pioneering Denver program, in which outreach nurses supervised outpatient therapy for "manifestly unreliable" tuberculosis patients. In describing the program in a seminal 1973 article in the *Journal of the American Medical Association,* Sbarbaro and Leonard Hudson observed that "no change in [patients'] living or drinking habits was required. The nurses' attributes included mature understanding and a non-punitive attitude toward alcoholic and sociopathic patients."[36] To phrase this another way, it mattered relatively little whether patients remained homeless, unemployed, or alcoholic after completing their prescribed treatment for tuberculosis. Indeed, demonstrating how distant the notion of treating "tuberculosis-alcoholism" had become, nurses were quite willing to meet alcoholic patients in bars or taverns if it increased the probability of success. The key to Denver's outpatient tuberculosis chemotherapy program was to acknowledge patients' social problems and to use this knowledge to better enable patients to complete their medical therapy.

If tuberculosis control in the United States since 1900 has thus become more narrowly medical, is it wrong to still speak of a social approach to the disease? In order to answer this question, it is necessary to merge the categories of "medical" and "social" kept distinct for much of this book. In her work on Typhoid Mary, the Irish immigrant detained for more than twenty years on New York City's North Brother Island, Judith Walzer Leavitt has argued that bacteriology and public health policy were not "scientific pursuits separated from the norms and structures of society."[37] Rather, attempts to control typhoid fever—through identification of carriers of the bacillus and scrutiny of their likelihood of transmitting the germ—were "determined by both scientific and social factors."[38] In other words, the adoption of Hill's "new public health" did not signal simply the triumph of a reductionist medical understanding of disease but rather the continuation of a broad approach to issues of prevention and treatment.

As with the control of typhoid fever, antituberculosis efforts have also been "characterized by broad social concerns."[39] Over time, Firland staff reined in their ambitious attempts to unearth and correct the root causes of medication noncompliance, increasingly emphasizing the narrower goal of getting patients to take their antibiotics. Yet this more direct strategy did not ignore the social context of tuberculosis. By aggressively pursuing medical cures, sanatorium physicians sought to eliminate the most correctable problem of many Skid Road patients: the endless cycle of worsening tuberculosis, sanatorium admission, and premature discharge. If Firland no longer explicitly confronted alcoholism or other social problems on the Skid Road, its staff nevertheless believed that successful medical treatment of tuberculosis was an achievable intervention that would make a concrete difference in the lives of Skid Road alcoholics.

This more limited notion of a "social intervention" also characterizes directly observed therapy. Rather than attempting to solve problems such as homelessness, drug addiction, or poverty, DOT seeks to improve the lives of patients by curing their tuberculosis and providing them with TLC. If some might criticize this approach as reviving an outdated paternalistic model in which doctor (or health care provider) knows best, supervised therapy may nevertheless represent the most practical intervention for noncompliant persons with a wide range of social problems. As Thomas R. Frieden, former head of the New York City Tuberculosis Control Bureau, has stated, "You have a patient who is HIV-positive, homeless, and drug addicted, and he develops tuberculosis. If the health department can successfully treat his tuberculosis, he may still be HIV-infected and still have problems with drugs and homelessness, but he will never have tuberculosis again—and that is one less thing for him to worry about."[40]

The widespread acceptance and success of DOT in the 1990s suggest two other important points. First, they belie the old belief that one must correct the underlying social causes of tuberculosis in order to prevent the spread of the disease. With the widespread diffusion of DOT across the United States, not only are patients with multiple social problems being cured, but overall rates of tuberculosis are falling. In 1996, for example, there were only 21,327 new cases of the disease nationwide, down from 26,673 in 1992. In New York City, which had 3,811 new cases in 1982, the total had declined dramatically to 2,053 by 1996.[41]

It is difficult to prove the connection between DOT, other treatment incentives, and the falling incidence of tuberculosis. Other possible explanations exist: for example, the declining number of new cases might also be attributable to better infection control measures implemented in hospitals and other congregate settings, such as homeless shelters.[42] In addition, because little improvement has been made in the general problems of homelessness, injection drug use, and poverty, the fall in tuberculosis incidence in the United States might prove transient. Nevertheless, the success achieved by treating active cases of the disease raises the question whether this strategy—rather than altering the living conditions of the poor—may be an effective method of tuberculosis prevention, as well.[43]

Such an argument ultimately may also apply to the Third World, where tuberculosis causes more adult deaths than any other disease. Recent data on DOT in underdeveloped countries (which is, after all, where supervised treatment began) suggest that mass-scale programs can generate up to 90 percent cure rates;[44] broad dissemination of DOT, therefore, might be expected to lower overall incidence of the disease. Such a strategy, however, may have its drawbacks. Logistically, given the combination of poverty, malnutrition, HIV infection, and substandard public health facilities in the Third World, it may be difficult to implement widespread DOT. Philosophically, the narrow focus on rectifying noncompliance may discourage practitioners from exploring the belief systems and social problems that influence how patients take medications. Tuberculosis workers have historically been among the strongest advocates for viewing disease in the context of individuals' lives. Such an emphasis should not be lost, even as more effective therapeutic strategies are implemented.

Second, in addressing the perennial debate over balancing civil liberties with protection of the public's health, a new equilibrium has been reached. In contrast with health officers in the 1950s, whose broad definition of a public health threat led them to rely too heavily on incarceration, modern officials have developed a system that discourages coercion by offering disadvantaged patients a variety of services. Yet DOT, while more responsive to the concerns of civil libertarians, has been most successful because it retains the same primary emphasis on protecting the community's health. Tuberculous persons who repeatedly do not comply—even if they remain homeless, drug addicted, or impoverished—can expect a series of increasingly restrictive measures that may ultimately culminate in forcible detention. The notion that all persons, regardless of their social circumstances, must comply with public health regulations exemplifies what the historian Nancy Tomes has termed "public health citizenship." In exchange for the state's implementation of programs to prevent the spread of disease, all of its citizens have a civic responsibility to submit to reasonable regulations and restrictions.[45]

Analogous concerns about the mutual obligations of health care providers and patients arise in cases of noncompliance that do not directly raise public health concerns. The biomedical ethics literature is filled with discussions of injection drug users who continue to use heroin or cocaine despite past heart-valve replacements and kidney failure patients who routinely miss scheduled dialysis sessions and then require emergency treatment.[46] In some instances, the reciprocal duties of patients are clearly stated. For example, methadone maintenance programs require that their clients, former heroin users, follow a series of strict guidelines.[47] With an eye toward cost control and resource allocation, some cardiac surgeons have favored a similar model that limits valve replacements for active drug users. Yet for the most part, both legal and ethical arguments favor the continued treatment of repeatedly noncompliant patients who are a danger to themselves. As the ethicist Ruth Macklin has argued, "There is no obvious and nondiscriminatory way to draw a line between people who contribute to their health or illness and those who do not."[48] Ironically, perhaps, noncompliance remains a more difficult problem in cases where officials do not have a public health justification for mandating treatment.

If society has thus established a type of quid pro quo in which public health departments and medical practitioners have an obligation not to abuse their authority and tuberculosis patients have some type of civic duty to comply, Firland also reminds us of the dangers of such a system. Modern tuberculosis control officers are not the first to promise to use forcible detention as a last resort. Seattle officials did so as well, yet the safeguards put in place were gradually ignored. So, too, the experience of Firland cautions us about the ramifications of labels such as "recalcitrant," "noncompliant," and even "nonadherent." Whether they are prescribing isoniazid, insulin, asthma inhalers, or triple-drug therapy for HIV disease,[49] clinicians and researchers continually seek to identify patient characteristics or behaviors that can successfully predict noncompliance with medical treatments. Yet overemphasizing the problem of noncompliance among specific populations, even if done with the best of intentions, may inadvertently stigmatize certain individuals and groups as necessarily uncooperative. Perhaps the most fruitful method of improving treatment completion is to acknowledge that all patients are potentially noncompliant[50] and thus deserve access to a broad range of facilitating interventions—such as simplified medical regimens, educational initiatives, better clinic facilities, financial incentives, and, if necessary, a program of supervised therapy.

Such historical lessons will be of particular importance if rates of tuberculosis in the United States continue their present decline. As in the past, better control of tuberculosis will almost certainly translate into decreases in both attention and funding.[51] In such a setting, the improvements made over the past decade may quickly disappear. Directly observed therapy programs may be cut back, leaving health officials without adequate resources to control tuberculosis—especially in poor and minority communities. Close legal examination of public health regulations may also wane, once again leaving disadvantaged persons susceptible to punitive action. The recent success of a narrower medical model of tuberculosis control should not obscure the potential for future visitations of the disease among society's most vulnerable populations.

Notes

MANUSCRIPT COLLECTIONS CITED

American Lung Association Archives, New York, New York (ALA Archives)
American Lung Association of New York Archives, New York, New York (ALA-NY Archives)
American Lung Association of Washington Archives, Seattle, Washington (ALA-W Archives)
Firland Sanatorium Medical Records, Washington State Department of Social and Health Services Warehouse, Tumwater, Washington
Joan K. Jackson, Personal Papers, Bethany, Connecticut
King County Medical Society Library, Seattle, Washington (KCMS Library)
Shoreline Historical Society, Seattle, Washington
University of Washington Archives, Seattle, Washington (UW Archives)
Washington State Archives, Olympia, Washington (WS Archives)

INTRODUCTION

1. Firland Sanatorium chart D16. In order to protect confidentiality, I have used a code, consisting of a letter and a number (e.g., A1, B2), when citing charts from Firland Sanatorium. While I do not intend to reveal the nature of my coding system, I have included my codes as a way to distinguish among patients. Identifiers, such as initials and ages, have been altered to prevent identification of the persons described.

2. René Dubos and Jean Dubos, *The White Plague: Tuberculosis, Man, and Society* (New Brunswick: Rutgers University Press, 1987), xxxvii. While the term *social disease* was (and is) more commonly associated with venereal disease, Dubos and Dubos used it to emphasize the connection between tuberculosis and poverty.

3. Robert Koch, "Aetiology of Tuberculosis" [1884], in Barbara G. Rosenkrantz, ed., *From Consumption to Tuberculosis: A Documentary History* (New York: Garland, 1994).

4. William Osler, "Discussion on the Advisability of the Registration of Tuberculosis" [1894], in Rosenkrantz, *From Consumption to Tuberculosis*, 317. See

also Barbara G. Rosenkrantz, "Introductory Essay: Dubos and Tuberculosis, Master Teachers," in Dubos and Dubos, *White Plague,* xvi.

5. Charles E. Rosenberg, "The Therapeutic Revolution: Medicine, Meaning, and Social Change in Nineteenth-Century America," in Morris J. Vogel and Charles E. Rosenberg, eds., *The Therapeutic Revolution: Essays in the Social History of American Medicine* (Philadelphia: University of Pennsylvania Press, 1979).

6. "Discussion on the Advisability," 317.

7. On the social construction of disease, see introduction to Peter Wright and Andrew Treacher, eds., *The Problem of Medical Knowledge: Examining the Social Construction of Medicine* (Edinburgh: Edinburgh University Press, 1982); Robert A. Aronowitz, "Lyme Disease: The Social Construction of Disease and Its Social Consequences," *Milbank Quarterly* 69 (1991): 79–112; Ludmilla Jordanova, "The Social Construction of Medical Knowledge," *Social History of Medicine* 8 (1995): 361–81; Charles E. Rosenberg, "Preface: Science in Play," in *No Other Gods: On Science and American Social Thought,* rev. ed. (Baltimore: Johns Hopkins University Press, 1997).

8. Charles E. Rosenberg has proposed an alternative model to social construction, which he terms "framing." According to Rosenberg, changing cultural, political, and medical factors lead societies to frame diseases differently over time. See Charles E. Rosenberg, "Disease in History: Frames and Framers," *Milbank Quarterly* 67, supp. 1 (1989): 1–15.

9. These quotations come from Henry E. Sigerist, *Man and Medicine: An Introduction to Medical Knowledge* (New York: Norton, 1932), 183; and Henry E. Sigerist, *Civilization and Disease* (Ithaca: Cornell University Press, 1944), 239. On Sigerist, see Elizabeth Fee, "Henry E. Sigerist: His Interpretations of the History of Disease and the Future of Medicine," in Charles E. Rosenberg and Janet Golden, eds., *Framing Disease: Studies in Cultural History* (New Brunswick: Rutgers University Press, 1992). For more on the history of "social medicine," see Dorothy Porter and Roy Porter, "What Was Social Medicine? An Historiographic Essay," *Journal of Historical Sociology* 1 (1989): 90–106; and Fee, "Henry E. Sigerist," 302–4.

10. Among the books on tuberculosis that explore these themes are Susan Sontag, *Illness as Metaphor* (New York: Farrar, Straus and Giroux, 1978); Sheila M. Rothman, *Living in the Shadow of Death: Tuberculosis and the Social Experience of Illness in American History* (New York: Basic Books, 1994); David S. Barnes, *The Making of a Social Disease: Tuberculosis in Nineteenth-Century France* (Berkeley: University of California Press, 1995). See also Richard H. Shryock, *National Tuberculosis Association, 1904–1954: A Study of the Voluntary Health Movement in the United States* (New York: NTA, 1957).

11. Dubos and Dubos, *The White Plague.*

12. Ibid., 224.

13. Barbara G. Rosenkrantz, *Public Health and the State: Changing Views in Massachusetts, 1842–1936* (Cambridge: Harvard University Press, 1972), 177–82; Michael E. Teller, *The Tuberculosis Movement: A Public Health Campaign in the*

Progressive Era (New York: Greenwood, 1988), 133–34; Barbara Bates, *Bargaining for Life: A Social History of Tuberculosis, 1876–1938* (Philadelphia: University of Pennsylvania Press, 1992), 333.

14. Rosenkrantz, *Public Health and the State,* 159.

15. Georgina D. Feldberg, *Disease and Class: Tuberculosis and the Shaping of Modern North American Society* (New Brunswick: Rutgers University Press, 1995).

16. See, for example, Teller, *The Tuberculosis Movement;* Bates, *Bargaining for Life;* Rothman, *Living in the Shadow of Death;* Mark Caldwell, *The Last Crusade: The War on Consumption, 1862–1954* (New York: Atheneum, 1988); F. B. Smith, *The Retreat of Tuberculosis in Twentieth-Century Britain, 1850–1950* (Oxford, England: Croom Helm, 1988); David McBride, *From TB to AIDS: Epidemics among Urban Blacks since 1900* (Albany: State University of New York Press, 1991); Katherine Ott, *Fevered Lives: Tuberculosis in American Culture since 1870* (Cambridge: Harvard University Press, 1996). Two books that venture into the post-antibiotic era, albeit briefly, are Feldberg, *Disease and Class;* and Linda Bryder, *Below the Magic Mountain: A Social History of Tuberculosis in Twentieth-Century Britain* (Oxford, England: Clarendon, 1988).

17. See Sontag, *Illness as Metaphor,* 35–36; Caldwell, *The Last Crusade,* 244–72; Smith, *The Retreat of Tuberculosis,* 246–47; J. Arthur Myers, *Invited and Conquered: Historical Sketch of Tuberculosis in Minnesota* (St. Paul: Minnesota Public Health Association, 1949), 616–24; Margaret E. Kidd Parsons, "White Plague and Double-Barred Cross in Atlanta, 1895–1945" (Ph.D. diss., Emory University, 1985), preface, 177; Frank Ryan, *The Forgotten Plague: How the Battle against Tuberculosis Was Won—and Lost* (Boston: Little, Brown, 1993), 342–64.

18. Historians have largely studied antituberculosis efforts in East Coast cities, such as New York and Philadelphia. One book that looks at tuberculosis in the West is Sheila Rothman's *Living in the Shadow of Death.* See also Jeanne L. Abrams, "Chasing the Cure: A History of the Jewish Consumptives' Relief Society of Denver" (Ph.D. diss., University of Colorado, 1983).

19. Carl Abbott, "Regional City and Network City: Portland and Seattle in the Twentieth Century," *Western Historical Quarterly* 23 (Aug. 1992): 293–322.

20. Although Seattle residents most often called these transients with tuberculosis "Skid Roaders" or "Skid Road alcoholics," this book also uses the more traditional term "vagrants." A *vagrant,* according to the American Heritage Dictionary, is "a person who wanders from place to place without a fixed home or livelihood" or "one who lives on the streets and constitutes a public nuisance, as a drunkard or a prostitute." Both of these phrases well describe the population that challenged tuberculosis officials both in Seattle and across the country.

21. Rothman, *Living in the Shadow of Death,* 191–93, 209–10; David F. Musto, "Popular and Public Health Responses to Tuberculosis in America after 1870," in Victoria A. Harden and Guenter B. Risse, eds., *AIDS and the Historian* (Washington, D.C.: U.S. Department of Health and Human Services, 1991), 14–20. There is an extensive historical literature on the use of coercion to control dis-

eases perceived as public health threats. See David F. Musto, "Quarantine and the Problem of AIDS," *Milbank Quarterly* 64, supp. 1 (1986): 97–117; Dorothy Porter and Roy Porter, "The Enforcement of Health: The British Debate," in Elizabeth Fee and Daniel M. Fox, eds., *AIDS: The Burdens of History* (Berkeley: University of California Press, 1986).

22. Historians are increasingly using medical records as primary documents. Such sources provide an illness narrative constructed by those who wrote in the charts, rather than "objective" information. See John Harley Warner, "Reconstructing Clinical Activities: Patient Records in Medical History," *Social History of Medicine* 5 (1992): 183–205; and Joel Howell, *Technology in the Hospital: Transforming Patient Care in the Early Twentieth Century* (Baltimore: Johns Hopkins University Press, 1995), 14–15.

23. *Annual Report, Firland Sanatorium, 1947* (Seattle: Firland Sanatorium, 1948), 12.

24. Use of the term *noncompliant* has recently been criticized as inappropriately implying that patients who do not follow medical recommendations are in error. Many authors now prefer the adjective *nonadherent* to describe persons either unable or unwilling to take prescribed therapy. Although this book uses the more common term *noncompliant,* it also explores the impact of such language on clinical decision making.

25. Dubos and Dubos, *White Plague,* 225.

26. I am drawing on Rosenberg's notion of "framing disease" here. See note 8, above.

27. Cedric Northrop, "Field Activities Report for January 1954," WS Archives, Health Department Administrative Files, box 6, folder "Tuberculosis Control, 1953–54."

28. Examples of "social control" literature include Ivan Illich, *Medical Nemesis: The Expropriation of Health* (New York: Pantheon Books, 1976); Michel Foucault, *Discipline and Punish: The Birth of the Prison* (New York: Pantheon Books, 1977); and David J. Rothman, *Conscience and Convenience: The Asylum and Its Alternatives in Progressive America* (Boston: Little, Brown, 1980).

29. Allan M. Brandt, *No Magic Bullet: A Social History of Venereal Disease in the United States since 1880* (New York: Oxford University Press, 1987).

30. Karen Brudney and Jay Dobkin, "Resurgent Tuberculosis in New York City: Human Immunodeficiency Virus, Homelessness, and the Decline of Tuberculosis Control Programs," *American Review of Respiratory Disease* 144 (1991): 745–49.

31. Two works that explore these issues are Paula A. Treichler, "AIDS, Gender, and Biomedical Discourse: Current Contests for Meaning," in Fee and Fox, *AIDS: The Burdens of History;* and Paula A. Treichler, "AIDS, HIV, and the Cultural Construction of Reality," in Gilbert Herdt and Shirley Lindenbaum, eds., *The Time of AIDS: Social Analysis, Theory, and Method* (Newbury Park, Calif.: Sage Publications, 1992).

32. Rosenkrantz, "Introductory Essay," xxxii.

33. Thomas R. Frieden, "Tuberculosis and Social Change," *American Journal of Public Health* 84 (1994): 1721-23; Mindy T. Fullilove, Rebecca Young, Paula G. Panzer, and Philip Muskin, "Psychosocial Issues in the Management of Tuberculosis," *Journal of Law, Medicine, and Ethics* 21 (1993): 324–31.

34. George A. Annas, "Control of Tuberculosis: The Law and the Public's Health," *New England Journal of Medicine* 328 (1993): 585–88; Lawrence O. Gostin, "Controlling the Resurgent Tuberculosis Epidemic: A Fifty-State Survey of TB Statutes and Proposals for Reform," *Journal of the American Medical Association* 269 (1993): 255–61.

35. Christine Cassel, John LaPuma, and Lance K. Stell, "The Noncompliant Substance Abuser," *Hastings Center Report* 21 (Mar.-Apr. 1991): 30–32.

ONE. SETTING THE STAGE

1. Roger Sale, *Seattle: Past to Present* (Seattle: University of Washington Press, 1976), 12, 35.

2. Murray Morgan, *Skid Road: An Informal Portrait of Seattle* (Seattle: University of Washington Press, 1982), 159–64.

3. Sale, *Seattle,* 54, 55; Richard C. Berner, *Seattle 1900–1920: From Boomtown, Urban Turbulence, to Restoration* (Seattle: Charles Press, 1991), 28–29.

4. Sale, *Seattle,* 50, 67–68; Berner, *Seattle 1900–1920,* xv, 30–32.

5. Janice L. Reiff, "Urbanization and the Social Structure: Seattle, Washington, 1852-1910" (Ph.D. diss., University of Washington, 1981), 5.

6. There is considerable disagreement as to whether the term *skid road* originated in Seattle. Seattle's Skid Road was probably the best known. See Berner, *Seattle 1900–1920,* 56–62; Sale, *Seattle,* 57–58; Monica Sone, *Nisei Daughter* (Seattle: University of Washington Press, 1979), 8, 57–58; James F. Rooney, "Societal Forces and the Unattached Male: An Historical Review," in Howard M. Bahr, ed., *Disaffiliated Man: Essays and Bibliography on Skid Row, Vagrancy, and Outsiders* (Toronto: University of Toronto Press, 1970), 13–22.

7. On Western skid rows, see Rooney, "Societal Forces," 14-16; Jim Marshall, *Swinging Doors* (Seattle: Frank McCaffrey, 1949), 218. On skid row more broadly, see Jacqueline P. Wiseman, *Stations of the Lost: The Treatment of Skid Row Alcoholics* (Englewood Cliffs, N.J.: Prentice-Hall, 1970); and Leonard U. Blumberg, Thomas E. Shipley Jr., and Stephen F. Barsky, *Liquor and Poverty: Skid Row as a Human Condition* (New Brunswick, N.J.: Rutgers Center of Alcohol Studies, 1978).

8. Morgan, *Skid Road,* 129–30.

9. John Dos Passos, *The 42nd Parallel* (New York: New American Library, 1979), 92.

10. Morgan, *Skid Road,* 9.

11. Ibid.

12. Berner, *Seattle 1900–1920,* 60–76; Sone, *Nisei Daughter,* 109–24; Emmett Watson, *Digressions of a Native Son* (Seattle: Pacific Institute, 1982), 12.

13. Quoted in Lee Forrest Pendergrass, "Urban Reform and Voluntary Asso-

ciation: A Case Study of the Seattle Municipal League" (Ph.D. diss., University of Washington, 1972), 65.

14. Quoted in Norman H. Clark, *The Dry Years: Prohibition and Social Change in Washington,* rev. ed. (Seattle: University of Washington Press, 1988), 111. See also xiii, 108–27.

15. Ibid., 113, 116.

16. Bryce E. Nelson, "Good Schools: The Development of Public Schooling in Seattle, 1901–1922" (Ph.D. diss., University of Washington, 1981), abstract. Progressive reform in Seattle had its origins in Populism. See Robert D. Saltvig, "The Progressive Movement in Washington" (Ph.D. diss., University of Washington, 1966), 180–203, 486–94.

17. Berner, *Seattle 1900–1920,* 109–11; Pendergrass, "Urban Reform," 18–22; Saltvig, "Progressive Movement," 112–15; Mansel G. Blackford, "Reform Politics in Seattle during the Progressive Era, 1902–1916," *Pacific Northwest Quarterly* 59 (Oct. 1968): 177–85. On the "organizational synthesis," see "The Progressive Movement: Liberal or Conservative?" in Gerald N. Grob and George A. Billias, eds., *Interpretations of American History: Patterns and Perspectives,* vol. 2, *Since 1877,* 6th ed. (New York: Free Press, 1992), 225–28.

18. Berner, *Seattle 1900–1920,* 141–49, 175–77; Sale, *Seattle,* 68–78.

19. Nancy M. Rockafellar, "Public Health in Progressive Seattle, 1876–1919" (master's thesis, University of Washington, 1986), 39.

20. Rockafellar, "Public Health," 42–43, 115–19; Sale, *Seattle,* 68–78; Reimert T. Ravenholt and Sanford P. Lehman, "History, Epidemiology, and Control of Typhoid Fever in Seattle," *Medical Times* 92 (Apr. 1964): 342–52. In the text, I refer to the Department of Health and Sanitation as the Department of Health.

21. Rockafellar, "Public Health," 66, 101–6. On "scientific sanitation" in Seattle, see *Report of the Department of Health and Sanitation, 1911* (Seattle: Lowman and Hanford, 1912). See also Judith W. Leavitt, *The Healthiest City: Milwaukee and the Politics of Health Reform* (Princeton: Princeton University Press, 1982), 214–23.

22. Quoted in Rockafellar, "Public Health," 103. See also *Report of the Department of Health and Sanitation, 1911.*

23. Rockafellar, "Public Health," 102–6; Franz Schneider, "A Survey of the Activities of Municipal Health Departments in the United States," *American Journal of Public Health* 6 (1916): 1–17.

24. *Report of the Department of Health and Sanitation, 1911.*

25. Department of Commerce and Labor, Bureau of the Census, *Special Reports: Mortality Statistics, 1900 to 1904* (Washington, D.C.: GPO, 1906), xxxvii. The phrase "captain of all these men of death" first appeared in John Bunyan, *The Life and Death of Mr. Badman* [1680] (London: Oxford University Press, 1929).

26. Otto Trott, M.D., interview with author, May 4, 1993.

27. René Dubos and Jean Dubos, *The White Plague: Tuberculosis, Man, and Society* (New Brunswick: Rutgers University Press, 1987), 69–76. On the significance of the nosological change from "consumption" to "tuberculosis," see

preface to Barbara G. Rosenkrantz, ed., *From Consumption to Tuberculosis: A Documentary History* (New York: Garland, 1994).

28. Dubos and Dubos, *The White Plague,* 94–110, 104; Barbara G. Rosenkrantz, "Introductory Essay: Dubos and Tuberculosis, Master Teachers," in Dubos and Dubos, *The White Plague,* xviii–xxiii; Henry Bowditch, "Consumption in America" [1869], in Rosenkrantz, *From Consumption to Tuberculosis.*

29. Katherine Ott, "The Intellectual Origins and Cultural Form of Tuberculosis in the United States, 1870–1925" (Ph.D. diss., Temple University, 1991), 279.

30. "Highlights of Annual Meeting Talks: Miss Anna R. Moore," *Health Notes* 8 (May–June 1952): 2–3; "Early Days of Tuberculosis," *Health Notes* 12 (Jan.–Feb. 1957): 3. *Health Notes,* the journal of the Anti-Tuberculosis League of King County (ATLKC), may be found in the Pacific Northwest Collection at the University of Washington Library, Seattle.

31. "Grover versus Zook," *Seattle Mail and Herald,* Nov. 11, 1905, 1.

32. Dr. Ringle to Dr. Northrop, "Law of 1909 Regarding Examination before Marriage," Sept. 21, 1948, WS Archives, Department of Health, Director's Office, RS 2 Disease File, box 8, folder 160.

33. On eugenics, see Martin S. Pernick, *The Black Stork: Eugenics and the Death of "Defective" Babies in American Medicine and Motion Pictures since 1915* (New York: Oxford University Press, 1996); Daniel J. Kevles, *In the Name of Eugenics* (New York: Knopf, 1985). Very little literature on the eugenics movement in Washington state exists.

34. "Women's Round Table," *Seattle Mail and Herald,* June 8, 1901, 9. See also "Tuberculosis in Washington," *Pacific Coast Journal of Tuberculosis* 1 (June 1908): 6–7.

35. Three western states, California, Colorado, and New Mexico, had begun some antituberculosis efforts in response to the influx of "health seekers" during the late 1800s. See Sheila M. Rothman, *Living in the Shadow of Death: Tuberculosis and the Social Experience of Illness in American History* (New York: Basic Books, 1994), 131–75, 190–91; J. E. Baur, *The Health-Seekers of Southern California* (San Marino, Calif.: Huntington Library, 1959).

36. Barbara Bates, *Bargaining for Life: A Social History of Tuberculosis, 1876–1938* (Philadelphia: University of Pennsylvania Press, 1992), 22.

37. On Biggs' efforts, see Charles-Edward A. Winslow, *The Life of Hermann Biggs, M.D., D.Sc., LL.D.: Physician and Statesman of the Public Health* (Philadelphia: Lea and Febiger, 1929), 131–52. On the rampant tuberculosis in New York's tenements, see Ernest Poole, *The Plague in Its Stronghold* (New York: Committee on the Prevention of Tuberculosis of the Charity Organization Society, 1903).

38. Rockafellar, "Public Health," 58; Sanford P. Lehman, *The Road to Health: A Short History of the Seattle–King County Department of Public Health* (Seattle, 1954).

39. For the history of the NTA, see Richard H. Shryock, *National Tuberculosis Association, 1904–1954: A Study of the Voluntary Health Movement in the United States* (New York: NTA, 1957).

40. Clarke A. Chambers, *Seedtime of Reform: American Social Service and Social Action, 1918–1933* (Minneapolis: University of Minnesota Press, 1963), 15; Allen F. Davis, *Spearheads for Reform: The Social Settlements and the Progressive Movement, 1890–1914* (New York: Oxford University Press, 1967), 27–29; Michael B. Katz, *In the Shadow of the Poorhouse: A Social History of Welfare in America* (New York: Basic Books, 1986), 58–84.

41. Katz, *In the Shadow*, 68–72; the quote appears on 71. For an alternative assessment that notes how tuberculosis work drew on religious imagery, see JoAnne Brown, "Playing the Game: Tuberculosis, Medievalist Nostalgia, and the Great War," paper presented at the annual meeting of the Organization of American Historians, Atlanta, Apr. 1994.

42. "Report of the Anti-Tuberculosis League" [1910?], included in the Minutes of the Executive Committee of the ATLKC, Aug. 5, 1959, ALA-W Archives.

43. "Just One Crisis after Another," *Health Notes* 9 (Jan.–Feb. 1953): 5. On demonstration projects, see Shryock, *National Tuberculosis Association*, 173.

44. "Local Sanitarium Needed," *Pacific Coast Journal of Tuberculosis* 1 (Aug. 1908): 14–15.

45. William K. McKibben to J. V. Smith, May 14, 1931, ALA-W Archives, folder "Historical Material."

46. McKibben to Smith, May 14, 1931.

47. Paul Dorpat, "TB Legacy. In 1909, 1,000 Seattleites Battled the Disease," *Pacific Magazine* (of the *Seattle Times* and *Seattle Post-Intelligencer*), Nov. 18, 1990, 32–33. See also *Report of the Department of Health and Sanitation, 1927* (Seattle: Lowman and Hanford, 1928), 43.

48. *Report of the Department of Health and Sanitation, 1911.*

49. Lehman, *The Road to Health.* On the vote, see Helen Ross, "Need for Aid in Fight against the Plague," *Town Crier*, Mar. 12, 1912, 11.

50. *Report of the Department of Health and Sanitation, 1911.*

51. *Report of the Washington State Board of Health upon House Bill 211, of the Eleventh Legislature, 1909* (Olympia, Wash.: E. L. Boardman, 1911), abstract. In finding that "the state has a social and economic duty to perform in relation to the tuberculosis question," the 1909 report reached conclusions similar to those of the Seattle commission in 1911. Public health advocates, such as the nineteenth-century British sanitarian Edwin Chadwick, had long stressed the economic benefits of preventive health work.

52. *Report of the Washington State Board of Health on H.B. 211*, abstract.

53. *Report of the Department of Health and Sanitation, 1916* (Seattle: Lowman and Hanford, 1917), 149–50.

54. McKibben to Smith, May 14, 1931.

55. "Some Historical Highlights of the Tuberculosis Program in Washington," n.d., ALA-W Archives, folder "Sanatoria, Washington."

56. *Report of the Department of Health and Sanitation, 1911.* Similarly, see Christen Quevli, "Report on Tuberculosis," *Northwest Medicine* 14 (1915): 268.

57. "Your Health Department: Division of Tuberculosis Control," *Seattle's Health and Sanitation* 21 (Mar. 1928), 4.

58. On the sanatorium movement, see, for example, Dubos and Dubos, *The White Plague,* 173–81; Rothman, *Living in the Shadow of Death,* 132–60; Mark Caldwell, *The Last Crusade: The War on Consumption, 1862–1954* (New York: Atheneum, 1988), 67–126; Robert Taylor, *Saranac: America's Magic Mountain* (Boston: Houghton Mifflin, 1986).

59. *Annual Report and Survey: Seattle Department of Health and Sanitation, 1939–1943* (Seattle, 1944), 167.

60. *Report of the Department of Health and Sanitation, 1912–1914* (Seattle: Lowman and Hanford, 1915); *Report of the Department of Health and Sanitation, 1915* (Seattle: Lowman and Hanford, 1916), 20; *Report of the Department of Health and Sanitation, 1918–1919* (Seattle: Lowman and Hanford, 1920), 56.

61. The Pulmonary Hospital opened in 1910, followed by Laurel Beach in 1921 and Morningside in 1928.

62. *Beginnings, Progress, and Achievement in the Medical Work of King County, Washington* (Seattle, [1931?]), 95.

63. This statistic is from 1918, in which 100 of 343 patients were listed as wanderers. See *Report of the Department of Health, 1918–1919,* 100–101.

64. On Salvarsan, see Harry F. Dowling, *Fighting Infection: Conquests of the Twentieth Century* (Cambridge: Harvard University Press, 1977), 91–95.

65. "Fresh Air," lesson 5 in *Firland Lessons* (Seattle, [1935?]), KCMS Library; *Firland: A Story of Firland Sanatorium* (Seattle: Firland Sanatorium, 1936), 33.

66. *Firland,* 31–45; *Report of the Department of Health and Sanitation, 1925* (Seattle: Lowman and Hanford, 1926), 10–11; Michael E. Teller, *The Tuberculosis Movement: A Public Health Campaign in the Progressive Era* (New York: Greenwood, 1988), 85–94.

67. *Report of the Department of Health and Sanitation, 1916,* 65. The "basis of selection" for admission to Firland was the following:

1. Stage of disease (advanced receiving preference)
2. Financial condition (the poor receiving preference)
3. Social condition, the number of children dependent or exposed, calls for preferential treatment

68. S. Adolphus Knopf, *Report to the United States Government on Tuberculosis, with Some Therapeutic and Prophylactic Suggestions* (New York, 1933), 37–39; Louis E. Siltzbach, *Clinical Evaluation of the Rehabilitation of the Tuberculous: Experience at Altro Work Shops, 1915–1939* (New York: NTA, 1944); H. A. Pattison, *Rehabilitation of the Tuberculous* (Livingston, N.Y.: Livingston Press, 1949), 180–88.

69. *Report of the Department of Health and Sanitation, 1916,* 68. For more on the classification system for tuberculosis, see Shryock, *National Tuberculosis As-*

sociation, 165–67; *Diagnostic Standards of the National Tuberculosis Association* (New York: NTA, 1920).

70. *Report of the Department of Health and Sanitation, 1915*, 56; *Report of the Department of Health and Sanitation, 1916*, 65. This view of advanced disease was widely shared at this time. For more on the issue of early versus late diagnosis of tuberculosis, see Teller, *The Tuberculosis Movement*, 85–89.

71. *Report of the Department of Health and Sanitation, 1912–1914.*

72. *Report of the Washington State Board of Health upon H.B. 211*, 41.

73. *Report of the Department of Health and Sanitation, 1918–1919*, 61.

74. Stith discussed this change in philosophy in the 1927 annual report: "Experience showed that segregation of advanced cases did not control infection in the community, for the reason that most of them came under observation only after they had been positively tuberculous for many months, or years" (*Report of the Department of Health and Sanitation, 1927*, 44).

75. *Report of the Department of Health and Sanitation, 1926* (Seattle: Lowman and Hanford, 1927), 12. See also *Report of the Department of Health and Sanitation, 1918–1919*, 62; *Report of the Department of Health and Sanitation, 1929* (Seattle: Lowman and Hanford, 1930), 65. The issue of how scarce resources should be allocated—whether to the sickest or to those most likely to recover—became an explicit focus of medicine after the growth of bioethics in the 1970s. The allocation of sanatorium beds during the early twentieth century is an interesting, and often neglected, precedent to these later discussions. See David J. Rothman, *Strangers at the Bedside: How Law and Bioethics Transformed Medical Decision Making* (New York: Basic Books, 1991), 148–56.

76. *Report of the Department of Health and Sanitation, 1923* (Seattle: Lowman and Hanford, 1924), 40.

77. Ibid. Sanatoriums across the United States at this time were increasingly emphasizing the admission of earlier cases. See, for example, Bates, *Bargaining for Life*, 272; and Teller, *The Tuberculosis Movement*, 83–89.

78. Lee Powers to the Honorable Board of Commissioners of King County and the Honorable City Council of the City of Seattle, Aug. 14, 1943, WS Archives, Department of Health, Director's Office, RS 2 Disease File, box 8, folder 189.

79. "An Interested Taxpayer Asks," *Pep* 24 (Mar. 1937): 9.

80. Betty MacDonald, *The Plague and I* (Philadelphia: J. B. Lippincott, 1948), 56.

81. *Report of the Department of Health and Sanitation, 1916*, 67. On "order" in the nineteenth-century almshouse and hospital, see Charles E. Rosenberg, *The Care of Strangers: The Rise of America's Hospital System* (New York: Basic Books, 1987), 34–43; and David J. Rothman, *The Discovery of the Asylum: Social Order and Disorder in the New Republic* (Boston: Little, Brown, 1990), 180–205.

82. *Report of the Department of Health and Sanitation, 1916*, 67.

83. Ibid., 68, 71. "Arrested disease" was defined as "All constitutional symptoms and expectoration with bacilli absent for a period of six months; the physical signs to be those of a healed lesion; roentgen findings to be compatible with

the physical exams." When these findings were present for only three months, the disease was considered to be "apparently arrested." See *Standards for the Diagnosis, Classification, and Disposition of Cases of Pulmonary and Glandular Tuberculosis*, 7th ed. (New York: NTA, 1926), 21.

84. *Report of the Department of Health and Sanitation, 1912–1914.*

85. On Biggs and Riverside Hospital, see Rothman, *Living in the Shadow of Death*, 192–93, 209. For similar sentiments, see John P. C. Foster, "Detention Institutes for Ignorant and Vicious Consumptives," *Transactions of the First Annual Meeting of the National Association for the Prevention and Study of Tuberculosis* 1 (May 1905): 333–38.

86. Hermann M. Biggs, "The Administrative Control of Tuberculosis," *Medical News* 84 (Feb. 20, 1904): 337–45, 341.

87. *Report of the Department of Health and Sanitation, 1916*, 23.

88. Cedric Northrop, John H. Fountain, and Daniel W. Zahn, "The Practical Management of the Recalcitrant Tuberculous Patient," *Public Health Reports* 67 (1952): 894–98, 895.

89. Nancy M. Rockafellar, "Making the World Safe for the Soldiers of Democracy: Patriotism, Public Health, and Venereal Disease Control on the West Coast, 1910–1919" (Ph.D. diss., University of Washington, 1990), 313, 318. For discussions of the historical relation of issues of war, disease, and gender, see Allan M. Brandt, *No Magic Bullet: A Social History of Venereal Disease in the United States since 1880* (New York: Oxford University Press, 1987); and Paula A. Treichler, "AIDS, Gender, and Biomedical Discourse: Current Contests for Meaning," in Elizabeth Fee and Daniel M. Fox, eds., *AIDS: The Burdens of History* (Berkeley: University of California Press, 1986).

90. Rockafellar, "Making the World Safe," 351.

91. Ibid., 326, 349–50.

92. Ibid., 324; Brandt, *No Magic Bullet*, 84–95.

93. Quoted in Rockafellar, "Making the World Safe," 332–33.

94. Ibid., 335.

95. Mrs. Trafford Huteson, chair of the ATLKC, to "Dear Sir," Nov. 28, 1919, UW Archives, Austin E. Griffiths Papers, box 9, folder 6. On the waning of antituberculosis measures after 1920, see Barron H. Lerner, " 'On What Authority Is This Being Done?' Tuberculosis Control, Poverty, and Coercion in Seattle, 1909–1973" (Ph.D. diss., University of Washington, 1996), 117–81.

96. *Report of the Department of Health and Sanitation, 1924* (Seattle: Lowman and Hanford, 1925), 15.

97. While this argument was often put forth in the early and middle years of the twentieth century, it did not generate much scholarly interest until the work of Thomas McKeown, a British professor of social medicine. Writing in the 1970s, McKeown explicitly claimed that improved nutrition and living conditions—as opposed to antituberculosis measures—had caused the marked decline of tuberculosis during the twentieth century. On the controversy this argument has produced, see Linda Bryder and Leonard G. Wilson, "Comments on 'The Historical

Decline of Tuberculosis in Europe and America: Its Causes and Significance,' by Leonard G. Wilson," *Journal of the History of Medicine and Allied Sciences* 46 (1991): 358–68; Nancy J. Tomes, "The White Plague Revisited," *Bulletin of the History of Medicine* 63 (fall 1989): 467–80.

98. *Report of the Department of Health and Sanitation, 1929,* 23. Changes in funding occurred much more slowly. Public health officials in Seattle continued to allocate most of their money for the control of tuberculosis and other infectious diseases.

99. The importance of fitness was a major theme of persons promoting eugenics at this time. See note 33, this chapter. The NTA used its Modern Health Crusade to publicize the dangers of malnutrition and poor health habits. See Shryock, *National Tuberculosis Association,* 170–73.

100. "Mr. Seattle Taxpayer Goes Shopping," 1934, ALA Archives, King County Association Correspondence File (587).

101. By 1929, for example, at least forty-six of the eighty-eight patients discharged from Firland had died. See *Report of the Department of Health and Sanitation, 1929,* 63.

102. Iago Galdston, "Humanism and Public Health," *Annals of Medical History,* 3d ser., 3 (1941): 513–23; Barbara G. Rosenkrantz, *Public Health and the State: Changing Views in Massachusetts, 1842–1936* (Cambridge: Harvard University Press, 1972), 177–82; Elizabeth Fee and Dorothy Porter, "Public Health and Professionalization: England and America in the Nineteenth Century," in Andrew Wear, ed., *Medicine in Society: Historical Essays* (Cambridge: Cambridge University Press, 1992).

103. This transition typified reform in Seattle during this era. See Carl Abbott, "Regional City and Network City: Portland and Seattle in the Twentieth Century," *Western Historical Quarterly* 23 (1992): 293–322, 306. Judith W. Leavitt has also documented this transformation of public health departments into largely bureaucratic entities. See Leavitt, *The Healthiest City,* 240.

104. Richard C. Berner, *Seattle 1921–1940: From Boom to Bust* (Seattle: Charles Press, 1992), 301–13, 370–71.

105. Teller, *The Tuberculosis Movement,* 47–48. For examples of activism in this era, see David McBride, *From TB to AIDS: Epidemics among Urban Blacks since 1900* (Albany: State University of New York Press, 1991), 58–67. See also the comments of Bailey B. Burritt and Louis I. Dublin in the *Report by the Committee on Tuberculosis and Public Health of the State Charities Aid Association* (New York: 1937), 12–16.

TWO. THE WAR YEARS

1. Quoted in Gustav Schmidt, *Review of the Fight against Tuberculosis in Wisconsin and Elsewhere, 1898–1946* (Milwaukee: North American Press, 1946), 37–38.

2. Kendall Emerson, "Renaissance," *Journal-Lancet* 60 (1940): 144.

3. Quoted in Stuart Whitehouse, "City Appeals Rule That Sanatorium Is Not Legal Expense," *Seattle Star,* Oct. 11, 1938, 1.

4. *Annual Report and Survey, Seattle Department of Health and Sanitation, 1939–1943* (Seattle, 1944), 154. The mortality from tuberculosis in Seattle in 1937 was 56.5 persons per 100,000 population.

5. Mary Dempsey to Kenneth B. Olson, Aug. 4, 1944, ALA Archives, Washington State Department of Public Health File (704). Aside from Firland, which was run by the city of Seattle, other sanatoriums in Washington, like Morningside, were county institutions.

6. Dorothy Northrop Hupp, interview with author, July 8, 1992.

7. Curriculum vitae of Cedric Northrop, n.d., ALA Archives, Washington State Department of Public Health File (704).

8. On the evolving use of skin testing and chest X-ray screening, see Robert G. Bloch, "Roentgenological Group Examinations for Pulmonary Tuberculosis," *American Review of Tuberculosis* 37 (1938): 174–99; K. M. Soderstrom, "The Tuberculin Test: Changing Concepts and Uses," *Northwest Medicine* 39 (1940): 329–31.

9. Calvin F. Schmid, *Social Trends in Seattle* (Seattle: University of Washington Press, 1944), 302, 320; Howard A. Droker, "Seattle Race Relations during the Second World War," *Pacific Northwest Quarterly* 67 (Oct. 1976): 163–74.

10. *Annual Report and Survey, 1939–1943,* 153; Kenneth Stave, "Firland: A Story of Achievement," *Pep* 31 (May 1944): 11. On the growth of Seattle in this era, see Gerald D. Nash, *The American West Transformed: The Impact of the Second World War* (Lincoln: University of Nebraska Press, 1985), 79–81.

11. *Public Health in Seattle, 1946: Report of the Department of Public Health, City of Seattle* (Seattle, 1947), 52; Emil E. Palmquist to Herman E. Hilleboe, Jan. 24, 1947, UW Archives, Warren G. Magnuson Papers, box 65, folder 1.

12. *Annual Report and Survey, 1939–1943,* 153; Lee Powers to the Honorable Board of Commissioners of King County and the Honorable City Council of the City of Seattle, Aug. 14, 1943, WS Archives, Department of Health, Director's Office, RS 2 Disease File, box 8, folder 189.

13. *Pep* 30 (July 1943): 4–5.

14. *Annual Report and Survey, 1939–1943,* 148–50; Cedric Northrop, "Washington State Plan for Tuberculosis Control," 1945, WS Archives, Health Department Administrative Files, box 2, folder 156A.

15. This dispute actually represented an interesting chapter in the history of public health work in Seattle. Basically, the city and King County were debating whether hospitalization of poor patients at Firland should properly be considered a welfare or a public health function. See Barron H. Lerner, "'On What Authority Is This Being Done?' Tuberculosis Control, Poverty and Coercion in Seattle, 1909–1973" (Ph.D. diss., University of Washington, 1996), 134–41.

16. Northrop, "Washington State Plan"; Cedric Northrop, "Notes on Firland Sanatorium," May 11, 1952, Firland Memorabilia Collection, Shoreline Historical Society, Seattle.

17. Powers to Board of Commissioners of King County and City Council of Seattle, Aug. 14, 1943, and Aug. 20, 1943.

18. Powers to Board of Commissioners of King County and City Council of Seattle, Aug. 14, 1943; Stave, "Firland," 11; Washington State Department of Health, *Annual Report, 1945* (Olympia, 1946).

19. Northrop, "Washington State Plan."

20. Henry D. Chadwick, "Tuberculosis Survey of the State of Washington" (1944), ALA-W Archives; Cedric Northrop, "Tuberculosis Control in the State of Washington," *Northwest Medicine* 44 (1945): 174–78.

21. "From the Desk," *Pep* 29 (Jan. 1942): 11. On the use of military metaphors in tuberculosis control, see JoAnne Brown, "Playing the Game: Tuberculosis, Medievalist Nostalgia, and the Great War," paper presented at the annual meeting of the Organization of American Historians, Atlanta, Apr. 1994.

22. Joseph D. Wassersug, "Tuberculosis," *New England Journal of Medicine* 230 (1944): 45–57, and 231 (1944): 876–84; Tamara M. Haygood and Jonathan E. Briggs, "World War II Military Led the Way in Screening Chest Radiography," *Military Medicine* 157 (Mar. 1992): 113–16.

23. On the tuberculosis program of the Public Health Service, see Wassersug, "Tuberculosis," 231 (1944), 877; Herman E. Hilleboe, "The Tuberculosis Control Program of the United States Public Health Service," *American Journal of Roentgenology* 50 (1943): 214–18; Georgina Feldberg, *Disease and Class: Tuberculosis and the Shaping of Modern North American Society* (New Brunswick: Rutgers University Press, 1995), 177–81.

24. Bob Willey and Floyd Swartz, "A Man You Should Know," *Pep and Courage* 40 (Jan. 1952): 18–21. On Minnesota's tuberculosis program, see Leonard G. Wilson, "The Rise and Fall of Tuberculosis in Minnesota: The Role of Infection," *Bulletin of the History of Medicine* 66 (spring 1992): 16–52, 39–41.

25. Quote is from Wilson, "Rise and Fall," 41. See also Roberts Davies, "The Effect on Tuberculosis Mortality of a Complete Community Survey with Hospitalization of All Active Cases," *American Review of Tuberculosis* 54 (1946): 254–60.

26. Cedric Northrop, "What We Expect from X-Ray Programs: Industry—The Health Department," *Transactions of the National Tuberculosis Association* 43 (1947): 165–71, 170.

27. Roberts J. Davies, "The Prerequisites for a Successful Campaign of Tuberculosis Eradication," *Health Pilot* (of the Washington Tuberculosis Association) 29 (June 1947): 6–8, 11.

28. Eunice Bessette, "Firland, 1911 to 1946: The Story of an Institution Dedicated to the Cure and Eradication of Tuberculosis," *Pep* 34 (May 1946): 14. Of note, other health departments, such as that of New York City, operated aggressive X-ray screening programs despite a paucity of sanatorium beds.

29. *Public Health in Seattle, 1946,* 52, 56; Otto Case to Warren G. Magnuson, Mar. 17, 1947, and William F. Devin to Warren G. Magnuson, May 12, 1947, UW Archives, Warren G. Magnuson Papers, box 65, folder 1.

30. Roberts Davies to Warren G. Magnuson, June 9, 1947, UW Archives, Warren G. Magnuson Papers, box 65, folder 1.

31. H. E. Busch and George E. Nethercut to Warren G. Magnuson, May 14, 1947, UW Archives, Warren G. Magnuson Papers, box 65, folder 1.

32. Paul Patrick to Warren G. Magnuson, June 27, 1947, UW Archives, Warren G. Magnuson Papers, box 65, folder 1.

33. James R. Royse to Warren G. Magnuson, June 28, 1947, UW Archives, Warren G. Magnuson Papers, box 65, folder 1.

34. C. W. Doyle to Warren G. Magnuson, May 14, 1947, UW Archives, Warren G. Magnuson Papers, box 65, folder 1.

35. Thorbjorg D. Arnason, "Study of One Hundred Deaths from Tuberculosis in Persons over Forty-Five Years in Seattle, Washington, 1943" (master's thesis, University of Washington, 1945), 27–28.

36. Paul Hawley to Warren G. Magnuson, Aug. 4, 1947, UW Archives, Warren G. Magnuson Papers, box 65, folder 1.

37. W. C. Speidel Jr., "Sounding the Death Knell for Tuberculosis," *Free Enterprise* 4 (Dec. 1947): 1, 4.

38. Ibid., 4; *Public Health in Seattle and King County, 1949: Annual Report of the Seattle–King County Department of Public Health* (Seattle, 1950), 23.

39. Cora Stevens, letter to the editor of the *Seattle Times,* 1947. A copy of this letter can be found in Firland Memorabilia Collection, Shoreline Historical Society, Seattle.

40. According to Northrop, the other states without waiting lists were Minnesota (not surprisingly), North Dakota, and Connecticut. See curriculum vitae of Cedric Northrop, n.d.; *Evaluation of Health Conditions and Services: Seattle and King County, 1948* (Seattle: Health and Welfare Council of Seattle and King County, 1949), 5; "Encouraging Progress in Tuberculosis Fight," *Seattle Times,* Apr. 9, 1952, 6.

41. Cedric Northrop, "Field Report for June 1948" and "Field Report, April 1950," WS Archives, Department of Health, Director's Office, RS 2 Disease File, box 8, folder 160; Cedric Northrop, "Field Activities Report for May 1953," WS Archives, Department of Health, Director's Office, RS 2 Disease File, box 7, folder 784; "Need for Hospital Facilities for the Tuberculous," *Public Health Reports* 61 (1946): 1131–32.

42. F. B. Exner, J. R. Erwin, B. F. Francis, H. V. Hartzell, S. J. Hawley, Honoria Hughes, and Louise Speer, "Voluntary Continuous Photofluorographic Tuberculosis Case Finding," *Northwest Medicine* 51 (1952): 591–95.

43. U.S. Public Health Service (PHS), *Community-Wide Chest X-Ray Survey* (Washington, D.C.: GPO, 1952), 3.

44. "League Votes to Aid Fall X-Ray Survey. Decision Means Curtailment of Present Program; Pledge $61,000," *Health Notes* (of the Anti-Tuberculosis League of King County [ATLKC]) 4 (Apr. 1948): 1–3.

45. Minutes of the X-Ray Committee of the ATLKC, Jan. 13, 1948, and "Executive Secretary's Report," included in the Minutes of the Executive Committee

of the ATLKC, July 22, 1947, ALA-W Archives; Julie Miale, "Report on Mass X-Ray Surveys," *Health Pilot* 30 (Sept. 1948): 5–7, 10.

46. Minutes of the X-Ray Committee, Jan. 13, 1948, and Minutes of the Board of Directors of the ATLKC, Mar. 11, 1948, ALA-W Archives.

47. Nick Hughes, interview with author, Dec. 11 and 12, 1992. On Buchanan, see Marjorie Jones, "Descendant Seeks to Refute Untruths about Daniel Boone," *Seattle Times,* July 18, 1965, 4.

48. In addition to issues of gender, the shift of projects from lay to medical control also led to a devaluing of the efforts of the voluntary agencies. See Lerner, " 'On What Authority,' " 191–98. On women's associations, see Anne F. Scott, *Natural Allies: Women's Associations in American History* (Urbana: University of Illinois, 1991); Kathryn Kish Sklar, *Florence Kelley and the Nation's Work: The Rise of Women's Political Culture, 1830–1900* (New Haven: Yale University Press, 1995).

49. Minutes of the X-Ray Committee of the ATLKC, Jan. 29, 1948, ALA-W Archives. For more discussion of this issue, see Minutes of the Executive Committee of the ATLKC, Mar. 23, 1948, ALA-W Archives; Miss Beery to Holland Hudson, Oct. 1, 1948, ALA Archives, Washington State Field File (585 R).

50. James E. Perkins to Wayne Dick, Mar. 22, 1948, included with Minutes of the Board of Directors of the ATLKC, Mar. 27, 1948, ALA-W Archives.

51. "Tacoma, Spokane Prepare for Mass X-ray Surveys," *Health Commentator* (of the Washington State Department of Health) 4 (Jan. 1949): 1.

52. Northrop, "Notes on Firland Sanatorium"; *Final Report on Seattle Area Chest X-Ray Program Compiled By Program Director, General Chairman and Executive Committee* (Seattle, 1949).

53. Minutes of the Advisory Staff of the SACXRP (Seattle Area Chest X-Ray Program), Aug. 5 and 12, 1948, and Sept. 2, 1948, KCMS Library, SACXRP Records, vol. 1.

54. Minutes of the Advisory Staff of the SACXRP, Aug. 5, 1948, KCMS Library, SACXRP Records, vol. 1.

55. "Instructions for Hosts and Hostesses," included with Minutes of the Advisory Staff of the SACXRP, summer 1948, KCMS Library, SACXRP Records, vol. 1.

56. "Parade to Open X-Ray Program," *Seattle Times,* Sept. 7, 1948, 5. See also Richard C. Berner, *Seattle, 1921–1940: From Boom to Bust* (Seattle: Charles Press, 1992), 6–7; Carl Abbott, "Regional City and Network City: Portland and Seattle in the Twentieth Century," *Western Historical Quarterly* 23 (1992): 293–322.

57. "8,309 X-Rays Set Day Record Here," *Seattle Times,* Oct. 9, 1948; "X-Ray Campaign in Seattle Is Near Record," *Seattle Times,* Nov. 21, 1948; "X-Ray Here to Top Other Cities," *Seattle Times,* Dec. 8, 1948.

58. George M. Shahan to Mrs. William Roth, Jan. 14, 1949, KCMS Library, SACXRP Records, vol. 5, Correspondence of the SACXRP.

59. William F. Devin to Lawrence Bates, Jan. 17, 1949, KCMS Library, SACXRP Records, vol. 5, Correspondence of the SACXRP.

60. PHS, *Community-Wide Chest X-Ray Survey,* 3.

61. Berner, *Seattle, 1921–1940,* 7; Roger Sale, *Seattle: Past to Present* (Seattle: University of Washington Press, 1976), 189–91; William O'Neill, *American High: The Years of Confidence, 1945–1960* (New York: Free Press, 1986), 1–3.

62. Murray Morgan, *Skid Road: An Informal Portrait of Seattle* (Seattle: University of Washington Press, 1982), 219. See also Sale, *Seattle,* 196.

63. Minutes of the Location Planning Division of the SACXRP, Oct. 20, 1948, KCMS Library, SACXRP Records, vol. 1; " 'Skid' Civic Pride Reaches Heights for X-Rays," *Seattle Post-Intelligencer,* Nov. 20, 1948, 1, 9.

64. William D. Kirkpatrick to Earl A. Jacobs, Aug. 24, 1948, and Earl A. Jacobs to Mrs. P. Schonwald, Aug. 30, 1948, KCMS Library, SACXRP Records, vol. 5, Correspondence of the SACXRP.

65. "A Doctor Speaks His Mind: Bureaucratic Medicine Causes Dr. F. B. Exner of Seattle to 'See Red,' " *Seattle Times Sunday Magazine,* July 6, 1952, 4; "Dr. Frederick Exner, Radiologist, Dead at 76," *Seattle Times,* Dec. 18, 1976, D15.

66. F. B. Exner, "Remarks of the President," included in the Minutes of the Board of Directors of the ATLKC, Oct. 21, 1949, ALA-W Archives.

67. Walter T. Miller, M.D., interview with author, July 15, 1992.

68. "U.S. 'Lied' in X-Ray Surveys, Says Dr. Exner," *Seattle Times,* Apr. 27, 1950, 19.

69. "X-Ray Committee Report," included in the Minutes of the Board of Directors of the ATLKC, Feb. 18, 1948, ALA-W Archives; Miale, "Report on Mass X-Ray Surveys," 5.

70. Minutes of the X-Ray Committee of the ATLKC, Jan. 29, 1948, ALA-W Archives. On the limitations of using X-rays as diagnostic tools, see Barron H. Lerner, "The Perils of 'X-Ray Vision': How Radiographic Images Have Historically Influenced Perception," *Perspectives in Biology and Medicine* 35 (1992): 382–97.

71. "X-Ray Committee Report," Feb. 18, 1948; Julie Miale to Mr. Stone, Mar. 29, 1948, ALA Archives, Washington State Field Report File (585 R). On the professionalization of radiology, see Joel D. Howell, *Technology in the Hospital: Transforming Patient Care in the Early Twentieth Century* (Baltimore: Johns Hopkins University Press, 1995), 126–28; Bettyann Kevles, *Naked to the Bone: Medical Imaging in the Twentieth Century* (New Brunswick: Rutgers University Press, 1997), 77–96.

72. Donal Sparkman, M.D., interview with author, July 7, 1992.

73. *Public Health in Seattle and King County, 1948: Annual Report of the Seattle–King County Department of Public Health* (Seattle, 1949), 13; "127 in Firland as Result of X-Ray Survey," *Seattle Times,* Feb. 6, 1949, 18.

74. David M. Gould, "Nontuberculous Lesions Found in Mass X-Ray Surveys," *Journal of the American Medical Association* 127 (1945): 753–56.

75. Richard Carter, *The Gentle Legions* (Garden City, N.Y.: Doubleday, 1961), 155–58, 175–78; Daniel M. Fox, *Power and Illness: The Failure and Future of American Health Policy* (Berkeley: University of California Press, 1993), 171–85.

76. J. A. Kahl to Arthur B. Langlie, Oct. 29, 1954, UW Archives, Arthur B. Langlie Papers, pt. 1, box 32, folder 13.

77. "State Health Budget Totals $9,449,300," *Health Notes* 5 (Mar.–Apr. 1949): 1; "Here's Story behind Slash," *Health Commentator* 4 (May 1949): 2; "Legislative Needs for Tuberculosis Control," memorandum from Cedric Northrop to John Kahl, Jan. 17, 1950, WS Archives, Department of Health, Director's Office, RS 2 Disease File, box 8, folder 160.

78. "Material for Governor Langlie on a Fifteen-Minute Radio Talk," UW Archives, Arthur B. Langlie Papers, pt. 1, box 32, folder 13. Washington State also received roughly ninety-five thousand dollars annually from the federal government for its tuberculosis control programs.

79. George W. Scott, "Arthur B. Langlie: Republican Governor in a Democratic Age" (Ph.D. diss., University of Washington, 1971), 3–4.

80. Scott, "Arthur B. Langlie," 95. Langlie was elected governor on the Republican ticket.

81. Message of Monrad C. Wallgren, governor of Washington, to the Thirtieth Legislature, Jan. 15, 1947, 21–22; available at University of Washington Library, Seattle.

82. Inaugural message of Arthur B. Langlie, governor of Washington, to the Thirty-First Legislature, Jan. 12, 1949, 15; available at University of Washington Library, Seattle.

83. Scott, "Arthur B. Langlie," 170–200, 180. For more on Initiatives 172 and 178, see Clement A. Finch, "Academia at Last: University of Washington School of Medicine," in Nancy M. Rockafellar and James W. Haviland, eds., *From Saddlebags to Scanners: The First Hundred Years of Medicine in Washington State* (Seattle: Washington State Medical Association, 1989), 183.

84. Scott, "Arthur B. Langlie," 180. See also Jane Sanders, *Cold War on the Campus: Academic Freedom at the University of Washington, 1946–1964* (Seattle: University of Washington Press, 1979), 85–91.

85. Northrop, "Notes on Firland Sanatorium"; "TB Appropriation $1,400,000 Less Than Requested," *Health Notes* 5 (Mar.–Apr. 1949): 1; Roberts Davies, "Analysis of the King County Tuberculosis Hospital Problem in Relation to Financing Such Care," 1949, WS Archives, Department of Health, Director's Office, RS 2 Disease File, box 8, folder 160; "Status of Tuberculosis Hospitalization Funds," memorandum from Cedric Northrop to J. A. Kahl, May 12, 1950, WS Archives, Department of Health, Director's Office, RS 2 Disease File, box 8, folder 160.

86. Davies, "Analysis"; "Fund Lack Hits T.B. Program," *Seattle Times*, Apr. 1, 1949.

87. Minutes of the Executive Committee of the Washington Tuberculosis Association, Mar. 25, 1949, and Minutes of the Program Committee of the ATLKC, Mar. 29, 1949, ALA-W Archives.

88. J. A. Kahl to Dr. Jones, June 7, 1949, J. A. Kahl to Arthur B. Langlie, Sept. 13, 1949, R. C. Watts to All County Commissioners, Sept. 17, 1949, and J. B.

Gibson to Governor Langlie, Jan. 24, 1950, WS Archives, Department of Health, Director's Office, RS 2 Disease File, box 8, folder 160.

89. Miller, interview, July 15, 1992.

90. "Highlights of Annual Meeting of the Anti-Tuberculosis League: 'Health and Legislation'—Northrop," *Health Notes* 5 (Feb. 1949): 2.

91. Cedric Northrop, "Field Activities Report for April 1953," WS Archives, Department of Health, Director's Office, RS 2 Disease File, box 7, folder 784; "Major Accomplishments in Public Health since 1940," memorandum from Bernard Bucove to Joseph F. Hiddleston, May 21, 1956, UW Archives, Arthur B. Langlie Papers, pt. 1, box 17, folder 7. Generous allocations for tuberculosis control persisted well into the 1960s.

92. "Major Accomplishments in Public Health."

93. Florence Sabin, quoted in William P. Shepard, "Some Unmet Needs in Tuberculosis Control: A Challenge for the Future," *American Journal of Public Health* 38 (1948): 1370–80, 1370.

94. Ibid., 1371.

THREE. STILL A SOCIAL DISEASE

1. See, for example, Margaret E. Kidd Parsons, "White Plague and Double-Barred Cross in Atlanta, 1895–1945" (Ph.D. diss., Emory University, 1985), preface, 177; Mark Caldwell, *The Last Crusade: The War on Consumption, 1862–1954* (New York: Atheneum, 1988), 245–72; F. B. Smith, *The Retreat of Tuberculosis in Twentieth-Century Britain, 1850–1950* (Oxford, England: Croom Helm, 1988), 246–47; Susan Sontag, *Illness as Metaphor* (New York: Farrar, Straus and Giroux, 1978), 35–36; Frank Ryan, *The Forgotten Plague: How the Battle against Tuberculosis Was Won—and Lost* (Boston: Little, Brown, 1993), 342–64.

2. Georgina D. Feldberg, *Disease and Class: Tuberculosis and the Shaping of Modern North American Society* (New Brunswick: Rutgers University Press, 1995), 205–6; George W. Comstock, "Tuberculosis: Is the Past Once Again Prologue?" *American Journal of Public Health* 84 (1994): 1729–31, 1730.

3. Ryan, *The Forgotten Plague,* 327; Harry F. Dowling, *Fighting Infection: Conquests of the Twentieth Century* (Cambridge: Harvard University Press, 1977), 164–67; Harry M. Marks, *The Progress of Experiment: Science and Therapeutic Reform in the United States, 1900–1990* (Cambridge: Cambridge University Press, 1997). Waksman's account of the discovery of streptomycin can be found in Selman A. Waksman, *The Conquest of Tuberculosis* (Berkeley: University of California Press, 1964).

4. *Annual Report, Firland Sanatorium, 1947* (Seattle: Firland Sanatorium, 1948), 12.

5. Ryan, *The Forgotten Plague,* 326–29; Emil Bogen, "Streptomycin Treatment of Tuberculosis," *American Review of Tuberculosis* 56 (1947): 442–44.

6. Ellson F. White, "Streptomycin in Tuberculosis," *Pep and Courage* 36 (May 1948): 8.

7. Ryan, *The Forgotten Plague,* 284–88.

8. *Annual Report, Firland Sanatorium, 1947,* 13; Minutes of the Executive Committee of the ATLKC (Anti-Tuberculosis League of King County), Apr. 10, 1947, and July 22, 1947, ALA-W Archives; Minutes of the Joint Program Committee and X-Ray Committee of the ATLKC, Aug. 12, 1947, ALA-W Archives.

9. Minutes of the Joint Program and X-Ray Committee of the ATLKC, Aug. 12, 1947, ALA-W Archives.

10. Roberts Davies to Honoria Hughes, included in the Minutes of the Executive Committee of the ATLKC, July 15, 1947, ALA-W Archives.

11. "About the New Tuberculosis Drugs," *Pep and Courage* 40 (Apr. 1952): 29; Dowling, *Fighting Infection,* 167; Ryan, *The Forgotten Plague,* 330–32.

12. Harold F. Osborne, "Firland Will Try New Wonder Drug," *Seattle Times,* Apr. 20, 1952, 12.

13. Dowling, *Fighting Infection,* 168. On the incident at Sea View, see Caldwell, *The Last Crusade,* 266–68.

14. "About the New Tuberculosis Drugs," 29.

15. Erle Howell, "Learning While Recovering," *Pacific Parade Magazine* (of the *Seattle Times*), Feb. 26, 1952, 10.

16. Ibid. For other comments by Davies on the value of bed rest, see "Highlights of Annual Meeting Talks: Dr. Roberts Davies," *Health Notes* (of the ATLKC) 8 (May–June 1952): 2–3. See also John A. Sbarbaro, "Tuberculosis: A Portal through Which to View the Future," *American Review of Respiratory Diseases* 125 (supp.) (1982): 127–32.

17. Cedric Northrop, "Field Report for February 1953," and "Field Report for March 1954," WS Archives, Department of Health, Director's Office, RS 2 Disease File, box 7, folder 785a; Daniel Widelock, Lenore R. Peizer, and Sarah Klein, "Public Health Significance of Tubercle Bacilli Resistant to Isoniazid," *American Journal of Public Health* 45 (1955): 79–83.

18. *Annual Report, Firland Sanatorium, 1950* (Seattle: Firland Sanatorium, 1951), 4; *Annual Report, Firland Sanatorium, 1954* (Seattle: Firland Sanatorium, 1955), 7, 14.

19. *Annual Report, Firland Sanatorium, 1954,* 5, 6; Roberts J. Davies, "Your Questions about Tuberculosis Answered," *Pep: The Magazine of Firland* 42 (May 1954): 24.

20. Cedric Northrop to Inez Lewis, Sept. 7, 1955, UW Archives, Arthur B. Langlie Papers, pt. 1, box 36, folder 1.

21. Arthur B. Robins and Aaron D. Chaves, "The Place of Drug Therapy in the Management of Unhospitalized Tuberculosis Patients," *Annals of Internal Medicine* 47 (1957): 774–81. Other cities that relied heavily on outpatient treatment of tuberculosis included Cleveland, Pittsburgh, and Oakland.

22. Caldwell, *The Last Crusade,* 269–72.

23. *Public Health in Seattle and King County, 1948: Annual Report of the Seattle–King County Department of Public Health* (Seattle, 1949), 70; *Annual Report, Firland Sanatorium, 1949* (Seattle: Firland Sanatorium, 1950), 8; *Report of*

the Seattle–King County Department of Public Health, 1952–1955 (Seattle, 1956), 18; *Annual Report, Firland Sanatorium, 1954,* 16. Mortality across the country declined from thirty-three per 100,000 population in 1947 to twelve per 100,000 in 1953. See Godias J. Drolet and Anthony M. Lowell, "Whereto Tuberculosis? The First Seven Years of the Antimicrobial Era, 1947–1953," *American Review of Tuberculosis* 72 (1955): 419–52, 424.

24. In 1954, there were actually 581 new cases. See *Report of the Seattle–King County Department of Public Health, 1952–1955,* 18. The number of new cases was rising across the country. See Herbert R. Edwards and Godias J. Drolet, "The Implications of Changing Morbidity and Mortality Rates from Tuberculosis," *American Review of Tuberculosis* 61 (1950): 39–50.

25. Quoted in Richard Carter, *The Gentle Legions* (Garden City, N.Y.: Doubleday, 1961), 90.

26. U.S. Public Health Service (PHS), *The Arden House Conference on Tuberculosis* (Washington, D.C.: GPO, 1960), 1.

27. "Report of the Tuberculosis Hospitalization Evaluation Team," 1957, WS Archives, Department of Health, Director's Files, 1954–57, box 1, folder 60.

28. Howell, "Learning While Recovering," 10.

29. Letter to the editor of an unknown newspaper from Mrs. Wells, 1957, WS Archives, Department of Health, Director's Files, 1954–57, box 2, folder 86.1.

30. See, for example, George Eckley, "Evidence Suggesting Differential Effects of Various Drug Regimens in Pulmonary Tuberculosis," *Transactions of the Thirteenth Conference on the Chemotherapy of Tuberculosis* 13 (1954): 134–40.

31. *Annual Report, Firland Sanatorium, 1954,* 8–9.

32. Jane Sanders, *Cold War on the Campus: Academic Freedom at the University of Washington, 1946–1964* (Seattle: University of Washington Press, 1979), 175–76; Clement A. Finch, "Academia at Last: University of Washington School of Medicine," in Nancy M. Rockafellar and James W. Haviland, eds., *From Saddlebags to Scanners: The First Hundred Years of Medicine in Washington State* (Seattle: Washington State Medical Association, 1989), 177–79, 187–90.

33. Charles E. Rosenberg, *The Care of Strangers: The Rise of America's Hospital System* (New York: Basic Books, 1987), 333. For references to the term *tuberculosis hospital,* see, for example, "Report of the Tuberculosis Hospitalization Evaluation Team"; Esmond R. Long, "Tuberculosis in Modern Society," *Bulletin of the History of Medicine* 27 (July–Aug. 1953): 301–19, 315.

34. Floyd Swartz, "Five Chiefs on the Reservation," *Pep and Courage* 40 (Mar. 1952): 22.

35. J. Arthur Myers, *A History of the American College of Chest Physicians* (El Paso, Tex.: Guynes Printing, 1959). John F. Murray has noted that the number of board-certified chest physicians (or pulmonologists) began to rise dramatically only after 1965. See John F. Murray, "The White Plague: Down and Out, or Up and Coming," *American Review of Respiratory Disease* 140 (1989): 1788–95.

36. Richard Greenleaf, M.D., interview with author, Oct. 14, 1992.

37. George H. Hames, "Surgical Treatment of Pulmonary Tuberculosis," *Pep*

and Courage 40 (Apr. 1952): 6–8; Fred J. Jarvis, "New Work for the Scalpel," *Pep: The Magazine of Firland* 41 (Oct. 1953): 7–8.

38. Godias J. Drolet, "Collapse Therapy: Trends in Frequency and Type of Surgical Procedures in Treatment of Pulmonary Tuberculosis," *American Review of Tuberculosis* 47 (1943): 184–215.

39. *Annual Report, Firland Sanatorium, 1953* (Seattle: Firland Sanatorium, 1954), 13.

40. For example, Donald King reviewed 3,840 resections performed at Veterans' Administration hospitals in the early 1950s. See Donald S. King, "Present Status of the Treatment of Tuberculosis in Man," *Journal of the American Medical Association* 158 (1955): 829–31.

41. *Annual Report, Firland Sanatorium, 1953,* 15; Hames, "Surgical Treatment," 7–8.

42. On this debate, see Edward J. O'Brien, Arthur C. Miller, Paul T. Chapman, Koert Koster, and Paul V. O'Rourke, "The Present Chaos Regarding Resection of Residual Caseous Nodules in Pulmonary Tuberculosis," *Journal of Thoracic Surgery* 26 (1953): 441–46; Bernard J. Ryan, Edgar M. Medlar, and Edward S. Welles, "Simple Excision in the Treatment of Pulmonary Tuberculosis," *Journal of Thoracic Surgery* 23 (1952): 327–340.

43. Firland Sanatorium chart S28.

44. Firland Sanatorium chart S4.

45. Firland Sanatorium chart S28.

46. Paul A. Kirschner, "Tuberculoma of the Lung," *Journal of the Mount Sinai Hospital* 23 (1956): 506–11, 511.

47. E. N. Moyes, "Tuberculoma of the Lung," *Thorax* 6 (1951): 238–49, 238. See also R. Grenville-Mathers, "The Natural History of So-Called Tuberculomas," *Journal of Thoracic Surgery* 23 (1952): 251–52.

48. The connection between tuberculomas and residual caseous masses is made in Grenville-Mathers, "Natural History," 251; Kirschner, "Tuberculoma of the Lung," 510; "Discussion on the Management of Patients Suffering from Pulmonary Tuberculosis," *Proceedings of the Royal Society of Medicine* 50 (1957): 335–46, 337.

49. These phrases can be found in Kirschner, "Tuberculoma of the Lung," 509–10; L. E. Houghton, "Collapse Therapy and the Bronchus," *Tubercle* 31 (Mar. 1950): 50–62, 60. See also "Discussion on the Management of Patients," 336–38.

50. That is, the treatment of tuberculomas had less to do with their "objective" anatomical or physiological qualities than with the way in which physicians—in an era that emphasized the use of X-rays and chest surgery—conceptualized them. In this manner, tuberculomas exemplify how disease entities may be socially constructed. On the "surgical construction" of splenic anemia, see Keith Wailoo, *Drawing Blood: Technology and Disease Identity in Twentieth-Century America* (Baltimore: Johns Hopkins University Press, 1997), 46–72.

51. King, "Present Status," 829–31; James W. Raleigh, "The Randomized Re-

section of Closed Necrotic Lesions, Pilot Study VI," *Transactions of the Sixteenth Conference on the Chemotherapy of Tuberculosis* 16 (1957): 185–90.

52. *Annual Report, Firland Sanatorium, 1960* (Seattle: Firland Sanatorium, 1961), 11, 13.

53. Cedric Northrop, John H. Fountain, and Daniel W. Zahn, "The Practical Management of the Recalcitrant Tuberculous Patient," *Public Health Reports* 67 (1952): 894–98, 895.

54. See, for example, Jean Berman and Leo H. Berman, "The Signing Out of Tuberculous Patients," *The Family* 25 (Apr. 1944): 67–73; William B. Tollen, "Irregular Discharge: The Problem of Hospitalization of the Tuberculous," *Public Health Reports* 63 (1948): 1441–70; William B. Tollen, "Why Do Patients Go AWOL?" *Bulletin of the National Tuberculosis Association* 36 (July 1950): 101–2.

55. "Why Patients Leave against Advice," *Health Pilot* (of the Washington Tuberculosis Association) 33 (Jan. 1950): 10–11.

56. Tollen, "Irregular Discharge," 1441–70; Louis I. Dublin, "Function of the Health Officer in the Control of Tuberculosis among Veterans," *American Journal of Public Health* 33 (1943): 1425–29.

57. Evelyn N. Hadaway, "A Medical Social Study of Fifty-Four Tuberculosis Patients Who Left Firland Sanatorium against Medical Advice in 1952" (master's thesis, University of Washington, 1953), 10. In chapter 8, I return to this notion of a quid pro quo between patients and the state.

58. Quote is from Feldberg, *Disease and Class,* 90–91. See also 205–7; and Daniel W. Zahn, "Home Care in Seattle," *Bulletin of the National Tuberculosis Association* 42 (Jan. 1956): 11–12.

59. Roberts Davies, "Why People Die of Tuberculosis," *Health Pilot* 35 (Jan. 1952): 4–5, 4.

60. Ibid., 5.

61. Lenna G. Eby, "Tuberculosis and Family Problems: A Study of the Problems of 135 Parents and the Medical Social Worker's Participation in Planning for the Admission to the Tuberculosis Sanatorium" (master's thesis, University of Washington, 1950); Alice B. Jacobson and Betty D. Peterson, "A Study of Sixty-Four Tuberculous Patients with Emphasis on Their Social Problems" (master's thesis, University of Washington, 1951); Montell C. Parks, "Tuberculosis and Family Problems: A Study of Fifty Fathers Known to the Seattle–King County Health Department Tuberculosis Division" (master's thesis, University of Washington, 1952).

62. Hadaway, "A Medical Social Study," 3, 27–28; Barbara Dike, "A Study of Clinical Records to Determine Some of the Factors Involved in Irregular Discharges of Ninety-Four Patients Who Left Firland Sanatorium against Medical Advice during the Period of January 1, 1950, to June 30, 1950" (master's thesis, University of Washington, 1953), 35–36, 58.

63. *Annual Report, Firland Sanatorium, 1950,* 7.

64. Hadaway, "A Medical Social Study," 43, 45; Dike, "A Study of Clinical

Records," 46. While active tuberculosis was not necessarily infectious, it invariably required additional treatment. The distinctions between infectious, active, and inactive tuberculosis are discussed extensively in chapter 6.

65. Hadaway, "A Medical Social Study," 18, 23; Dike, "A Study of Clinical Records," 37, 39.

66. Hadaway, "A Medical Social Study," 23.

67. Dike, "A Study of Clinical Records," 22. See also Hadaway, "A Medical Social Study," 32.

68. Dike, "A Study of Clinical Records," 4–5, 31; Hadaway, "A Medical Social Study," 31.

69. Dike, "A Study of Clinical Records," 53. Tollen's studies of Veterans' Administration patients had yielded comparable percentages.

70. Hadaway, "A Medical Social Study," 41, 50.

71. Dike, "A Study of Clinical Records," 63.

72. Hadaway, "A Medical Social Study," 56–57.

73. For a review of this literature, see E. D. Wittkower, H. B. Durost, and W. A. R. Laing, "A Psychosomatic Study of the Course of Pulmonary Tuberculosis," *American Review of Tuberculosis* 71 (1955): 201–19.

74. Jules V. Coleman, Allan Hurst, and Ruth Hornbein, "Psychiatric Contributions to Care of Tuberculosis Patients," *Journal of the American Medical Association* 135 (1947): 699–703; Barbara M. Stewart, "Current Status and Future Directions of the Psychologist's Role in a Tuberculosis Hospital," in Phineas J. Sparer, ed., *Personality, Stress, and Tuberculosis* (New York: International Universities Press, 1956), 393–95.

75. Catherine E. Vavra and Edith D. Rainboth, *A Study of Patients' Attitudes toward Care at Firland Sanatorium, Seattle, Washington* (Seattle: Firland Sanatorium, 1955). The study received the World Health Organization award of merit.

76. Ibid., 2.

77. Ibid., iv, 41.

78. Ibid., 29, 33.

79. Julius A. Roth, *Timetables: Structuring the Passage of Time in Hospital Treatment and Other Careers* (Indianapolis: Bobbs-Merrill, 1963), 1–21.

80. Vavra and Rainboth, "A Study of Patients' Attitudes," iv.

81. Peggy Cyra, "The Story of Dr. Davies," *Pep: The Magazine of Firland* 42 (Oct. 1954): 14; "Bob Feller Visits Firland," *Firland Magazine* 45 (Aug. 1957): 10. Despite these changes, Firland still relied on a rigorous daily schedule and a long list of rules and regulations.

82. On the Patients' Council, see Bob Willey, "Patients' Council Confidential: What's It All About," *Pep and Courage* 39 (Sept. 1951): 12–13, 20–21.

83. Vavra and Rainboth, "A Study of Patients' Attitudes," iii.

84. Pauline Miller, *Medical Social Service in a Tuberculosis Sanatorium,* (Washington, D.C.: GPO, 1951), 12. The National Jewish Hospital, in Denver, Colorado, was actually the first tuberculosis institution to hire a full-time psy-

chologist, doing so in 1938. See Stewart, "Current Status and Future Directions," 388.

85. Stewart, "Current Status and Future Directions," 387–88; Gerald N. Grob, *From Asylum to Community: Mental Health Policy in Modern America* (Princeton: Princeton University Press, 1991), 5–23.

86. Doris Carrington, "A Study of Mothers Who Left the King County Tuberculosis Sanatorium against Medical Advice" (master's thesis, University of Washington, 1950), 18. "Many signouts," wrote another commentator, "are the result of emotional maladjustment or mental imbalance which might be corrected by a psychiatrist." See "Why Patients Leave against Advice," 11.

87. Gardner Middlebrook, "Tuberculosis: Some Aspects of Causation and Treatment in Human Beings," in Phineas J. Sparer, ed., *Personality, Stress, and Tuberculosis* (New York: International Universities Press, 1956), 13.

88. René Dubos and Jean Dubos, *The White Plague: Tuberculosis, Man, and Society* (New Brunswick: Rutgers University Press, 1987), vii.

89. Ibid., 224–25.

90. Wade Hampton Frost, "How Much Control of Tuberculosis?" *American Journal of Public Health* 27 (1937): 759–66.

91. "Death and Death Rates for Selected Causes By Age, Race, and Sex," *Vital Statistics of the United States* 35 (Nov. 27, 1950): 334. On the high rates of tuberculosis among the poor and minorities in Seattle and Washington, see Cedric Northrop, "Tuberculosis Control in the State of Washington," *Northwest Medicine* 44 (1945): 174–78; "1,121 Jackson Street Residents X-Rayed during Unit's 3rd Visit," *Health Notes* 4 (June 1948): 1–2.

92. Dubos and Dubos, *The White Plague*, 219–28; Long, "Tuberculosis in Modern Society," 311–13; Edwards and Drolet, "Implications of Changing Morbidity and Mortality," 39–50; Sophia Bloom, "Some Economic and Emotional Problems of the Tuberculosis Patient and His Family," *Public Health Reports* 63 (1948): 448–55.

93. See, for example, Thomas Parran, "Tuberculosis: A Time for Decision," *Public Health Reports* 68 (1953): 921–27; J. Yerushalmy, "The Increase in Tuberculosis Proportionate Mortality among Nonwhite Young Adults," *Public Health Reports* 61 (1946): 251–58; Anthony M. Lowell, *Socio-Economic Conditions and Tuberculosis Prevalence: New York City, 1949–1951* (New York: New York Tuberculosis and Health Association, 1956); James G. Stone, "Anti-Poverty-Anti-TB," *Bulletin of the National Tuberculosis Association* 51 (Nov. 1965): 2–3. On housing, see N. S. Keith, "How Can the Tuberculosis Association Assist in Improving Standards of Living through Housing," *Transactions of the National Tuberculosis Association* 47 (1951): 322–27.

94. Quote is from Miss Becht to Dr. Feldman, Oct. 9, 1953, ALA Archives, Committee on Social Research File (1137). See also Clarence W. Kehoe, "How Can the Tuberculosis Association Assist in Improving Standards of Living through Welfare Service," *Transactions of the National Tuberculosis Association* 47 (1951):

317–21; "Financial Assistance," *Bulletin of the National Tuberculosis Association* 43 (Jan. 1957): 7–8.

95. Feldberg, *Disease and Class,* 181.

96. Louise Shaffrath, "Social Service at Firland," *Pep and Courage* 38 (Feb. 1950): 7, 21.

97. Elizabeth Lunbeck, *The Psychiatric Persuasion: Knowledge, Gender, and Power in Modern America* (Princeton: Princeton University Press, 1994), 35–45.

98. Eby, "A Study of the Problems," 24–26.

99. Miss Beery to Holland Hudson, May 20, 1946, ALA Archives, Washington State Field Report File (585 R).

100. Jacobson and Peterson, "A Study of Sixty-Four Tuberculous Patients," 31, 36.

101. Roberts Davies, "Analysis of the King County Tuberculosis Hospital Problem in Relation to Financing Such Care," 1949, WS Archives, Department of Health, Director's Office, RS 2 Disease File, box 8, folder 160.

102. Cedric Northrop to John Kahl, Jan. 12, 1949, "Medical Social Services for Tuberculosis Patients," WS Archives, Department of Health, Director's Office, RS 2 Disease File, box 8, folder 160.

103. Shaffrath, "Social Service," 7, 21.

104. Middlebrook, "Tuberculosis: Some Aspects of Causation," 13. Indeed, some physicians saw isoniazid as a potential fix for a variety of complex sociomedical problems. Use of isoniazid for longer than two years, noted Theodore L. Badger, was indicated in cases of "refusal of surgical treatment, unsuitability for surgical treatment, a family history of tuberculosis, evidence of relapse before starting drugs, the intention of raising a family, old fibrotic cavitary disease persistently "negative," advanced disease that has done well with multiple drugs, diabetics, and those with silicotic disease or extensive exposure to silicotic dusts." See "Panel Two. The Hospital and Home: Respective Roles in Tuberculosis Management, Including the Chemotherapy of Tuberculosis," *American Review of Tuberculosis and Pulmonary Diseases* 80, pt. 2 (Oct. 1959): 22–45, 35.

105. Sidney Licht, foreword to William H. Soden, ed., *Rehabilitation of the Handicapped: A Survey of Means and Methods* (New York: Ronald Press, 1949), iii, iv. See also Herman E. Hilleboe, "Medical Aspects of the Rehabilitation of Persons with Tuberculosis," *War Medicine* 7 (Jan. 1945): 1–2; Daniel M. Fox, *Power and Illness: The Failure and Future of American Health Policy* (Berkeley: University of California Press, 1993), 62–63.

106. "Report of the Committee on Rehabilitation," *American Review of Tuberculosis* 56 (1947): 461–63, 461.

107. Alma V. Armstrong, "A Study of the Vocational Rehabilitation Problems of 1,361 Tuberculous Patients Referred for Counseling by Medical Staff to Educational and Vocational Counselors of the Anti-Tuberculosis League of King County between October 21, 1946, and September 1, 1950" (Ph.D. diss., University of Washington, 1953). Technically, a Firland physician was in charge of the rehabilitation program.

108. Holland Hudson, "Rehabilitation of the Tuberculous," in Soden, *Rehabilitation of the Handicapped,* 98; Ernest L. Beamish, "Vocational Rehabilitation at Firland," *Firland Magazine* 43 (Dec. 1955): 11–12.

109. *1946–1947 Annual Report of the Anti-Tuberculosis League of King County* (Seattle, 1947).

110. Hudson, "Rehabilitation of the Tuberculous," 96, 100–101; H. A. Pattison, *Rehabilitation of the Tuberculous* (Livingston, N.Y.: Livingston Press, 1949), 71–72.

111. Pattison, *Rehabilitation,* 173–209. The most celebrated aftercare program in the United States was New York City's Altro Work Shops. The mortality rates of Altro workers approached those of the general nontuberculous population.

112. Max Pinner, "Rehabilitation and Prognosis," *American Review of Tuberculosis* 56 (1947): 165–76, 166. Similarly, see I. D. Bobrowitz, "Rehabilitation of the Tuberculous: The Program of a Municipal Sanatorium," *American Review of Tuberculosis* 55 (1947): 43–48.

113. Bobrowitz, "Rehabilitation of the Tuberculous," 47 (emphasis added). See also Seymour M. Farber, "Rehabilitation as Part of Treatment," *Transactions of the National Tuberculosis Association* 43 (1947): 275–79.

114. Stuart Willis, "Rehabilitation from the Standpoint of the Tuberculosis Physician," *American Review of Tuberculosis* 62 (July 1950): 76–79; A. Ryrie Koch, "Our Neglected Patients?" *Bulletin of the National Tuberculosis Association* 43 (Mar. 1957): 43–44.

115. David T. Carr and Ezra V. Bridge, "Vocational Rehabilitation in Pulmonary Tuberculosis Today," *American Review of Tuberculosis and Pulmonary Diseases* 78 (1958): 647–49.

116. Karl H. Pfuetze and Marjorie M. Pyle, "Vocational Rehabilitation in Pulmonary Tuberculosis Today," *American Review of Tuberculosis and Pulmonary Diseases* 78 (1958): 649–50.

117. "Turning Point," *Pep and Courage* (Sept. 1951): 10, 16.

118. Mr. Stone to Members of the Committee on Social and Economic Problems, "Problems Imposed by Community Attitudes," Dec. 13, 1951, ALA Archives, Committee on Social Research File (1137). One commentator went so far as to call the means test an "implement of torture." See Daniel E. Jenkins to Mr. Roberts, Jan. 20, 1959, ALA Archives, Compulsory Isolation File (2708).

119. George J. Nelbach, "Social and Economic Hindrances to Program for Prevention of Tuberculosis," *California Medicine* 65 (supp.) (Aug. 1946): 24–25, 25.

120. Jenkins to Roberts, Jan. 20, 1959; Minutes of the Meeting of Social Research and Statistical Personnel, May 18, 1954, ALA Archives, Committee on Social Research File (1137).

121. Sydney Jacobs, "Report of the Social Research Committee to the National Tuberculosis Association Board of Directors," Feb. 13, 1958, ALA Archives, Committee on Social Research File (1137). See also Minutes of the Committee on Social Research, Feb. 14, 1957, and May 28, 1959, ALA Archives, Committee on Social Research File (1137).

122. Sydney Jacobs, "Panel Discussion: 'Social Research'" [1958], ALA Archives, Committee on Social Research File (1137).

FOUR. BEYOND THE GERM THEORY

1. David M. Kissen, *Emotional Factors in Pulmonary Tuberculosis* (London: Tavistock, 1958), ix–xi.

2. Clarence A. Neymann, "The Psychopathology of Tuberculosis," in Benjamin Goldberg, ed., *Clinical Tuberculosis,* vol. 2 (Philadelphia: F. A. Davis, 1935), M4–M6; René Dubos and Jean Dubos, *The White Plague: Tuberculosis, Man, and Society* (New Brunswick: Rutgers University Press, 1987), 44–66.

3. On diathesis, see Erwin H. Ackerknecht, "Diathesis: The Word and the Concept in Medical History," *Bulletin of the History of Medicine* 56 (fall 1982): 317–25; Georgina D. Feldberg, *Disease and Class: Tuberculosis and the Shaping of Modern North American Society* (New Brunswick: Rutgers University Press, 1995), 18.

4. Susan Sontag, *Illness as Metaphor* (New York: Farrar, Straus and Giroux, 1978), 26–36.

5. Dubos and Dubos, *The White Plague,* 225.

6. The term *psychosomatics* actually dates back to the work of an early-nineteenth-century German psychiatrist named Johann Christian Heinroth. See John J. Schwab, "Psychosomatic Medicine: Its Past and Present," *Psychosomatics* 26 (1985): 583–93, 584–86; and Franz Alexander, "The Development of Psychosomatic Medicine," *Psychosomatic Medicine* 24 (1962): 13–24, 17–18.

7. Schwab, "Psychosomatic Medicine," 589; Alexander, "Development," 19–20; Z. J. Lipowski, "Psychosomatic Medicine: Past and Present. Part I: Historical background," *Canadian Journal of Psychiatry* 31 (Feb. 1986): 2–7.

8. Eric Wittkower, "Twenty Years of North American Psychosomatic Medicine," *Psychosomatic Medicine* 22 (1960): 308–16; Robert C. Powell, "Helen Flanders Dunbar (1902–1959) and a Holistic Approach to Psychosomatic Problems. I: The Rise and Fall of a Medical Philosophy," *Psychiatric Quarterly* 49 (1977): 133–52, 135–36.

9. Alexander, "Development," 13–24; Franz Alexander, *Psychosomatic Medicine* (New York: Norton, 1950); J. W. Paulley, "Specificity Revisited and Updated," *Psychotherapy and Psychosomatics* 55 (Apr. 1991): 42–46.

10. Walter B. Cannon, *Bodily Changes in Pain, Hunger, Fear, and Rage* (New York: Appleton, 1915); Claude Bernard, *An Introduction to the Study of Experimental Medicine* (New York: Macmillan, 1927).

11. Lipowski, "Psychosomatic Medicine," 5–6; Harold G. Wolff, "A Concept of Disease in Man," *Psychosomatic Medicine* 24 (1962): 25–30, 29–30.

12. Richard H. Rahe, "Life Change, Stress Responsivity, and Captivity Research," *Psychosomatic Medicine* 52 (1990): 373–96, 374; Adolf Meyer, *Psychobiology: A Science of Man* (Springfield, Ill.: Charles C. Thomas, 1957).

13. Powell, "Helen Flanders Dunbar," 133–52; Helen Flanders Dunbar, *Mind and Body: Psychosomatic Medicine* (New York: Random House, 1947). For an ex-

cellent discussion of George Draper and "constitutional medicine," see Sarah W. Tracy, "George Draper and American Constitutional Medicine, 1916–1946: Reinventing the Sick Man," *Bulletin of the History of Medicine* 66 (spring 1992): 53–89.

14. Jerome Hartz, "Tuberculosis and Personality Conflicts," *Psychosomatic Medicine* 6 (1944): 17–22; Eric Wittkower, *A Psychiatrist Looks at Tuberculosis* (London: National Association for the Prevention of Tuberculosis, 1949), 86–142. See also Beatrice B. Berle, "Emotional Factors and Tuberculosis: A Critical Review of the Literature," *Psychosomatic Medicine* 10 (1948): 366–73, 370.

15. Gerald N. Grob, *From Asylum to Community: Mental Health Policy in Modern America* (Princeton: Princeton University Press, 1991), 16–23; Kyra Kester, "Shadows of War: The Historical Dimensions and Social Implications of Military Psychology and Veteran Counseling in the United States, 1860–1989" (Ph.D. diss., University of Washington, 1992).

16. Ian Stevenson, "Psychosomatic Medicine," *Harper's Magazine* 209 (July 1954): 34–37; Ian Stevenson, "As a Man Thinketh . . ." *Harper's Magazine,* 209 (Aug. 1954): 83–87. See also Calvin F. Schmid and Earle H. MacCannell, *Mortality Trends in the State of Washington* (Seattle: Washington State Census Board, 1955), 1.

17. See, for example, H. A. Pattison, *Rehabilitation of the Tuberculous* (Livingston, N.Y.: Livingston Press, 1949), 4.

18. Ezra Bridge, "Rehabilitation Difficulties," *American Review of Tuberculosis* 55 (1947): 379–81, 379.

19. Harold G. Wolff, *Headache and Other Head Pain* (New York: Oxford University Press, 1948.

20. Wolff, "A Concept of Disease," 29, 30; Stewart Wolf and Helen Goodell, *Harold G. Wolff's Stress and Disease,* 2d ed. (Springfield, Ill.: Charles C. Thomas, 1968), 3–4.

21. Stewart Wolf, M.D., interview with author, Mar. 14 and 16, 1995.

22. Thomas H. Holmes, Helen Goodell, Stewart Wolf, and Harold G. Wolff, *The Nose: An Experimental Study of Reactions within the Nose in Human Subjects during Varying Life Experiences* (Springfield, Ill.: Charles C. Thomas, 1950), 62–68, 110–12.

23. Emanuel Wolinsky, M.D., interview with author, May 13, 1994.

24. Wolf, interview, Mar. 14 and 16, 1995. Helen Flanders Dunbar had a similarly ambiguous arrangement, working as a psychiatrist "on assignment to the Department of Medicine" at Columbia-Presbyterian Medical Center.

25. Edmund R. Clarke Jr, Daniel W. Zahn, and Thomas H. Holmes, "The Relationship of Stress, Adrenocortical Function, and Tuberculosis," *American Review of Tuberculosis* 69 (1954): 351–69.

26. Hans Selye, "Recent Progress in Stress Research, with Reference to Tuberculosis," in Phineas J. Sparer, ed., *Personality, Stress, and Tuberculosis* (New York: International Universities Press, 1956). For more on general adaptation, see Hans Selye, *The Story of the Adaptation Syndrome* (Montreal: Acta, 1952).

27. Clarke, Zahn, and Holmes, "Relationship of Stress," 354–55.

28. Ibid., 365.

29. Selye, "Recent Progress," 52. Note that Selye was not implying that the combination of stress and high steroids actually "caused" tuberculosis. Rather, he posited that a person's immune system responded suboptimally in such a situation, causing greater susceptibility to tuberculosis.

30. Harold F. Osborne, "Fright Aids TB Care, Seattle Medics Report," *Seattle Times,* May 20, 1953, 19.

31. Richard Totman, *Social Causes of Illness* (New York: Pantheon Books, 1979), 108–9.

32. Norman G. Hawkins, Roberts Davies, and Thomas H. Holmes, "Evidence of Psychosocial Factors in the Development of Pulmonary Tuberculosis," *American Review of Tuberculosis and Pulmonary Diseases* 75 (1957): 768–80, 768.

33. Norman G. Hawkins, "A Research Application of Case Material in the Sociology of Tuberculosis" (master's thesis, University of Washington, 1953), 22–23.

34. Ibid., 22, 41.

35. Ibid., 58.

36. Thomas H. Holmes, "Multidiscipline Studies of Tuberculosis," in Phineas J. Sparer, ed., *Personality, Stress, and Tuberculosis* (New York: International Universities Press, 1956), 93–94.

37. Hawkins, Davies, and Holmes, "Evidence of Psychosocial Factors," 773–74; Holmes, "Multidiscipline Studies," 92–102.

38. Hawkins, Davies, and Holmes, "Evidence of Psychosocial Factors," 774–76; Holmes, "Multidiscipline Studies," 78–85.

39. What is most noticeable about these data is that nearly half of the Firland employees tested (eighteen of forty) were "pathologically disturbed," if one believes the validity of the Cornell Medical Index.

40. Holmes, "Multidiscipline Studies," 100.

41. Hawkins, Davies, and Holmes, "Evidence of Psychosocial Factors," 778.

42. Ibid., 777. Other discussions of methodological problems may be found in Hawkins, "A Research Application," 54; Totman, *Social Causes of Illness,* 112–14.

43. James E. Hart, "A Medical and Psychosocial Study of Tuberculous Patients Who Relapse to Infectious Sputum during Hospitalization" (M.D. thesis, University of Washington Medical School, 1959), 26–27, 81–82.

44. Ibid., 32–66.

45. Ibid., 81. See also 92–94.

46. Ibid., 104–10.

47. Thomas H. Holmes, Joy R. Joffe, Janet W. Ketcham, and Thomas F. Sheehy, "Experimental Study of Prognosis," *Journal of Psychosomatic Research* 5 (1961): 235–52.

48. Kerr L. White to Thomas H. Holmes, May 19, 1955, UW Archives, Thomas Holmes Papers, box 1, folder "General Correspondence, 12/54–9/55."

49. Kerr L. White, M.D., interview with author, Feb. 20, 1995.

50. Dubos and Dubos, *The White Plague,* 128; Herman E. Hilleboe, *Medical Social Service in Tuberculosis Control* (Washington, D.C.: Public Health Service, 1946); "Tuberculosis Infection Puzzling, Says Expert," *Seattle Times,* Jan. 24, 1957, 9.

51. Andres I. Karstens to Thomas Holmes, Jan. 29, 1953, UW Archives, Thomas Holmes Papers, box 2, folder "Adrenocortical Function 20-13."

52. Manny Wolinsky to Thomas H. Holmes, Sept. 25, 1953, UW Archives, Thomas Holmes Papers, box 1, folder "General Correspondence, 9/53–11/54."

53. Edith Heinemann, M.A., interview with author, Nov. 13, 1994.

54. A. Frans Koome to Thomas H. Holmes, Sept. 27, 1965, UW Archives, Thomas Holmes Papers, box 1, folder "General Correspondence, 6/65–3/66."

55. Roberts J. Davies, "The Doctor Answers," *Pep and Courage* 40 (Apr. 1952): 18; Roberts J. Davies, "Your Questions about Tuberculosis Answered," *Pep: The Magazine of Firland* 41 (May 1953): 9; Daniel W. Zahn, "Your Questions about Tuberculosis Answered," *Pep: The Magazine of Firland* 42 (Dec. 1954): 80.

56. For example, the 1972 graduating class presented Holmes with a special award for "untiring dedication to maintaining student voice, dignity, and participation." See curriculum vitae of Thomas H. Holmes, Jan. 1, 1985, UW Archives, Thomas Holmes Papers, box 1, folder "Biographical Features."

57. Thomas H. Holmes to William J. Grace, Feb. 26, 1954, UW Archives, Thomas Holmes Papers, box 1, folder "General Correspondence, 9/53–11/54"; Joan Jackson, letter to the author, Apr. 10, 1995.

58. Quoted in Holmes, Joffe, Ketcham, and Sheehy, "Experimental Study," 244.

59. Ibid.

60. Norman G. Hawkins, "Social Crisis as a Characteristic of Tuberculosis Etiology" (Ph.D. diss., University of Washington, 1956), i.

61. Holmes, "Multidiscipline Studies," 145–46.

62. M. Roy Schwarz to Thomas H. Holmes, June 5, 1964, UW Archives, Thomas Holmes Papers, box 1, folder "General Correspondence, 1/64–9/64"; and Marion Amundson to Raymond Sobel, March 16, 1966, UW Archives, Thomas Holmes Papers, box 1, folder "General Correspondence, 6/65–3/66"; Archibald Ruprecht, M.D., interview with author, Nov. 13, 1994.

63. Thomas H. Holmes to C. Balcom Moore, Dec. 28, 1960, UW Archives, Thomas Holmes Papers, box 1, folder "General Correspondence, 10/60–3/61."

64. On attitudes, see William J. Grace and David T. Graham, "Relationship of Specific Attitudes and Emotions to Certain Bodily Diseases," *Psychosomatic Medicine* 14 (1952): 243–51.

65. These quotes may be found in a document entitled "Verbal Statements of Attitudes," n.d. Collection of the author.

66. Hawkins, "Social Crisis," 48. In a sense, therefore, Holmes' work was the latest version of efforts that stressed the importance of the "soil" as opposed to the "seed" (see the introduction to this book). Other historical figures who minimized the importance of the tubercle bacillus are discussed in Feldberg, *Disease*

and Class, 43–55, 149–52; and David S. Barnes, *The Making of a Social Disease: Tuberculosis in Nineteenth-Century France* (Berkeley: University of California Press, 1995), 235–41.

67. Iago Galdston, *Beyond the Germ Theory: The Roles of Deprivation and Stress in Health and Disease* (New York: Health Education Council, 1954). See also Charles E. Rosenberg, "Explaining Epidemics," in Charles E. Rosenberg, ed., *Explaining Epidemics and Other Studies in the History of Medicine* (Cambridge: Cambridge University Press, 1992). Rosenberg classifies psychosomatics as an approach to epidemic diseases that stresses the importance of "configuration" as opposed to "contamination."

68. Feldberg, *Disease and Class,* 182–83, 197.

69. Phineas J. Sparer, introduction to Phineas J. Sparer, ed., *Personality, Stress, and Tuberculosis* (New York: International Universities Press, 1956), 4.

70. Ibid., 4–5. See also Iago Galdston, "Tuberculosis Causality," *Journal of the Michigan State Medical Society* 48 (1949): 1391.

71. Sparer, introduction, 5–6.

72. Harry Klonoff, "An Exploratory Study of the Effect of Short-Term Group Psychotherapy on Attitudes of Tubercular Patients" (Ph.D. diss., University of Washington, 1954), 60.

73. Hart, "Medical and Psychosocial Study," 111.

74. Thomas H. Holmes, "Life Situations, Emotions, and Disease," *Psychosomatics* 19 (1978): 747–54, 754. Similarly, a 1964 lecture given by Holmes was entitled "How to Be Sick Successfully."

75. Grob, *From Asylum to Community,* 134–39; Paul Starr, *The Social Transformation of American Medicine* (New York: Basic Books, 1982), 189–94.

76. James T. Patterson, *America's Struggle against Poverty, 1900–1985* (Cambridge: Harvard University Press, 1986), 94–96.

77. Velma T. Joyner to Thomas Holmes, July 23, 1965, UW Archives, Thomas Holmes Papers, box 1, folder "General Correspondence, 6/65–3/66."

78. On blaming the victim, see Linda Bryder, *Below the Magic Mountain: A Social History of Tuberculosis in Twentieth-Century Britain* (Oxford, England: Clarendon, 1988), 112–29; Nancy Krieger and Mary Bassett, "The Health of Black Folk: Disease, Class, and Ideology in Science," in Sandra Harding, ed., *The "Racial" Economy of Science: Toward a Democratic Future* (Bloomington: Indiana University Press, 1993), 165–68.

79. Barron H. Lerner, "Can Stress Cause Disease? Revisiting the Tuberculosis Research of Thomas Holmes, 1949–1961," *Annals of Internal Medicine* 124 (1996): 673–80.

80. Arthur Bobroff to Thomas Holmes, Feb. 13, 1961, UW Archives, Thomas Holmes Papers, box 1, folder "General Correspondence, 10/60–3/61."

FIVE. VAGRANTS AS PATIENTS

1. Hill Williams, "Seattle Described as 'End of Line' for Migrant Alcoholics," *Seattle Times,* Aug. 12, 1959, 40.

2. "Progress Report on Tentative Plans for Firland Tuberculous-Alcoholism Treatment Program," WS Archives, Health Department Administrative Files, box 5, folder "Treatment for Tuberculous Alcoholic, Firland." On the social construction of disease, see the introduction to this book.

3. Frances Farmer, *Will There Really Be a Morning?* (New York: Putnam, 1972), 29.

4. See Ronald P. Roizen, "The American Discovery of Alcoholism, 1933–1939" (Ph.D. diss., University of California at Berkeley, 1991), preface, 288; and Jay L. Rubin, "Shifting Perspectives on the Alcoholism Movement, 1940–1955," *Journal of Studies on Alcohol* 40 (1979): 376–86.

5. Elvin M. Jellinek, *The Disease Concept of Alcoholism* (Piscataway, N.J.: Alcohol Research Documentation, 1960). On the concurrent medicalization of drug addiction and crime during this era, see Peter Conrad and Joseph W. Schneider, *Deviance and Medicalization: From Badness to Sickness* (Philadelphia: Temple University Press, 1992), 110–44, 215–40. The role of business and the media in promoting these new disease concepts is analyzed in John C. Burnham, *Bad Habits: Drinking, Smoking, Taking Drugs, Gambling, Sexual Misbehavior, and Swearing in American History* (New York: New York University Press, 1993), 50–85.

6. Robert Straus, "Alcohol and the Homeless Man," *Quarterly Journal of Studies on Alcohol* 7 (1946): 360–404, 364. For more on "loss of control," see Elvin M. Jellinek, "Phases of Alcohol Addiction," *Quarterly Journal of Studies on Alcohol* 13 (1952): 673–84. For an alternative viewpoint, see Robin Room, "Dependence and Society," *British Journal of Addiction* 80 (1985): 133–39.

7. Bill Pittman, *A.A.: The Way It Began: The History of Alcoholism Treatment in America* (Seattle: Glen Abbey Books, 1988); Leonard Blumberg and William Pittman, *Beware the First Drink! The Washington Temperance Movement and Alcoholics Anonymous* (Seattle: Glen Abbey Books, 1991).

8. "Summer School of Alcohol Studies, Yale University," *Quarterly Journal of Studies on Alcohol* 3 (1943): 704–9; E. M. Jellinek, "Establishment of Diagnostic and Guidance Clinics for Inebriates in Connecticut (Yale Plan Clinics)," *Quarterly Journal of Studies on Alcohol* 4 (1943): 496–507; Richard M. Earle, "Prevention of Alcoholism in the United States and the National Council on Alcoholism: 1944–1950," *International Journal of the Addictions* 17 (1982): 679–702, 680–84.

9. E. M. Jellinek, "Phases in the Drinking History of Alcoholics: Analysis of a Survey Conducted by the Official Organ of Alcoholics Anonymous," *Quarterly Journal of Studies on Alcohol* 7 (1946): 1–88. See also Conrad and Schneider, *Deviance and Medicalization,* 90–94.

10. Jellinek, "Establishment of Diagnostic and Guidance Clinics," 497, 502–7. See also Edwin M. Lemert, "Alcoholism and the Sociocultural Situation," *Quarterly Journal of Studies on Alcohol* 17 (1956): 306–17; and David J. Myerson, "The Study and Treatment of Alcoholism: A Historical Perspective," *New England Journal of Medicine* 257 (1957): 820–25.

11. Marty Mann, "What TB Associations Can Do about Alcoholism," *Bulletin*

of the National Tuberculosis Association 45 (Apr. 1959): 58–59; Earle, "Prevention of Alcoholism," 684–86; Mr. Sloma to Mr. Susman, Mar. 17, 1960, ALA Archives, Alcoholism File (2725). The NCA actually was initially called the National Committee for Education on Alcoholism.

12. Harry G. Levine, "The Discovery of Addiction: Changing Conceptions of Habitual Drunkenness in America," *Journal of Studies on Alcohol* 39 (1978): 143–74; Robin Room, "Governing Images and the Prevention of Alcohol Problems," *Preventive Medicine* 3 (Mar. 1974): 11–23; Room, "Dependence and Society." See also Conrad and Schneider, *Deviance and Medicalization,* 79–85; and William F. Bynum, "Chronic Alcoholism in the First Half of the Nineteenth Century," *Bulletin of the History of Medicine* 42 (Mar.–Apr. 1968): 160–85.

13. Roizen, "American Discovery of Alcoholism."

14. "Hospitalization of Patients with Alcoholism," *Journal of the American Medical Association* 162 (1956): 750. See also Blumberg and Pittman, *Beware the First Drink,* 204; Earle, "Prevention of Alcoholism," 692; and G. Lolli, "Alcoholism as a Medical Problem," *Bulletin of the New York Academy of Medicine* 31 (1955): 876–85.

15. Raymond G. McCarthy, "Public Health Approach to the Control of Alcoholism," *American Journal of Public Health* 40 (1950): 1412–17; Dan Morse, "Alcohol and Tuberculosis," *Bulletin of the National Tuberculosis Association* 42 (Oct. 1956): 157–58; Mark Keller and Vera Effron, "Rate of Alcoholism in the U.S.A.," *Quarterly Journal of Studies on Alcoholism* 19 (1958): 316–19; Hill Williams, "State Opens Battle against Alcoholism in Seattle," *Seattle Times,* Aug. 11, 1959, 19; introduction to David L. Strug, S. Priyadarsini, and Merton M. Hyman, eds., *Alcohol Interventions: Historical and Sociocultural Approaches* (New York: Haworth, 1986), 6.

16. S. Harvard Kaufman, "Alcoholism: A Symptom of Emotional Illness," *Health Commentator* (of the Washington State Department of Health) 3 (Feb. 1948): 6.

17. Williams, "State Opens Battle," 19; James T. Golder, "Seattle's Dubious Distinction: Alcoholic Rate" (letter to the editor), *Seattle Times,* Feb. 12, 1958, 12; National Committee for the Prevention of Alcoholism, "Seattle Ranks High in Alcoholism," *Firland Magazine* 47 (Nov. 1959): 15.

18. Calvin F. Schmid, *Social Trends in Seattle* (Seattle: University of Washington Press, 1944), 331; Gerald D. Nash, *The American West Transformed: The Impact of the Second World War* (Lincoln: University of Nebraska Press, 1985), 37–55, 214.

19. Williams, "Seattle Described as 'End of Line,'" 40; Joan K. Jackson, "Some Problems Involved in Helping the Skid Road Patient Adjust to the Hospital," May 14, 1957, Joan K. Jackson, Personal Papers.

20. This term is referenced in Harold W. Demone and John C. Smith, "Experiences in Alcoholic Rehabilitation," in NIMH, *The Alcoholic Tuberculous Patient and the Community* (Bethesda, Md.: NIMH, 1959), 99. See also Williams, "Seattle

Described as 'End of Line,'" 40; and Archibald L. Ruprecht, "The Doctor's Responsibility to the Alcoholic," *Postgraduate Medicine* 32 (July 1962): 56–68, 57.

21. Joan K. Jackson, Ronald J. Fagan, and Roscoe C. Burr, "The Seattle Police Department Rehabilitation Project for Chronic Alcoholics," *Federal Probation* 22 (June 1958): 36–41.

22. Joan K. Jackson and Ralph Connor, "The Skid Road Alcoholic," *Quarterly Journal of Studies on Alcohol* 14 (1953): 468–86, 469.

23. Ibid., 470.

24. Ibid., 483. See also Joan K. Jackson and Thomas H. Holmes, "Alcoholism and Tuberculosis," *Human Organization* 16 (winter 1958): 41–43.

25. Calvin F. Schmid and Wayne W. McVey Jr., *Growth and Distribution of Minority Races in Seattle, Washington* (Seattle: University of Washington Press, 1964), 1. On the exclusion of minorities and women from skid row studies, see Howard M. Bahr, *Skid Row: An Introduction to Disaffiliation* (New York: Oxford University Press, 1973), 105, 175–221.

26. Alice W. Solenberger, *One Thousand Homeless Men* (New York: Charities Publication Committee, 1911); Nels Anderson, *The Hobo* (Chicago: University of Chicago Press, 1923). An article celebrating the hobo lifestyle is Walter B. Pitkin, "Hobo Paradise on the Pacific," *Coronet* 20 (May 1946): 80–82.

27. Bahr, *Skid Row,* 36, 99, 100; Howard M. Bahr, ed., *Disaffiliated Man: Essays and Bibliography on Skid Row, Vagrancy, and Outsiders* (Toronto: University of Toronto, 1970), 28–33.

28. Lawrason Brown and Joseph T. Eagan, "Alcohol and Tuberculosis," *American Review of Tuberculosis* 27 (1933): 217–46, 242. For more on alcoholism and tuberculosis, see F. W. B., "Tuberculosis and Alcoholism," *Diseases of the Chest* 7 (Feb. 1941): 38, 61.

29. S. Adolphus Knopf, quoted in Michael E. Teller, *The Tuberculosis Movement: A Public Health Campaign in the Progressive Era* (New York: Greenwood, 1988), 103.

30. Quoted in Brown and Eagan, "Alcohol and Tuberculosis," 218, 219.

31. Herbert W. Jones Jr., Jean Roberts, and John Brantner, "Incidence of Tuberculosis among Homeless Men," *Journal of the American Medical Association* 155 (1954): 1222–23.

32. Cedric Northrop, "Finding Tuberculosis," *Today's Health* 32 (Oct. 1954): 38–39, 56–58, quote on 58. See also Demone and Smith, "Experiences," 88.

33. "Mobile X-Ray Unit to Visit Jackson St.," *Seattle Times,* Mar. 21, 1954, 25; "Reductions in Mass X-Rays Planned," *Seattle Times,* Nov. 21, 1957, 11.

34. Brown and Eagan, "Alcohol and Tuberculosis," 226.

35. Barbara Dike, "A Study of Clinical Records to Determine Some of the Factors Involved in Irregular Discharges of Ninety-Four Patients Who Left Firland Sanatorium against Medical Advice during the Period of January 1, 1950, to June 30, 1950" (master's thesis, University of Washington, 1953), 23; Evelyn N. Hadaway, "A Medical Social Study of Fifty-Four Tuberculosis Patients Who Left

Firland Sanatorium against Medical Advice in 1952" (master's thesis, University of Washington, 1953), 32.

36. Dike, "A Study of Clinical Records," 54, 61.

37. *Annual Report, Firland Sanatorium, 1950* (Seattle: Firland Sanatorium, 1951), 6. See also Roberts Davies, "Why People Die of Tuberculosis," *Health Pilot* (of the Washington Tuberculosis Association) 35 (Jan. 1952): 4–5.

38. Joan K. Jackson, "Alcoholism and Tuberculosis," June 15, 1957, Jackson Papers.

39. Joan K. Jackson, "The Problem of Alcoholic Tuberculous Patients," in Phineas J. Sparer, ed., *Personality, Stress, and Tuberculosis* (New York: International Universities Press, 1956), 504; U.S. Department of Health, Education, and Welfare (HEW), *Toward Intensive Treatment for the Tuberculous Alcoholic Patient: Proceedings of a Workshop* (Washington, D.C.: HEW, 1962), 50–52.

40. Norman G. Hawkins, "Skid Road: A Health Challenge," *Journal-Lancet* 77 (1957): 153–56.

41. Jackson, "The Problem of Alcoholic Tuberculous Patients," 504–38; Joan K. Jackson, "Progress Report: Research on Alcoholism and Tuberculosis," Oct. 15, 1956, Jackson Papers; Emily B. Fergus and Joan K. Jackson, "The Tuberculous Alcoholic before and during Hospitalization," *American Review of Tuberculosis and Pulmonary Diseases* 79 (1959): 659–62.

42. Joan K. Jackson, "N.W. Nursing Conference," Nov. 15, 1957, Jackson Papers.

43. Jackson, "The Problem of Alcoholic Tuberculous Patients," 508.

44. Jackson, "Alcoholism and Tuberculosis" (1957); Jackson and Holmes, "Alcoholism and Tuberculosis," 41.

45. Joan K. Jackson, "Psychosocial Studies in the Natural History of Tuberculosis: Summary and Conclusions," Nov. 1, 1957, UW Archives, Thomas Holmes Papers, box 2, folder "Psychosocial Studies in the Natural History of Tuberculosis, 9/1/55 to 10/31/57."

46. Joan K. Jackson, "Research on Alcoholism and Tuberculosis," Apr. 11, 1958, Jackson Papers.

47. Ibid. See also Jackson, "Psychosocial Studies."

48. Jackson, "Research on Alcoholism and Tuberculosis."

49. Shadel, founded in 1935, relied on so-called aversion therapy, in which patients would be given an emetic agent in conjunction with alcohol to discourage drinking. See Frederick Lemere, Walter L. Voegtlin, William R. Broz, and Paul O'Hollaren, "Conditioned Reflex Treatment of Alcoholism," *Northwest Medicine* 41 (1942): 88–89.

50. Jackson, "Some Problems."

51. Joan K. Jackson, "Alcoholism and Tuberculosis" [1960?], Jackson Papers.

52. Jackson, "Alcoholism and Tuberculosis" [1960?]. See also Jackson, "Alcoholism and Tuberculosis" (1957).

53. Fergus and Jackson, "Tuberculous Alcoholic," 661.

54. Ibid., 659–61; Joan K. Jackson, "Some Aspects of the Sanatorium Adjust-

ment Difficulties of White Male Skid Road Alcoholic Tuberculous Patients," in Phineas J. Sparer, ed., *Personality, Stress, and Tuberculosis* (New York: International Universities Press, 1956), 539–72.

55. Jackson, "N.W. Nursing Conference."

56. Jackson, "Some Problems"; Jackson, "Research on Alcoholism and Tuberculosis."

57. Firland Sanatorium chart C1. See also charts C18, D19. The quote regarding the sanatorium subculture comes from Arnold S. Linsky, M. Edith Heinemann, and Karen M. Sorenson, "Problems of the Alcoholic Tuberculous Patient: A Study of Attitudes of the Non-Hospitalized Alcoholic-Tuberculous, the Non-Alcoholic Tuberculous, and the Nurse," *Nursing Research* 14 (winter 1965): 33–36, 33.

58. Elmer Bendiner, *The Bowery Man* (New York: Thomas Nelson and Sons, 1961), 101.

59. Jackson, "Alcoholism and Tuberculosis" [1960?].

60. Fergus and Jackson, "Tuberculous Alcoholic," 662.

61. Joan K. Jackson, interview with author, June 10, 1994; Ronald J. Fagan and Arnold S. Linsky, *Hospital Change and Resistance to Change in the Treatment of Alcoholism-Tuberculosis: The Experiences of One Tuberculosis Hospital* (Seattle, 1966), 14, 15. On milieu therapy, see Gerald N. Grob, *From Asylum to Community: Mental Health Policy in Modern America* (Princeton: Princeton University Press, 1991), 139–46.

62. John F. Allen, "Medics Hit for Scorning Alcoholics," *San Francisco Examiner*, Apr. 12, 1958, 6; "Alcoholism Tours," n.d., Joan K. Jackson Papers.

63. Daniel W. Zahn, "Sheehy of Innis Arden," *Firland Magazine* 43 (Sept. 1955): 5–6. See also author's interviews with Marcelle F. Dunning, M.D., Oct. 9, 1992, Katherine M. Anderson, R.N., June 11, 1993, and Charlotte A. Rose, R.N., July 1, 1993.

64. Joan K. Jackson, "Some Characteristics of Tuberculous Alcoholics," May 8, 1957, Jackson Papers.

65. See, for example, "Alcoholics Anonymous," *Pep and Courage* 38 (Oct. 1950): 4, 21; J. B., "You're an Alcoholic, Hey!" *Firland Magazine* 44 (July 1956): 22; "The Miracle of Alcoholics Anonymous," *Firland Magazine* 45 (Oct. 1957): 6; Verne H., "To the Alcoholic at Firland," *Firland Magazine* 48 (May 1960): 11; Francis H., "Just in Case You Didn't Know," *Firland Magazine* 50 (Sept. 1962): 5.

66. "Alcoholics Take but Don't Give," *Firland Magazine* 45 (Dec. 1957): 33; Thomas F. Sheehy Jr., "Informally Speaking," *Firland Magazine* 47 (Feb. 1959): 3; Helen B. Anthony, "Editorial," *Firland Magazine* 48 (Mar. 1960): 1. On disulfiram, see Daniel J. Feldman, "The Treatment of Chronic Alcoholism: A Survey of Current Methods," *Annals of Internal Medicine* 44 (1956): 78–87, 81, 82.

67. "Firland Sanatorium Takes a Bold Look at Its Tuberculous Alcoholic Problem," *Rehabilitation Events* (of the National Tuberculosis Association) 2 (Dec. 1956): 4. See also A. Ryrie Koch to Mr. Stone, Sept. 12, 1956, ALA Archives, Washington State Field Report File (585 R).

68. See the December 1956 issue of *Rehabilitation Events;* Demone and Smith, "Experiences," 92–95.

69. "Help for the Alcoholic Woman," *Firland Magazine* 46 (Mar. 1958): 10; "76 Physicians Attend Postgraduate Course on Alcoholism at University," *Washington's Health* (of the Washington State Department of Health) 3 (June–July 1960): 3, 7; "Roundup: Anti-Tuberculosis League of King County," Mar. 1963, ALA Archives, Honoria Hughes File (587 Special). Father James Royce offered the country's first college course on alcoholism at Seattle University beginning in 1949.

70. Williams, "State Opens Battle," 19; Joan K. Jackson, "Actions and Recommendations to Date," Nov. 29, 1962, Jackson Papers.

71. Williams, "State Opens Battle," 19; *Programs on Alcoholism Research, Treatment, and Rehabilitation in the United States and Canada,* 1956, ALA Archives, Alcoholism File (2725); Bernard Bucove, "Alcoholism: Old Problem, New Program," *Washington's Health* (of the Washington State Department of Health) 3 (June–July 1960): 2.

72. Poll results are available in the Washington State Health File in Special Collections at the University of Washington Library. See also Norman H. Clark, *The Dry Years: Prohibition and Social Change in Washington,* rev. ed. (Seattle: University of Washington Press, 1988), 250.

73. Quoted in James E. Hart, "A Medical and Psychosocial Study of Tuberculous Patients Who Relapse to Infectious Sputum during Hospitalization" (M.D. thesis, University of Washington Medical School, 1959), 76. Similarly, see Alf Nygren, "A Patient's Point of View," *Firland Magazine* 44 (Mar. 1956): 6–7.

74. Archibald L. Ruprecht, M.D., interview with author, Nov. 13, 1994. For Ruprecht's writings on the subject of alcoholism, see Ruprecht, "The Doctor's Responsibility," 56–68.

75. A. Ryrie Koch, "Our Neglected Patients?" *Bulletin of the National Tuberculosis Association* 43 (Mar. 1957): 43–44, 44. See also "Alcohol and Bacilli Bad Mixture," *Health Notes* (of the Anti-Tuberculosis League of King County [ATLKC]) 12 (fall 1956): 1–2; "Alcohol Big Problem When Added to TB," *Health Notes* 13 (spring 1957): 1–2.

76. Honoria Hughes and Clayton T. Knowles, "Jobs for the 'Hard Core' TB Patient," *Bulletin of the National Tuberculosis Association* 45 (Jan. 1959): 5–6. On a more successful program in Boston, see David L. Myerson, "The 'Skid Row' Problem: Further Observations on a Group of Alcoholic Patients, with Emphasis on Interpersonal Relations and the Therapeutic Approach," *New England Journal of Medicine* 254 (1956): 1168–73.

77. Howery, quoted in Hughes and Knowles, "Jobs," 6.

78. Jackson, "Research on Alcoholism and Tuberculosis." See also Hale Pragoff, "Adjustment of Tuberculosis Patients One Year after Discharge," *Public Health Reports* 77 (1962): 671–79, 677, 678; and Barbara S. Wilbur, David Salkin, and Harold Birnbaum, "A Critical Evaluation of the Therapeutic Community Approach to the Tuberculous Alcoholic," in HEW, *Toward Intensive Treatment.*

79. Firland Sanatorium charts C16, D4, D7, D14.

80. George Stevenson, letter to the editor, *Firland Magazine* 48 (July 1960): 8.

81. "Discussion," in NIMH, *Alcoholic Tuberculous Patient and the Community*, 27.

82. Dan Morse, "Alcohol and Tuberculosis," *Peoria Fluoroscope* 23 (Nov. 1955). See also Donald J. Ottenberg, "The Physician's Role in the Treatment of Tuberculosis-Alcoholism," in HEW, *Toward Intensive Treatment*, 11.

83. Pauline Miller, *Medical Social Service in a Tuberculosis Sanatorium* (Washington, D.C.: GPO, 1951), 19.

84. Donald J. Ottenberg, "TB on Skid Row," *Bulletin of the National Tuberculosis Association* 42 (June 1956): 85–86, 86.

85. The relation of alcoholism to antituberculosis efforts is discussed in a series of memorandums from 1956 to 1961 in the "Alcoholism" file (2725) at the ALA Archives.

86. "Meet the New Board Members," *Health Notes* 14 (fall 1958): 2.

87. Jackson, "Getting Drunk Isn't All," *Firland Magazine* 45 (Nov. 1957): 24.

88. This quote is actually a paraphrase of Sigerist's writings that appears in Elizabeth Fee, "Henry E. Sigerist: His Interpretations of the History of Disease and the Future of Medicine," in Charles E. Rosenberg and Janet Golden, eds., *Framing Disease: Studies in Cultural History* (New Brunswick: Rutgers University Press, 1992), 304. Sigerist defined alcoholism as a "disease of misery." On alcoholism and poverty, see David S. Barnes, *The Making of a Social Disease: Tuberculosis in Nineteenth-Century France* (Berkeley: University of California Press, 1995), 236, 237.

SIX. TEMPORARILY DETAINED

1. David F. Musto, "Quarantine and the Problem of AIDS," *Milbank Quarterly* 64, supp. 1 (1986): 97–117, 98.

2. Edgar A. Jonas, "Law Enforcement in the Control of Tuberculosis," *American Journal of Public Health* 13 (1923): 113–18; Allan Brandt, *No Magic Bullet: A Social History of Venereal Disease in the United States since 1880* (New York: Oxford University Press, 1987), 92–95; Naomi Rogers, *Dirt and Disease: Polio before FDR* (New Brunswick: Rutgers University Press, 1992), 30–44, 106–37; George Rosen, *A History of Public Health*, rev. ed. (Baltimore: Johns Hopkins University Press, 1993), 251–54.

3. Dorothy Porter and Roy Porter, "The Enforcement of Health: The British Debate," in Elizabeth Fee and Daniel M. Fox, eds., *AIDS: The Burdens of History* (Berkeley: University of California Press, 1986), 107.

4. Allan M. Brandt, "AIDS: From Social History to Social Policy," in Fee and Fox, *AIDS: The Burdens of History*, 151.

5. Musto, "Quarantine," 109–12; Alan M. Kraut, *Silent Travelers: Germs, Genes, and the "Immigrant Menace"* (New York: Basic Books, 1994); Howard Markel, *Quarantine! East European Jewish Immigrants and the New York City Epidemics of 1892* (Baltimore: Johns Hopkins University Press, 1997).

6. See, for example, David J. Rothman, *The Discovery of the Asylum: Social*

Order and Disorder in the New Republic (Boston: Little, Brown, 1990); and David J. Rothman, *Conscience and Convenience: The Asylum and Its Alternatives in Progressive America* (Boston: Little, Brown, 1980), 324–421.

7. Erving Goffman, *Asylums: Essays on the Social Situation of Mental Patients and Other Inmates* (Garden City, N.Y.: Anchor Books, 1961), 6. For an alternative interpretation of social control within the institutional setting, see Michel Foucault, *Discipline and Punish: The Birth of the Prison* (New York: Pantheon Books, 1977). See also Elizabeth Lunbeck, *The Psychiatric Persuasion: Knowledge, Gender, and Power in Modern America* (Princeton: Princeton University Press, 1994).

8. Sheila M. Rothman, *Living in the Shadow of Death: Tuberculosis and the Social Experience of Illness in American History* (New York: Basic Books, 1994), 191–93. North Brother was the island where Typhoid Mary would later be quarantined.

9. One exception was California, which began a program of detention in 1931. See Edward Kupka, "Compulsory Hospitalization of Recalcitrant Tuberculous Patients," *California and Western Medicine* 59 (July 1943): 43–45. On tuberculosis and the law, see James A. Tobey, *Public Health Law,* 2d ed. (New York: Commonwealth Fund, 1939), 149–61.

10. Cedric Northrop, John H. Fountain, and Daniel W. Zahn, "The Practical Management of the Recalcitrant Tuberculous Patient," *Public Health Reports* 67 (1952): 894–98, 895, 896.

11. Ibid.

12. See, for example, Ezra Bridge, "The Recalcitrant Patient," *Bulletin of the National Tuberculosis Association* 35 (Sept. 1949): 119–20; Roberts Davies, "Isolating the Recalcitrants," *Bulletin of the National Tuberculosis Association* 40 (June 1954): 121–22; and Maurice Campagna and Harry B. Greenberg, "Recalcitrant Patients with Pulmonary Tuberculosis," *Journal of the Louisiana State Medical Society* 116 (1964): 262–67.

13. Anton Chekhov, "Ward Number Six" [1892], in *Seven Chekhov Stories* (London: Oxford University Press, 1974).

14. Davies, "Isolating the Recalcitrants," 121; Northrop, Fountain, and Zahn, "Practical Management," 896; M. A. Linell, "The Detention Ward and Its Place in the Control and Treatment of Tuberculosis," *American Review of Tuberculosis and Pulmonary Diseases* 74 (1956): 410–16, 411, 412.

15. Roberts J. Davies, "The Prerequisites for a Successful Campaign of Tuberculosis Eradication," *Health Pilot* (of the Washington Tuberculosis Association) 29 (June 1947): 6–8, 11.

16. Washington State Department of Health, *Annual Report, 1949* (Seattle, 1950), 9.

17. Linell, "Detention Ward," 415. See also Dan Morse, "Alcohol and Tuberculosis," *Bulletin of the National Tuberculosis Association* 42 (Oct. 1956): 157–58, 158.

18. Karl Fischel, "The Prognostic and Social Significance of Cavities in Pulmonary Tuberculosis," *American Review of Tuberculosis* 24 (1931): 461–78, 463.

19. Linda Bryder, *Below the Magic Mountain: A Social History of Tuberculosis*

in Twentieth-Century Britain (Oxford, England: Clarendon, 1988), 253–56. Alcoholic patients were expected to continue antibiotics after surgery. The operation, however, ostensibly improved their chances if they proved insufficiently compliant.

20. Firland Sanatorium chart S2.

21. Firland Sanatorium chart S27.

22. Firland Sanatorium chart C8.

23. Paul Starr, *The Social Transformation of American Medicine* (New York: Basic Books, 1982), 3–9; John C. Burnham, "American Medicine's Golden Age: What Happened to It?" *Science* 215 (Mar. 1982): 1475–77. Major postwar accomplishments included the introduction of antibiotics and the polio vaccine.

24. Firland Sanatorium chart B4. On alcoholism among northwest Indian and Eskimo populations, see Edwin M. Lemert, *Alcohol and the Northwest Coast Indians* (Berkeley: University of California Press, 1954).

25. Waldo Mills, interview with author, Oct. 1, 1992. This saying, obviously, was an exaggeration. Not all patients with these characteristics received surgery. Divorced patients were cited because they were believed to be less compliant; school teachers obviously posed a potential infectious risk.

26. Irving Kass, Terumasa Miyamoto, John Denst, George J. Wittenstein, William F. Russell Jr., Gardner Middlebrook, and Sidney H. Dressler, "The Residual Lesion in Pulmonary Tuberculosis Requiring Surgery: A Review of One Hundred Sputum-Negative Patients Consecutively Operated On," *New England Journal of Medicine* 262 (1960): 315–20. The authors listed as indications for surgery such vaguely defined criteria as "social irresponsibility" and "ethnic predisposition to progressive tuberculosis." Similarly, see A. L. Paine and Z. Matwichuk, "Five- to Seventeen-Year End-Results in 402 Patients with Pulmonary Resection for Tuberculosis," *American Review of Respiratory Disease* 90 (1964): 760–70.

27. Firland Sanatorium chart S14.

28. Cedric Northrop to Mr. Blomquist, Jan. 15, 1957, ALA Archives, Washington State Department of Public Health File (704); "Drinking by Patients Big Problem, Says Firland Director," *Seattle Times*, Sept. 1, 1960, 1.

29. Firland Sanatorium chart C2.

30. Firland Sanatorium chart C15.

31. Daniel Widelock, Lenore R. Peizer, and Sarah Klein, "Public Health Significance of Tubercle Bacilli Resistant to Isoniazid," *American Journal of Public Health* 45 (1955): 79–83. Most commentators believed that drug-resistant strains of the tubercle bacillus were less virulent than standard strains. On the need for prolonged therapy, see Daniel W. Zahn, "Home Care in Seattle," *Bulletin of the National Tuberculosis Association* 42 (Jan. 1956): 11–12.

32. Cedric Northrop, "Field Activities Report for April 1953," WS Archives, Department of Health, Director's Office, RS 2 Disease File, box 7, folder 784.

33. A. P. to To Whom It May Concern, n.d., UW Archives, WCLU (American Civil Liberties Union of Washington) Papers, box 25, folder 11-19.

34. Firland Sanatorium chart F8. By this time, alcoholic patients were more often kept until their sputum had been negative for six months. Some, therefore, did not stay an entire year.

35. See table 2, "TB Admissions by Diagnosis of Alcoholism at Time of Admission, by Sanatoria, and by Year, 1963–1967," Oct. 10, 1967, WS Archives, DSHS (Department of Social and Health Services) 300 Files, box 42, folder "Patient Census."

36. Thomas F. Sheehy Jr., "Informally Speaking," *Firland Magazine* 45 (Mar. 1957): 3. The AMA (against medical advice) rate was obviously helped by the overall decreasing length of stay.

37. Northrop, Fountain, and Zahn, "Practical Management," 895.

38. *Diagnostic Standards and Classification of Tuberculosis* (New York: NTA, 1940), 21, 22.

39. *Diagnostic Standards and Classification of Tuberculosis* (New York: NTA, 1950), 36, 37.

40. Firland Sanatorium chart A7; emphasis added.

41. Firland Sanatorium chart C4; emphasis added. For another discussion of infectiousness as the criterion for quarantine, see *Public Health in Seattle, 1949, 1950, 1951: Report of the Seattle–King County Department of Public Health* (Seattle, 1952), 20.

42. Firland Sanatorium chart A2.

43. Ibid.

44. Ibid.

45. Firland Sanatorium chart S8. See also charts C2 and S15.

46. Firland Sanatorium chart C1. See also charts C6, C7, C24, D14, D18, and D20.

47. Firland Sanatorium chart A10.

48. Firland Sanatorium chart A11. The two charts without any discussion of the reason for transfer are A3 and A4. See also the Firland Daily Census Logs, Washington State DSHS Warehouse, Tumwater, Washington.

49. William J. Curran, "Civil Commitment of Alcoholics: A Legal Survey," in *National Conference on Legal Issues in Alcoholism and Alcohol Usage* (Bethesda, Md.: National Institute of Mental Health, 1965). See especially 40–42, 48–51.

50. Northrop, Fountain, and Zahn, "Practical Management," 895, 896; Walter T. Miller, M.D., interview with author, July 15, 1992; Ronald J. Fagan and Sue M. Berger, *A Partial Evaluation of the Firland Alcoholism Program with a Profile of Alcoholic and Non-Alcoholic Patients at First Admission* (Seattle, 1964), 24.

51. These letters of quarantine appear in the Firland patient charts. See also Miller interview, July 15, 1992.

52. Northrop, Fountain, and Zahn, "Practical Management," 898.

53. Linell, "Detention Ward," 413; Firland Sanatorium charts C22, D12, D16.

54. Davies, "Isolating the Recalcitrants," 121, 122; Linell, "Detention Ward," 411. The use of progressively longer sentences was borrowed from the criminal

justice system. See Nicholas N. Kittrie, *The Right to Be Different: Deviance and Enforced Therapy* (Baltimore: Johns Hopkins University Press, 1971), 267.

55. Linell, "Detention Ward," 411. Patients discharged from Ward Six included Firland Sanatorium charts B3, B5, C2, C8, C15, C18, and C24. In one 1957 case (chart C27) a physician even noted that a patient on Ward Six was "no public health hazard."

56. Firland Sanatorium chart A7. For a similar anecdote, see Davies, "Isolating the Recalcitrants," 121.

57. Firland Sanatorium chart C4.

58. *The Firland Patients' Information Booklet* (Seattle: Firland Sanatorium, 1958), 21.

59. Linell, "Detention Ward," 411; "Doctor's Report: Only 20 Per Cent at Firland Diagnosed as Alcoholics," *Seattle Times*, Sept. 2, 1960, 6. At times employees smuggled in liquor for patients. See Charlotte A. Rose, R.N., interview with author, July 1, 1993.

60. Linell, "Detention Ward," 415. The phrase "utter chaos" comes from the Miller interview, July 15, 1992.

61. Northrop, Fountain, and Zahn, "Practical Management," 896; Miller, interview, July 15, 1992.

62. Firland Sanatorium chart C8.

63. Firland Sanatorium chart D20.

64. Firland Sanatorium chart D14.

65. Others have characterized tuberculosis sanatoriums as "total institutions." See Bryder, *Below the Magic Mountain*, 200–214; Goffman, *Asylums*, 4; Rothman, *Living in the Shadow*, 227.

66. Erving Goffman used the term "rationalization" to describe how institutional requirements are framed in terms of the needs of inmates. See Goffman, *Asylums*, 46, 47. On physicians' disciplinary authority, see Lunbeck, *Psychiatric Persuasion*, 81–96.

67. Thomas F. Sheehy Jr., "Informally Speaking," *Firland Magazine* 46 (May 1958): 4–5.

68. Louis E. Siltzbach, "Relapse and Rehabilitation in the Era of Anti-Tuberculosis Drugs," *Journal of the Mount Sinai Hospital* 23 (1956): 628–40, 635; Eugene Low, "Relapse Rate in a Two- to Eleven-Year Follow-Up Study of Patients with Pulmonary Tuberculosis Treated with and without Antimicrobials and Discharged from 1946 through 1955," *American Review of Tuberculosis and Pulmonary Diseases* 79 (1959): 612–21; John Crofton, "Tuberculosis Undefeated," *British Medical Journal*, no. 5200 (1960): 679–87.

69. "Panel Three: The Problem of Relapse of Tuberculous Lesions under Chemotherapy and Following Treatment; The Duration of Drug Treatment; The Pathology of Healing Tuberculous Lesions; Bacteriologic Problems," *American Review of Tuberculosis and Pulmonary Diseases* 80, pt. 2 (Oct. 1959): 46–71, 50, 51.

70. Thomas F. Sheehy Jr., "Relapse Experience of Optimally Treated Patients,"

May 21, 1959, WS Archives, Wallace Lane Papers. Similarly, see Gertrude M. Willis, "The Tuberculous Patient at Home: The Sanatorium on Trial," *American Review of Tuberculosis* 76 (1957): 1049–62, 1050.

71. Sheehy, "Relapse Experience." Obviously, there was a great deal of overlap between the alcoholic population and patients who left against advice.

72. Thomas F. Sheehy Jr. to Bernard Bucove, Oct. 6, 1959, WS Archives, Wallace Lane Papers.

73. "Doctor's Report," 6; Davies, "Isolating the Recalcitrants," 121.

74. Fagan and Berger, *A Partial Evaluation,* 19; "New Mexico Reports on Questionnaire Survey," *Rehabilitation Events* (of the National Tuberculosis Association) 6 (Mar. 1960): 1, 2.

75. Byron F. Francis, "Policies Covering the Operation of the Detention Ward at Firland Sanatorium, 1960," WS Archives, DSHS 300 Files, box 40, folder "Firland (1968)."

76. "New Mexico Reports," 1; "Report on Compulsory Isolation in the United States, December 1955," ALA Archives, Compulsory Isolation File (2708).

77. The three states were California, Virginia, and North Carolina. The three cities were Pittsburgh, New York, and the District of Columbia. For more on these programs, see Robert Glass, "Forcible Detention of Patients with Active Tuberculosis," *Public Health Reports* 74 (1959): 399–404; Mack I. Shanholtz, "Quarantine and/or Enforced Isolation for Tuberculosis in Virginia," *Virginia Medical Monthly* 94 (1967): 376–77. The use of prison facilities was questioned in Edward Kupka and Marion R. King, "Enforced Legal Isolation of Tuberculosis Patients," *Public Health Reports* 69 (1954): 351–59, 354, 355.

78. Legal proceedings are discussed in Bridge, "The Recalcitrant Patient," 119, 120; James F. Bell, "Ohio Recalcitrants," *Bulletin of the National Tuberculosis Association* 41 (Dec. 1955): 117–18; John H. Gross, "Compulsory Isolation of the Uncooperative Tuberculosis Patient: The Experience in the State of Georgia," *American Review of Tuberculosis* 77 (1958): 506–10.

79. "Report on Compulsory Isolation"; N. J. Swearingen, "Laws Regarding Tuberculosis Hospital Care and Isolation of Patients," Sept. 1953, and F. E. Hesse, "Control of the Recalcitrant Tuberculosis Patient: Legislation and Practice, 1954," ALA Archives, Compulsory Isolation File (2708).

80. The term "communicable" appears in Bell, "Ohio Recalcitrants," 117; the term "infectious" is used in Kupka and King, "Enforced Legal Isolation," 353; "open" cases are discussed in Andrew L. Banyai and Anthony V. Cadden, "Compulsory Hospitalization of Open Cases of Tuberculosis," *American Review of Tuberculosis* 50 (1944): 136–46, 136.

81. William L. Potts and Ollie M. Goodloe, "Compulsory Hospital Isolation of the Recalcitrant Positive-Sputum Patient (with Analysis of an Extremely Successful Enforcement Plan)," *Ohio State Medical Journal* 48 (1952): 25–31.

82. Shanholtz, "Quarantine and/or Enforced Isolation," 376.

83. Hesse, "Control of the Recalcitrant Tuberculosis Patient"; Kupka and King, "Enforced Legal Isolation," 353; Stuart Willis, "The Case for Forcible Hos-

pitalization of the Recalcitrant Tuberculosis Patient," *Rhode Island Medical Journal* 42 (Oct. 1959): 650, 652, 654–55, quote on 654.

84. Thomas F. Sheehy Jr., Informally Speaking," *Firland Magazine* 45 (Feb. 1957): 3–4. See also Cedric Northrop, "Field Report for May 1954," WS Archives, Department of Health, Director's Office, RS 2 Disease File, box 7, folder 785a.

85. Northrop, Fountain, and Zahn, "Practical Management"; Davies, "Isolating the Recalcitrants"; Linell, "Detention Ward"; Cedric Northrop, "Compulsory Isolation," *Bulletin of the National Tuberculosis Association* 42 (Nov. 1956): 149–50.

86. Northrop, "Field Report for May 1954."

87. "The Recalcitrant Tuberculosis Patient," *Journal of the American Medical Association* 167 (1958): 74.

88. Ruth B. Taylor, "Patients Who Disregard Medical Recommendations," *Public Health Reports* 71 (1956): 904–7, 906.

89. Donald J. Ottenberg, "The Physician's Role in the Treatment of Tuberculosis-Alcoholism," in U.S. Department of Health, Education, and Welfare (HEW), *Toward Intensive Treatment for the Tuberculous Alcoholic Patient: Proceedings of a Workshop* (Washington, D.C.: HEW, 1962), 12. See also Harry A. Wilmer, "Pity, Sympathy, and Empathy: I Have Been a Stranger in a Strange Land," in Phineas J. Sparer, ed., *Personality, Stress, and Tuberculosis* (New York: International Universities Press, 1956), 249, 250.

90. Sidney H. Dressler, "The Case against Compulsory Isolation of the Recalcitrant Tuberculous," *Rhode Island Medical Journal* 42 (1959): 651, 653, quote on 651.

91. Donald J. Ottenberg, "Experiences in Tuberculosis Control," in National Institute of Mental Health (NIMH), *The Alcoholic Tuberculous Patient and the Community* (Bethesda, Md.: NIMH, 1959), 75.

92. James P. Spradley, *You Owe Yourself a Drunk: An Ethnography of Urban Nomads* (Boston: Little, Brown, 1970), 159.

93. The Washington state Supreme Court had upheld the 1966 ruling of the Seattle Superior Court judge Henry W. Cramer. See *City of Seattle v. Wayne J. Hill*, WCLU news release, June 8, 1966, UW Archives, WCLU Papers, box 41, folder "Treatment of Alcoholics, 1965–1967." The Washington case anticipated the 1968 ruling of the U.S. Supreme Court in *Powell v. Texas* that public drunkenness was still a crime. See Kittrie, *The Right to Be Different*, 276–89.

94. Cedric Northrop, "Unfinished Business in Tuberculosis Control," Dec. 12, 1949, WS Archives, Department of Health, Director's Office, RS 2 Disease File, box 8, folder 160.

95. Joan K. Jackson, "A Social Science View," in NIMH, *Alcoholic Tuberculous Patient and the Community*, 48. This discussion draws on recent historical writings that stress that "objective" language may actually reflect and promote the agenda of those who employ it. See JoAnne Brown, "Professional Language: Words That Succeed," *Radical History Review* 34 (1986): 33–51. On the term "noncompliance" in particular, see James A. Trostle, "Medical Compliance as

an Ideology," *Social Science and Medicine* 27 (1988): 1299–1308; and Barron H. Lerner, "From Careless Consumptives to Recalcitrant Patients: The Historical Construction of Noncompliance," *Social Science and Medicine* 45 (1997): 1423–31.

96. Joan K. Jackson, "Common Denominators in Alcoholism and Tuberculosis: Social Aspects," 1959, Joan K. Jackson, Personal Papers. See also Joan K. Jackson, "Research on Alcoholism and Tuberculosis," Apr. 11, 1958, Jackson Papers; Howard M. Bahr, *Skid Row: An Introduction to Disaffiliation* (New York: Oxford University Press, 1973), 44–47. For a modern commentary on inadvertent blaming of the victim, see Paul Farmer, "Social Scientists and the New Tuberculosis," *Social Science and Medicine* 44 (1997): 347–58.

SEVEN. "A JAIL IN EVERY SENSE OF THE WORD"

1. Washington State Department of Health and Sanitation, "Objectives of Tuberculosis Hospital Survey Team," Mar. 21, 1957, WS Archives, DSHS (Department of Social and Health Services) 300 Files, box 42, folder "Consolidation (History)."

2. A. S. to Arthur B. Langlie, Mar. 20, 1954, WS Archives, Health Department Administrative Files, box 6, folder "T.B. Control, 1953–59."

3. N. D. to Albert Rosellini, Feb. 28, 1957, WS Archives, Department of Health, Director's Files, 1954–57, box 2, folder 86.1.

4. Doris Hilberry, "In Memory of Dr. Zahn," *Firland Magazine* 45 (May 1957): 13. See also Duke Dugent, "The Patients' Council," *Firland Magazine* 45 (Jan. 1957): 8.

5. Doris Hilberry and Duke Dugent to the editor of the *Spokane Chronicle,* Jan. 15, 1957, WS Archives, Department of Health, Director's Files, 1954–57, box 1, folder 59.

6. Ibid.

7. Doris Hilberry to Albert Rosellini, Jan. 21, 1957, WS Archives, Department of Health, Director's Files, 1954–57, box 1, folder 59.

8. A Group of Firland Patients to the editor of the *Seattle Times,* Nov. 11, 1956, UW Archives, WCLU (American Civil Liberties Union of Washington) Papers, box 25, folder 11-19.

9. A. P. to To Whom It May Concern, n.d., UW Archives, WCLU Papers, box 25, folder 11-19.

10. Hilberry to Rosellini, Jan. 21, 1957.

11. These quotes may be found in Thomas F. Sheehy Jr., "Informally Speaking," *Firland Magazine* 45 (Feb. 1957): 3–4, and Thomas F. Sheehy Jr., "Informally Speaking," *Firland Magazine* 47 (May 1959): 4–5. Sheehy's language is criticized in A Group of Firland Patients to the editor of the *Seattle Times,* Nov. 11, 1956; Hilberry and Dugent to the editor of the *Spokane Chronicle,* Jan. 15, 1957.

12. A. P. to To Whom It May Concern, n.d.

13. Hilberry and Dugent to the editor of the *Spokane Chronicle,* Jan. 15, 1957.

14. Harvey Hurtt to Governor Albert Rosellini, Mar. 28, 1957, WS Archives, Department of Health, Director's Files, 1954–57, box 2, folder 86.1.

15. Cedric Northrop to Bernard Bucove, Feb. 19, 1957, WS Archives, Department of Health, Director's Files, 1954–57, box 2, folder 86.1.

16. Mason Morisset, "The American Civil Liberties Union of Washington," summer 1965, 3–8, UW Archives, Leonard Schroeter Papers, box 13, unmarked folder; Doug Honig and Laura Brenner, *On Freedom's Frontier: The First Fifty Years of the American Civil Liberties Union in Washington State* (Seattle: ACLU of Washington, 1987). The WCLU was actually the Seattle chapter until 1952.

17. Minutes of the Board of Directors of the American Civil Liberties Union of Washington, Feb. 7, 1957, and Dec. 5, 1957, UW Archives, WCLU Papers, box 15, folder 5.

18. Minutes of the Board of Directors of the American Civil Liberties Union of Washington, Aug. 1, 1957, UW Archives, WCLU Papers, box 15, folder 5.

19. Honig and Brenner, *On Freedom's Frontier,* 38, 39; David J. Rothman and Sheila M. Rothman, *The Willowbrook Wars: A Decade of Struggle for Social Justice* (New York: Harper and Row, 1984), 50–57.

20. Honig and Brenner, *On Freedom's Frontier,* 30–32; Morisset, "The American Civil Liberties Union of Washington," 13–15, 58–60; Rothman and Rothman, *Willowbrook Wars,* 53; Melvin Rader, *False Witness* (Seattle: University of Washington Press, 1969). The WCLU eventually won the case, which was decided by the U.S. Supreme Court in 1964.

21. Morisset, "The American Civil Liberties Union of Washington," 76–80.

22. Ibid., 78–79; Minutes of the Board of Directors of the American Civil Liberties Union of Washington, July 11, 1957, UW Archives, Leonard Schroeter Papers, box 13, folder "Board Minutes, 1954–1962."

23. Morisset, "The American Civil Liberties Union of Washington," 80–81.

24. Erving Goffman, *Asylums: Essays on the Social Situation of Mental Patients and Other Inmates* (Garden City, N.Y.: Anchor Books, 1961), 51–53; Julius A. Roth, *Timetables: Structuring the Passage of Time in Hospital Treatment and Other Careers* (Indianapolis: Bobbs-Merrill, 1963), 52–56.

25. Notices of modified quarantine appear in the Firland Sanatorium charts. See also *This Is Firland* (Seattle: Firland Sanatorium, 1958), 21.

26. Firland Sanatorium chart C1.

27. Firland Sanatorium chart S14. For similar requests, see charts A11, C22, and D14.

28. Firland Sanatorium chart C18.

29. Firland Sanatorium chart C6.

30. Firland Sanatorium chart E3.

31. Barney Harvey, "Homicide Charged: Woman Sobs at News Her Auto Killed Two," *Seattle Times,* Sept. 1, 1960, 1; Ken Fleming, "Young Mother, Tot Die: Tragic Car Crash Ends Couple's Happy Story," *Seattle Post-Intelligencer,* Sept. 1, 1960, 1, 12.

32. Letter to the editor, *Firland Magazine* 44 (June 1956): 8–9.

33. Joan K. Jackson, "Some Problems Involved in Helping the Skid Road Patient Adjust to the Hospital," May 14, 1957, Joan K. Jackson, Personal Papers.

34. Quote is from Firland Sanatorium chart D16. See also M. A. Linell, "The Detention Ward and Its Place in the Control and Treatment of Tuberculosis," *American Review of Tuberculosis and Pulmonary Diseases* 74 (1956): 410–16, 411; Ronald J. Fagan and Arnold S. Linsky, *Hospital Change and Resistance to Change in the Treatment of Alcoholism-Tuberculosis: The Experiences of One Tuberculosis Hospital* (Seattle, 1966), 9–10; Joan K. Jackson, interview with author, June 10, 1994.

35. Cedric Northrop, "Field Report for March 1954," WS Archives, Department of Health, Director's Office, RS 2 Disease File, box 7, folder 785a.

36. Firland Sanatorium chart C11. See also Fagan and Linsky, *Hospital Change and Resistance to Change*, 9–10.

37. Joan K. Jackson and Ralph Connor, "The Skid Road Alcoholic," *Quarterly Journal of Studies on Alcohol* 14 (1953): 468–86, 476.

38. Firland Sanatorium chart C5.

39. David J. Pittman and C. Wayne Gordon, *The Revolving Door: A Study of the Chronic Police Case Inebriate* (New York: Free Press, 1958).

40. Firland Sanatorium chart D12.

41. Linell, "Detention Ward," 411.

42. Daniel W. Zahn, "Informally Speaking," *Firland Magazine* 44 (Mar. 1956): 13; Kay Anderson, R.N., interview with author, June 11, 1993; Walter T. Miller, M.D., interview with author, July 15, 1992.

43. Donald J. Ottenberg, "Experiences in Tuberculosis Control," in National Institute of Mental Health (NIMH), *The Alcoholic Tuberculous Patient and the Community* (Bethesda, Md.: NIMH, 1959), 75.

44. "Report on Luncheon Meeting with Dr. Donald Ottenberg with Medical Staff, Firland," Feb. 12, 1962, WS Archives, Health Department Administrative Files, box 5, folder "Treatment for Tuberculous Alcoholic, Firland."

45. Rothman and Rothman, *Willowbrook Wars*, 50–57; David J. Bodenhamer, *Fair Trial: Rights of the Accused in American History* (New York: Oxford University Press, 1992), 99–125.

46. Sue M. Berger to Byron F. Francis, Aug. 27, 1964, WS Archives, Wallace Lane Papers.

47. Fagan and Linsky, *Hospital Change and Resistance to Change*, 7.

48. Washington State Department of Health, "A Study of Factors Affecting Tuberculosis Sanatoria Costs," May 1964, WS Archives, DSHS 300 Files, box 42, unmarked folder. See also Earl Rubington, "Legal Commitment and Hospital Behavior," *Mental Hygiene* 53 (1969): 41–53, 51; Julius A. Roth, "The Treatment of the Sick," in John Kosa, Aaron Antonovsy, and Irving K. Zola, eds., *Poverty and Health: A Sociological Analysis* (Cambridge: Harvard University Press, 1969), 236–38.

49. Data had shown only that longer duration of antibiotic therapy decreased relapses.

50. Berger to Francis, Aug. 27, 1964. The twelve-month rule was also ques-

tioned in Richard M. Hudson, "A Study of Tuberculous Skid Road Alcoholics" (master's thesis, University of Washington, 1963), 69–71, 79.

51. Hudson, "A Study of Tuberculous Skid Road Alcoholics," 52–53.

52. Les Hill, quoted in "The Man on the Ward," *Firland Magazine* 50 (Nov. 1962): 19.

53. "Ward 6," *Firland Magazine* 51 (Feb. 1963): 8.

54. "San Landers: Advice to Those Who Land in the San," *Firland Magazine* 53 (Feb. 1965): 9.

55. "Smile . . . You're on SAN-Did Camera," *Firland Magazine* 50 (Dec. 1962): 12.

56. Firland Sanatorium chart S40; Burnice Calhoun, R.N., interview with author, Sept. 18, 1992; Jonathan Ostrow, M.D., interview with author, Oct. 5, 1992.

57. Rothman and Rothman, *Willowbrook Wars*, 83–89.

58. Firland Sanatorium charts D5 and D16.

59. Firland Sanatorium chart D6.

60. Firland Sanatorium chart D12.

61. Firland Sanatorium chart D16. This quote actually comes from a physician's summary of the hearing with Judge Elston.

62. Firland Sanatorium charts F3 and F4; Harlan Strickett to Miss Boyd, Apr. 7, 1971, ALA Archives, Washington State Field Report File (585 R).

63. Firland Sanatorium chart S40.

64. *1967 Session Laws of the State of Washington*, Regular Session, Fortieth Legislature (Olympia, 1967), 277–87.

65. These percentages come from a review of the charts of the fifty-five men detained on Ward Six between January 1, 1967, and June 30, 1967. The numbers of African Americans and Native Americans in Seattle did increase considerably between 1950 and 1960.

66. Michelle McClellan, "The Emergence of the Female Alcoholic in American Medical Literature, 1930–1960," paper presented at the annual meeting of the American Historical Association, Chicago, Jan. 1995. See also Charlotte A. Rose, R.N., interview with author, July 1, 1993.

67. This quotation comes from a psychiatrist discussing the infamous Seattle kidney failure patient Ernie Crowfeather. See Renee C. Fox and Judith P. Swazey, *The Courage to Fail: A Social View of Organ Transplants and Dialysis* (Chicago: University of Chicago Press, 1974), 293–94.

68. Firland Sanatorium chart B14.

69. Joan K. Jackson, Byron F. Francis, and Ronald J. Fagan, "The Conference: Its Background and Goals," in U.S. Department of Housing, Education, and Welfare (HEW), *Toward Intensive Treatment for the Tuberculous Alcoholic Patient: Proceedings of a Workshop* (Washington, D.C.: HEW, 1962), 1.

70. Ibid.

71. John E. Bell, "Summarization of Group Discussion and Conference Evaluation," in HEW, *Toward Intensive Treatment*, 40–44.

72. David F. Musto, *The American Disease: Origins of Narcotic Control* (New York: Oxford University Press, 1987), 237–39.

73. Emmett Watson, "Ron Fagan Reclaimed His Life, Others from Alcohol," *Seattle Times*, June 2, 1987, B1.

74. Emmett Watson, *Digressions of a Native Son* (Seattle: Pacific Institute, 1982), 131.

75. Watson, "Ron Fagan," B1; Watson, *Digressions*, 128–38. Fagan eventually became the founder-director of the Cedar Hills Alcoholic Treatment Center in King County.

76. "Progress Report on Tentative Plans for Firland Tuberculous-Alcoholism Treatment Program," WS Archives, Health Department Administrative Files, box 5, folder "Treatment for Tuberculous Alcoholic, Firland."

77. Fagan and Linsky, *Hospital Change and Resistance to Change*, 11; see also 14–21; Joan K. Jackson, "Evaluation of Visits with the Consultants" [1962?], Jackson Personal Papers.

78. Ronald J. Fagan and Sue M. Berger, *A Partial Evaluation of Firland Alcoholism Program with a Profile of Alcoholic and Non-Alcoholic Patients at First Admission* (Seattle, 1964), 8–9.

79. Fagan and Linsky, *Hospital Change and Resistance to Change*, 27.

80. Ibid. See also Jackson, "Evaluation of Visits"; Archibald Ruprecht, M.D., interview with author, Nov. 13, 1994.

81. Fagan and Linsky, *Hospital Change and Resistance to Change*, 31, 37. For more on the continued stigmatization of alcoholics, see Howard M. Bahr, *Skid Row: An Introduction to Disaffiliation* (New York: Oxford University Press, 1973), 53–55, 63, 64; and Edith Heinemann and Robert J. Rhodes, "How Nurses View the Tuberculous Alcoholic Patient," *Nursing Research* 16 (1967): 361–65.

82. Jackson, "Evaluation of Visits."

83. Ottenberg, "Experiences in Tuberculosis Control," 74–75.

84. Helen S. Marshall, M.D., interview with author, Dec. 14, 1992. See also Fagan and Linsky, *Hospital Change and Resistance to Change*, 31, 37.

85. "Progress Report on Tentative Plans for Firland Tuberculous-Alcoholism Treatment Program," WS Archives, Health Department Administrative Files, box 5, folder "Treatment for Tuberculous Alcoholic, Firland."

86. Byron F. Francis, "Firland's Plans for Treatment of Tuberculosis-Alcoholism," in HEW, *Toward Intensive Treatment*, 32.

87. The phrase "socially marginal" comes from Fagan and Linsky, *Hospital Change and Resistance to Change*, 1.

88. Samuel Butler, *Erehwon and Erehwon Revisited* [1872] (New York: Modern Library, 1927), 106–7.

89. Ibid., 110.

90. For an overview of social control, see Peter Conrad and Joseph W. Schneider, *Deviance and Medicalization: From Badness to Sickness* (Philadelphia: Temple University Press, 1992), 17–37. Authors who nuance social control theories include Nancy Tomes, *A Generous Confidence: Thomas Story Kirkbride and*

the Art of Asylum-Keeping, 1840–1883 (New York: Cambridge University Press, 1984); and Gerald N. Grob, "The History of the Asylum Revisited: Personal Reflections," in Mark S. Micale and Roy Porter, eds., *Discovering the History of Psychiatry* (New York: Oxford University Press, 1994), especially 275–77.

91. David J. Rothman, *Conscience and Convenience: The Asylum and Its Alternatives in Progressive America* (Boston: Little, Brown, 1980), 419. See also 337–60.

92. Ostrow, interview, Oct. 5, 1992.

93. Nancy M. Rockafellar, "Making the World Safe for the Soldiers of Democracy: Patriotism, Public Health, and Venereal Disease Control on the West Coast, 1910–1919" (Ph.D. diss., University of Washington, 1990), 332.

94. For provocative discussions about the proper role of historians in judging the medical and public health practices of earlier eras, see David J. Rothman, "Radiation" (book review), *Journal of the American Medical Association* 276 (1996): 421–23; and Sherwin B. Nuland, "Hate in the Time of Cholera" (book review), *New Republic,* May 26, 1997, 32–37.

95. Sheila M. Rothman, *Living in the Shadow of Death: Tuberculosis and the Social Experience of Illness in American History* (New York, Basic Books, 1994), 227.

96. Firland Sanatorium chart F4.

97. Nancy J. Tomes, "The White Plague Revisited," *Bulletin of the History of Medicine* 63 (fall 1989): 467–80.

98. Message of Arthur B. Langlie, governor of Washington, to the Thirty-fifth Legislature, Olympia, Washington, Jan. 15, 1957, 15–17, available at University of Washington Library, Seattle; "Washington's Tuberculosis Fight Cited," *Firland Magazine* 49 (Sept. 1961): 6.

99. Joan K. Jackson, interview with author, Dec. 5, 1992; Joan K. Jackson, letter to the author, July 2, 1994. This contrast is also emphasized in James P. Spradley, *You Owe Yourself a Drunk: An Ethnography of Urban Nomads* (Boston: Little, Brown, 1970), 59–60, 159–60.

100. Firland sanatorium charts B1, D7, and D10; Helen S. Marshall, M.D., interview, Sept. 2, 1992. For a Ward Six patient praising Firland, see Jack Stumpf, "A Patient Speaks," *Firland Magazine* 45 (Oct. 1957): 12–13.

101. Ostrow, interview, Oct. 5, 1992; Mr. Eisenberg to A. Ryrie Koch, Aug. 22, 1957, ALA Archives, Washington State Department of Public Health File (704).

102. "Discussion," in NIMH, *Alcoholic Tuberculous Patient and the Community,* 29, 30.

103. Jackson, interview, Dec. 5, 1992.

104. Jackson, "Evaluation of Visits." Others favoring a "control ward" included Bell, "Summarization," 41; John C. Smith and Harold W. Demone, "Measurement of the Tuberculosis-Alcoholism Problem in Massachusetts and Steps to Control It," *American Review of Respiratory Disease* 84 (1961): 263–67. See also "Discussion," in NIMH, *Alcoholic Tuberculous Patient and the Community,* especially 111, 120.

105. Jackson, interview, June 10, 1994.

106. The limited number of alcoholism treatment programs for tuberculosis patients is discussed in Robert J. Rhodes, George H. Hames, and Michael D. Campbell, "The Problem of Alcoholism among Hospitalized Tuberculous Patients: Reports of a National Questionnaire Survey," *American Review of Respiratory Disease* 99 (1969): 440–42. For ongoing rehabilitation efforts, see Smith and Demone, "Measurement," 263–67; Barbara S. Wilbur, David Salkin, and Harold Birnbaum, "A Critical Evaluation of the Therapeutic Community Approach to the Tuberculous Alcoholic," in HEW, *Toward Intensive Treatment;* and Hale Pragoff, "Adjustment of Tuberculosis Patients One Year after Discharge," *Public Health Reports* 77 (1962): 671–79.

107. Ronald J. Miller, *The Demolition of Skid Row* (Lexington, Mass.: Lexington Books, 1982), 23–25.

108. "What TB Associations Are Doing in the War on Poverty," *Bulletin of the National Tuberculosis Association* 51 (Nov. 1965): 14–15. See also John J. Hanlon, "An Attack against Poverty Is an Assault on Preventable Disease," *Bulletin of the National Tuberculosis Association* 51 (Nov. 1965): 9–11.

109. Miller, *Demolition,* 16–17. Medicaid, passed in 1965, did not originally cover tuberculosis.

110. Spradley, *You Owe Yourself a Drunk,* 260; Griffith Edwards, Jim Orford, Stella Egert, Sally Guthrie, Ann Hawker, Celia Hensman, Martin Mitcheson, Edna Oppenheimer, and Colin Taylor, "Alcoholism: A Controlled Trial of 'Treatment' and 'Advice,'" *Journal of Studies on Alcohol* 38 (1977): 1004–31.

111. J. Thomas Millington, "III. The Missing Links in Alcoholism Control," *American Journal of Public Health* 57 (1967): 967–71; Frank A. Seixas, "The Prevention of Alcoholism: Guest Editor's Introduction," *Preventive Medicine* 3 (Mar. 1974): 1–4.

112. Walsh McDermott, Kirby S. Howlett Jr., James W. Raleigh, and Robert L. Yeager, "Study of Tuberculosis Care in New York City, 1961," ALA-NY Archives.

113. Thomas S. Szasz, *Law, Liberty, and Psychiatry* (New York: Collier Books, 1963), 57–71; E. Fuller Torrey, *Out of the Shadows: Confronting America's Mental Illness Crisis* (New York: John Wiley and Sons, 1997).

114. Leonard D. Hudson and John A. Sbarbaro, "Twice Weekly Tuberculosis Chemotherapy," *Journal of the American Medical Association* 223 (1973): 139–43. On Madras, see Tuberculosis Chemotherapy Centre, Madras, "Concurrent Comparison of Home and Sanatorium Treatment of Pulmonary Tuberculosis," *Bulletin of the World Health Organization* 21, no. 1 (1959): 51–144. See also Ronald Bayer and David Wilkinson, "Directly Observed Therapy for Tuberculosis: History of an Idea," *Lancet* 345 (1995): 1545–48.

115. Harlan Stricklett to Miss Boyd, Apr. 7, 1971, ALA Archives, Washington State Field Report File (585 R); Al Dieffenbach, "Plan for Local Treatment of Tuberculosis Is Given Support," *Seattle Times,* July 13, 1973, A4.

116. *Public Health in Seattle and King County, 1949: Annual Report of the Seattle–King County Department of Public Health* (Seattle, 1950), 70–71; Seattle–King County Department of Public Health, *Annual Report, 1972* (Seattle, 1973), 3.

117. Hans L. Rieder, George M. Cauthen, George M. Comstock, and Dixie E. Snider Jr., "Epidemiology of Tuberculosis in the United States," *Epidemiological Reviews* 11 (1989): 79–98, 92–93.

118. Hill Williams, "Seattle Medicine: Tuberculosis Program Shows No Area Is Free," *Seattle Times*, Jan. 8, 1964, 11.

119. Richard Carter, *The Gentle Legions* (Garden City, N.Y.: Doubleday, 1961), 84–87; Peter Maas, "Where Does Your Charity Dollar Go?" *Look*, Mar. 15, 1960, 40–46. Regarding Seattle, see Miss Boyd to Mr. Stone and Miss Ostwald, July 13, 1962, ALA Archives, Washington State Field Report File (585 R); and Richard Greenleaf, M.D., interview with author, Oct. 14, 1992.

120. Harold Laws, M.D., interview with author, Oct. 1, 1992.

121. Daniel E. Jenkins, "NTA Has Changed Its Name," *Bulletin of the National Tuberculosis and Respiratory Disease Association* 54 (Apr. 1968): 2.

122. "Food Handlers No Longer Need Chest X-Rays," *Seattle Times*, Jan. 24, 1973, E12.

123. Stricklett to Boyd, Apr. 7, 1971; Guilda M. Albert to Miss Ostwald, Dec. 11, 1970, ALA Archives, Washington State Field Report File (585 R).

124. Stricklett to Boyd, Apr. 7, 1971; R. W. Baker, "Brief of House Bill," May 28, 1971, KCMS Library, folder "Tuberculosis Summary, 6 Years, 1969–1974."

125. "Last Tuberculosis Patient at Firland to Be Moved," *Seattle Times*, Oct. 30, 1973, A7.

EIGHT. AN EPIDEMIC RETURNS

1. Cedric Northrop, "Notes on Firland Sanatorium," May 11, 1952, Shoreline Historical Society, Seattle.

2. Geoffrey Cowley, Elizabeth Ann Leonard, and Mary Hager, "Tuberculosis: A Deadly Return," *Newsweek*, Mar. 16, 1992, 52–57.

3. Thomas R. Frieden, Paula I. Fujiwara, Rita M. Washko, and Margaret A. Hamburg, "Tuberculosis in New York City: Turning the Tide," *New England Journal of Medicine* 333 (1995): 229–33.

4. *Tuberculosis in New York City 1992: Information Summary* (New York: New York City Department of Health, 1993), table 1.

5. Michael F. Cantwell, Dixie E. Snider Jr., George M. Cauthen, and Ida M. Onorato, "Epidemiology of Tuberculosis in the United States, 1985 through 1992," *Journal of the American Medical Association* 272 (1994): 535–39; Barron Lerner, "The White Plague: As Tuberculosis Makes a Comeback It's Time to Re-learn Lessons from Seattle's Past Programs," *Seattle Weekly*, Jan. 5, 1994, 17.

6. Thomas R. Frieden, Timothy Sterling, Ariel Pablos-Mendez, James O. Kilburn, George M. Cauthen, and Samuel W. Dooley, "The Emergence of Drug-Resistant Tuberculosis in New York City," *New England Journal of Medicine* 328 (1993): 521–26; Alan B. Bloch, George M. Cauthen, Ida M. Onorato, Kenneth G. Dansbury, Gloria D. Kelly, Cynthia R. Driver, and Dixie E. Snider Jr., "Nationwide Survey of Drug-Resistant Tuberculosis in the United States," *Journal of the American Medical Association* 271 (1994): 665–71.

7. Karen Brudney and Jay Dobkin, "Resurgent Tuberculosis in New York City: Human Immunodeficiency Virus, Homelessness, and the Decline of Tuberculosis Control Programs," *American Review of Respiratory Disease* 144 (1991): 745–49; Barron H. Lerner, "New York City's Tuberculosis Control Efforts: The Historical Limitations of the 'War on Consumption,'" *American Journal of Public Health* 83 (1993): 758–66.

8. J. Randall Curtis, Thomas M. Hooton, and Charles M. Nolan, "New Developments in Tuberculosis and HIV Infection: An Opportunity for Prevention," *Journal of General Internal Medicine* 9 (1994): 286–94.

9. Marc van Leuven, Mark De Groot, Karen P. Shean, Ulrich O. von Oppell, and Paul A. Willcox, "Pulmonary Resection as an Adjunct in the Treatment of Multiple Drug-Resistant Tuberculosis," *Annals of Thoracic Surgery* 63 (1997): 1368–72.

10. Brudney and Dobkin, "Resurgent Tuberculosis."

11. Mireya Navarro, "Gauging Threat of Recalcitrant TB Patients," *New York Times,* Apr. 14, 1992, A1, A17; *Petitioners v. Antoinette R., Also Known as Marie C., Also Known as Chastity C., Respondent,* 165 Misc. 2d 1014; 630 N.Y.S. 2d 1008; 1995 N.Y. Misc. LEXIS 392.

12. Rosemary G. Reilly, "Combating the Tuberculosis Epidemic: The Legality of Coercive Tuberculosis Measures," *Columbia Journal of Law and Social Problems* 27 (1993): 101–49, 121–25; Ronald Bayer and Laurence Dupuis, "Tuberculosis, Public Health, and Civil Liberties," *Annual Review of Public Health* 16 (1995): 307–26, 310–11, 319–20.

13. Julie Emery and Warren King, "Tuberculosis Patient Is Fighting the State's Power to Quarantine," *Seattle Times–Seattle Post-Intelligencer,* Jan. 19, 1986, B4; Julie Emery and Warren King, "TB Patient Wins Case over State," *Seattle Times,* Feb. 10, 1986, B1.

14. Bayer and Dupuis, "Tuberculosis," 313–22; Nancy N. Dubler, Ronald Bayer, Seth Landesman, and Amanda White, "Tuberculosis in the 1990s: Ethical, Legal, and Public Policy Issues in Screening, Treatment, and the Protection of Those in Congregate Facilities," in *The Tuberculosis Revival: Individual Rights and Societal Obligation in a Time of AIDS* (New York: United Hospital Fund, 1992); George J. Annas, "Control of Tuberculosis: The Law and the Public's Health," *New England Journal of Medicine* 328 (1993): 585–88; Lawrence O. Gostin, "Controlling the Resurgent Tuberculosis Epidemic: A Fifty-State Survey of TB Statutes and Proposals for Reform," *Journal of the American Medical Association* 269 (1993): 255–61.

15. Ronald Bayer and David Wilkinson, "Directly Observed Therapy for Tuberculosis: History of an Idea," *Lancet* 345 (1995): 1545–48.

16. "Ray Finally Takes the Cure," in *Health of the City: Focus on Tuberculosis* (New York: New York City Department of Health, 1995), 51. See also Paula I. Fujiwara, Christina Larkin, and Thomas R. Frieden, "Directly Observed Therapy in New York City," *Clinics in Chest Medicine* 18 (Mar. 1997): 135–48; and C. Patrick Chaulk and Diana S. Pope, "The Baltimore City Health Department Program of

Directly Observed Therapy for Tuberculosis," *Clinics in Chest Medicine* 18 (Mar. 1997): 149–54.

17. Ronald Bayer, Catherine Stayton, Moise Desvarieux, Cheryl Healton, and Sheldon Landesman, "Directly Observed Therapy and Treatment Completion for Tuberculosis in the United States, 1990–1994," unpublished manuscript (1997, courtesy of Ronald Bayer).

18. Stephen E. Weis, Philip C. Slocum, Francis X. Blais, Barbara King, Mary Nunn, Burgis Matney, Enriqueta Gomez, and Brian H. Foresman, "The Effect of Directly Observed Therapy on the Rates of Drug Resistance and Relapse in Tuberculosis," *New England Journal of Medicine* 330 (1994): 1179–84; C. Patricia Chaulk, Kristina Moore-Rice, Rosetta Rizzo, and Richard E. Chaisson, "Eleven Years of Community-Based Directly Observed Therapy for Tuberculosis," *Journal of the American Medical Association* 274 (1995): 945–51.

19. Stephen E. Weis, "Universal Directly Observed Therapy: A Treatment Strategy for Tuberculosis," *Clinics in Chest Medicine* 18 (Mar. 1997): 155–63, 156. See also Dubler, Bayer, Landesman, and White, "Tuberculosis in the 1990s," 24, 25; Michael D. Iseman, David L. Cohn, and John A. Sbarbaro, "Directly Observed Treatment of Tuberculosis: We Can't Afford Not to Try It," *New England Journal of Medicine* 328 (1993): 576–78.

20. Rebecca Voelker, " 'Shoe Leather Therapy' Is Gaining on TB," *Journal of the American Medical Association* 275 (1996): 743–44, 744.

21. Carol J. Pozsik, "Compliance with Tuberculosis Therapy," *Medical Clinics of North America* 77 (1993): 1289–1301, 1297.

22. Mireya Navarro, "Confining Tuberculosis Patients: Weighing Rights versus Health Risks," *New York Times,* Nov. 21, 1993, 1, 45; Donna Leusner, "State Drawing Plans to Quarantine Uncooperative Tuberculosis Patients," *Newark (N.J.) Star-Ledger* Apr. 28, 1994, 14; "Quarantine Center Proposed for Recalcitrant Tuberculosis Patients," *San Francisco Chronicle,* June 14, 1994, 17; *TB Times* (of the New York City Department of Health) 9 (summer 1996).

23. Gabriel Feldman, Prem Srivastava, Edward Eden, and Thomas R. Frieden, "Detention until Cure as a Last Resort: New York City's Experience with Involuntary In-Hospital Detention of Persistently Nonadherent Tuberculosis Patients," *Seminars in Respiratory and Critical Care Medicine* 18 (1997): 493–501. For similar percentages, see Tom Oscherwitz, Jacqueline P. Tulsky, Steve Roger, Stan Sciortino, Ann Alpers, Sarah Royce, and Bernard Lo, "Detention of Persistently Nonadherent Tuberculosis Patients," *Journal of the American Medical Association* 278 (1997): 843–46.

24. See the amended version of Section 11.47 of the New York City Health Code, Mar. 31, 1993.

25. William J. Burman, David L. Cohn, Cornelis A. Rietmeijer, Franklyn N. Judson, John A. Sbarbaro, and Randall R. Reves, "Short-Term Incarceration for the Management of Noncompliance with Tuberculosis Treatment," *Chest* 112 (July 1997): 57–62.

26. Linda Singleton, Marie Turner, Ruth Haskal, Sue Etkind, Maria Tricarico,

and Edward Nardell, "Long-Term Hospitalization for Tuberculosis Control: Experience with a Medical-Psychosocial Inpatient Unit," *Journal of the American Medical Association* 278 (1997): 838–42.

27. Barron H. Lerner, "Temporarily Detained: Tuberculous Alcoholics in Seattle, 1949–1960," *American Journal of Public Health* 86 (1996): 257–65.

28. Oscherwitz et al., "Detention of Persistently Nonadherent Tuberculosis Patients," 844.

29. Brudney and Dobkin, "Resurgent Tuberculosis"; Andrew R. Zolopa, Judith A. Hahn, and Robert Gorter, "HIV and Tuberculosis Infection in San Francisco's Homeless Adults: Prevalence and Risk Factors in a Representative Sample," *Journal of the American Medical Association* 272 (1994): 455–61.

30. Paul Starr, *The Social Transformation of American Medicine* (New York: Basic Books, 1982), 191.

31. Hibbert W. Hill, *The New Public Health* (New York: MacMillan, 1916), 19.

32. Arthur J. Rubel and Linda C. Garro, "Social and Cultural Factors in the Successful Control of Tuberculosis," *Public Health Reports* 107 (1992): 626–36; Mindy T. Fullilove, Rebecca Young, Paula G. Panzer, and Philip Muskin, "Psychosocial Issues in the Management of Tuberculosis," *Journal of Law, Medicine, and Ethics* 21 (1993): 324–31; Esther Sumartojo, "When Tuberculosis Treatment Fails: A Social Behavioral Account of Patient Adherence," *American Review of Respiratory Disease* 147 (1993): 1311–20.

33. Lerner, "New York City's Tuberculosis Control Efforts," 758–66; Karen Brudney and Jay Dobkin, "A Tale of Two Cities: Tuberculosis Control in Nicaragua and New York City," *Seminars in Respiratory Infections* 6 (1991): 261–72; Victor W. Sidel, Ernest Drucker, and Steven C. Martin, "The Resurgence of Tuberculosis in the United States: Societal Origins and Societal Responses," *Journal of Law, Medicine, and Ethics* 21 (1993): 303–16; Thomas R. Frieden, "Tuberculosis and Social Change," *American Journal of Public Health* 84 (1994): 1721–23; Paul Farmer, "Social Scientists and the New Tuberculosis," *Social Science and Medicine* 44 (1997): 347–58.

34. *Public Hearing of the Proposed Amendment to Section 11.47 of the New York City Health Code*, Dec. 3, 1992, 40–41; see also 115–21.

35. Voelker, " 'Shoe Leather Therapy,' " 744.

36. Leonard D. Hudson and John A. Sbarbaro, "Twice Weekly Tuberculosis Chemotherapy," *Journal of the American Medical Association* 223 (1973): 139–43, 140.

37. Judith Walzer Leavitt, "Letter to the Editor," *Isis* 86 (1995): 617–18, 617.

38. Ibid. Leavitt was responding to J. Andrew Mendelsohn, " 'Typhoid Mary Strikes Again: The Social and Scientific in the Making of Modern Public Health," *Isis* 86 (1995): 268–77. See also Leavitt, " 'Typhoid Mary' Strikes Back: Bacteriological Theory and Practice in Early-Twentieth-Century Public Health," *Isis* 83 (1992): 608–29, 608–9, and *'Typhoid Mary': Captive to the Public's Health* (Boston: Beacon Press, 1996).

39. Leavitt, " 'Typhoid Mary' Strikes Back," 609.

40. Thomas R. Frieden, M.D., interview with author, May 14, 1997. For an argument favoring the institutionalization of certain mentally ill patients for their own good, see E. Fuller Torrey, *Out of the Shadows: Confronting America's Mental Illness Crisis* (New York: John Wiley and Sons, 1997).

41. *Bureau of Tuberculosis Control, New York City Department of Health: Information Summary* (New York: New York City Department of Health, 1997), 8. The number of annual cases in Seattle, which rose from 84 in 1984 to 131 in 1995, declined in 1996, to 128. See "Tuberculosis in Seattle–King County, 1996: World TB Day, March 24, 1997," unpublished manuscript (1997, courtesy of Charles Nolan).

42. Steven C. Martin, Peter S. Arno, Steven M. Sayfer, and Ernest Drucker, "The Performance of the Public Health System of New York City and the Resurgence of Tuberculosis," unpublished manuscript (1996, courtesy of Steven Martin).

43. Bayer, Stayton, Desvarieux, Healton, and Landesman, "Directly Observed Therapy."

44. "Results of Directly Observed Short-Course Chemotherapy in 112,842 Chinese Patients with Smear-Positive Tuberculosis: China Tuberculosis Control Collaboration," *Lancet* 347 (1996): 358–62.

45. Nancy J. Tomes, *The Gospel of Germs: Men, Women, and the Microbe in American Life* (Cambridge: Harvard University Press, 1998). For a similar discussion on the responsibilities of HIV-positive persons, see Ronald Bayer, "AIDS Prevention: Sexual Ethics and Responsibility," *New England Journal of Medicine* 334 (1996): 1540–42. I am indebted to Ron Bayer and Mark Barnes for their thoughts on the subject of public health and civic duty.

46. Christine Cassel, John LaPuma, and Lance K. Stell, "The Noncompliant Substance Abuser," *Hastings Center Report* 21 (Mar.–Apr. 1991): 30–32; David Orentlicher, "Denying Treatment to the Noncompliant Patient," *Journal of the American Medical Association* 265 (1991): 1579–82.

47. M. Kidorf, M. L. Stitzer, R. K. Brooner, and J. Goldberg, "Contingent Methadone Take-Home Doses Reinforce Adjunct Therapy Attendance of Methadone Maintenance Patients," *Drug and Alcohol Dependence* 36 (1994): 221–26.

48. Ruth Macklin, *Enemies of Patients* (New York: Oxford University Press, 1993), 123.

49. Deborah Sontag and Lynda Richardson, "Doctors Withhold HIV Pill Regimen from Some," *New York Times*, Mar. 2, 1997, A1.

50. Stephen A. Eraker, John P. Kirscht, and Marshall H. Becker, "Understanding and Improving Patient Compliance," *Annals of Internal Medicine* 100 (1984): 258–68.

51. Lee B. Reichman, "The U-Shaped Curve of Concern," *American Review of Respiratory Disease* 144 (1991): 743, 744.

Index

Page numbers in italics refer to figures.

Library of Congress Cataloging-in-Publication Data
Lerner, Barron H.
Contagion and confinement : controlling tuberculosis along the Skid Road / Barron H. Lerner.
p. cm.
Includes bibliographical references and index.
ISBN 0-8018-5898-4 (alk. paper)
1. Firland Sanitorium (Seattle, Wash.) — History. 2. Tuberculosis — Hospitals — Washington (State) — Seattle — History. I. Title.
RC309.W2L47 1998
362.1′96995′009797772 — dc21 98-5700
CIP